This book is due for return not later than the
last date stamped below, unless recalled sooner.

Immunogenicity of Biopharmaceuticals

Biotechnology: Pharmaceutical Aspects

Immunogenicity of Biopharmaceuticals

Marco van de Weert
University of Copenhagen
Copenhagen, Denmark

Eva Horn Møller
University of Copenhagen
Copenhagen, Denmark

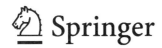

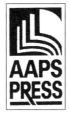

Editors

Marco van de Weert
University of Copenhagen
Copenhagen, Denmark
mvdw@farma.ku.dk

Eva Horn Møller
University of Copenhagen
Copenhagen, Denmark
ehm@farma.ku.dk

ISBN: 978-0-387-75840-4   e-ISBN: 978-0-387-75841-1

Library of Congress Control Number: 2007941403

Preface

The last few decades have seen a rapid rise in novel drugs that mimic the compounds found in the body, such as peptides, proteins, oligonucleotides, certain therapeutic vaccines and genes. These products, especially when derived from biotechnological processing, are commonly referred to as "biopharmaceuticals", although the classification as biopharmaceuticals differs slightly between Europe and the USA. Currently, these compounds constitute about 50% of all new drugs in pre-clinical development and about 25–30% of all new approved drugs.

Biopharmaceuticals are strikingly different from low molecular weight drugs. Their delicate and complex nature, as well as their poor absorption through biological membranes, renders them a tough challenge for the scientist that wants to develop a rugged therapeutic for the market. As a result, delivery of these compounds is usually by injection or infusion, and the formulation is often unique for each new biopharmaceutical. Some of the analytical and formulation challenges of biopharmaceuticals have been addressed in two previous volumes in these series (volume II: Lyophilization of Biopharmaceuticals and volume III: Methods for Structural Analysis of Protein Pharmaceuticals).

Biopharmaceuticals also introduce another challenge, usually absent for low molecular weight drugs, which is the ability to provoke an unwanted immune response. This immune response not only can reduce the effectiveness of the therapy, but can also lead to serious and life-threatening side-effects. Most biopharmaceuticals are to some extent immunogenic, and as a result the regulatory agencies insist that for protein pharmaceuticals potential antidrug antibody formation is studied during drug development.

As many patents are expiring for first-generation biopharmaceuticals, biogeneric products (also termed biosimilars) are approaching the market. The risk of an immune response is a major concern in development of these biosimilars, especially since biopharmaceuticals are often too complex to characterize in full detail. Minor differences between two products may, however, lead to a big difference in immunogenicity, which may not be picked up in small clinical trials of short duration.

The focus of this book is this potential unwanted immune response to biopharmaceuticals. The book is essentially divided into three parts: The first five chapters give a general overview of the nature, causes and (clinical) implications of immunogenicity of biopharmaceuticals, as well as of the prediction and analysis of immunogenicity. The next six chapters present specific cases of immune responses to biopharmaceuticals. The final chapter contains a discussion on risk management of potential unwanted immunogenicity during the drug development process.

The reader will note that the primary focus in all but one chapter is on unwanted immunogenicity of protein pharmaceuticals. This is due to the fact that these constitute the vast majority of biopharmaceutical products and that experience with other biopharmaceuticals is very limited. However, we believe that the concepts discussed in this book will be valid for non-protein biopharmaceuticals also.

Regrettably, this book cannot give a definite answer to the question what factors cause unwanted immunogenicity, and what to do about it. Our insights into many of the mechanisms are still too limited to provide a clear answer. However, the book outlines the present state of knowledge and provides some potential explanations and caveats.

The book should assist those working in early drug development of biopharmaceuticals and allow them to define potential areas of concern as early as possible. It will also serve the formulation scientist, who is responsible for preparing a stable and safe product. Awareness of some of the risk factors for immunogenicity development can aid in preventing future failure of the product. Pharmacologists and clinicians working with biopharmaceuticals may also benefit from this book, as it gives potential explanations for several observations and provides discussions on the methodology used to determine and quantify the immune response. Finally, the book will be of interest to academics, from M.Sc. upwards, working with biopharmaceuticals. It shows that there is still much to learn in this area, and it contains a number of warnings for those developing novel biopharmaceuticals and advanced drug delivery systems.

The editors hope that this book will contribute to the development of better and safer biopharmaceuticals. We also hope that this book can promote a concerted effort in elucidating the important risk factors that lead to immunogenicity.

Marco van de Weert
Eva Horn Møller

Contents

Contributors

John R. Bartholomew
Section of Vascular Medicine, Department of Cardiovascular Medicine, Cleveland Clinic, Cleveland, OH, United States of America
E-mail: *barthoj@ccf.org*

Klaus Bendtzen
Institute for Inflammation Research (IIR), Rigshospitalet National University Hospital, BioMonitor ApS, Copenhagen, Denmark
E-mail: *kben@mail.dk*

Antonio Bertolotto
Centro di Riferimento Regionale Sclerosi Multipla, Hospital San Luigi, Orbassano, Turin, Italy
E-mail: *sclerosi.multipla@sanluigi.piemonte.it*

Carmel A. Celestin
Section of Vascular Medicine, Department of Cardiovascular Medicine, Cleveland Clinic, Cleveland, OH, United States of America
E-mail: *celestc@ccf.org*

Paul Chamberlain
bioLOGICA Consulting, France
E-mail: *paul.chamberlain@biologicaconsulting.com*

Gilbert Deray
Groupe Hospitalier Pitié-Salpêtrière, Paris, France
E-mail: *gilbert.deray@psl.ap-hop-paris.fr*

Silke Ehrenforth
Global Development, Novo Nordisk A/S, Bagsværd, Denmark
E-mail: *sieh@novonordisk.com*

Camilla Foged
Department of Pharmaceutics and Analytical Chemistry, Faculty of Pharmaceutical Sciences, University of Copenhagen, Copenhagen, Denmark
E-mail: *cfo@farma.ku.dk*

Lisbeth Bjerring Jensen
Global Development, Antibody Analysis, Novo Nordisk A/S, Måløv, Denmark
E-mail: *lbjj@novonordisk.com*

Arno Kromminga
Institute for Immunology, Clinical Pathology, Molecular Medicine (IPM), Hamburg, Germany
E-mail: *arno.kromminga@gmx.de*

Simona Malucchi
Centro di Riferimento Regionale Sclerosi Multipla, Hospital San Luigi, Orbassano, Turin, Italy
E-mail: *sclerosi.multipla@sanluigi.piemonte.it*

Henriette Mersebach
Global Development, Novo Nordisk A/S, Bagsværd, Denmark
E-mail: *httm@novonordisk.com*

Eva Horn Møller
Department of Pharmaceutics and Analytical Chemistry, Faculty of Pharmaceutical Sciences, University of Copenhagen, Copenhagen, Denmark
E-mail: *ehm@farma.ku.dk*

Erwin L Roggen
Novozymes AS, Bagsværd, Denmark
E-mail: *elro@novozymes.com*

Stephanie Seremetis
Global Development, Novo Nordisk A/S, Bagsværd, Denmark
E-mail: *sest@novonordisk.com*

Fannie Smith
Global Development, Novo Nordisk A/S, Bagsværd, Denmark
E-mail: *fsm@novonordisk.com*

Thomas Sparre
Global Development, Novo Nordisk A/S, Bagsværd, Denmark
E-mail: *tspa@novonordisk.com*

Meena Subramanyam
Biogen Idec, Inc., Cambridge, MA, United States of America
E-mail: *meena.subramanyam@biogenidec.com*

Anne Sundblad
Department of Medicine, Division of Hematology, Karolinska University Hospital and Institute, Stockholm, Sweden
E-mail: *anne.sundblad@ki.se*

Robin Thorpe
Biotherapeutics group, National Institute for Biological Standards and
Control, Blanche Lane, South Mimms, Potters Bar, United Kingdom
E-mail: *rthorpe@nibsc.co.uk*

Marco van de Weert
Department of Pharmaceutics and Analytical Chemistry, Faculty of
Pharmaceutical Sciences, University of Copenhagen, Copenhagen,
Denmark
E-mail: *mvdw@farma.ku.dk*

Meenu Wadhwa
Biotherapeutics group, National Institute for Biological Standards and
Control, Blanche Lane, South Mimms, Potters Bar, United Kingdom
E-mail: *mwadhwa@nibsc.ac.uk*

Immune Reactions Towards Biopharmaceuticals – a General, Mechanistic Overview

Camilla Foged and Anne Sundblad

1.1. Introduction

Our immune system constitutes a natural defense that has evolved during millions of years to protect eukaryotes from the invasion of pathogenic microorganisms that could otherwise cause life-threatening infectious disease. This defense is a complex system that functions via the concerted action of a variety of components identified to date. Although certain basic aspects of immunological functions have been partly clarified, regarding for example the mechanisms leading to tolerance or immunity, we lack an understanding of regulatory mechanisms, and many immuno-biological questions are still to be answered (reviewed in Zinkernagel 2000).

Biopharmaceuticals (proteins, peptides and nucleic acids) represent a rapidly growing class of drugs expected to constitute an increasing part of marketed future pharmaceuticals. One of the major challenges in applying biopharmaceuticals for medical purposes is to ensure that they either circumvent recognition by the immune system or specifically stimulate or inhibit the targeted immune reactions in the case of immunoregulatory drugs. It is therefore essential to clarify the question regarding the potential of a biopharmaceutical to either be accepted as self-molecules by the immune system or alternatively lead to an induction of a specific or non-specific immune response and if so, by which mechanism (reviewed by Schellekens 2005). Addressing problems related to the immunogenicity of biophar-maceuticals requires the concerted efforts of distinct disciplines, among them medical immunology and pharmaceutical sciences, which represent an expanding research area in the field of drug development.

The scope of this chapter is to provide the reader with a general overview of the immune system with emphasis on the mechanisms responsible for induction of innate and adaptive immune responses towards foreign molecules including biopharmaceuticals and the mechanisms maintaining a state of immunological tolerance. The chapter does not provide a comprehensive review of the immune system. The aim is rather to introduce some of the basic immunological mechanisms that may be involved when a biopharmaceutical induces unintended serious immunological side effects.

1.1.1. The Innate Immune System

The immune system is classically viewed as composed of two arms (Table 1.1 and Figure 1.1): the innate and the adaptive immune system (Vivier and Malissen 2005). The innate immune system constitutes the first line of host defense that rapidly recognizes and responds to a microbial invasion. The innate is more ancient than the adaptive immune system, and it is mainly composed of phagocytic cells like macrophages and dendritic cells (DCs) that ingest and kill pathogens, together with the complement system.

The innate immune system depends on germ-line encoded receptors that have evolved to recognize highly conserved pathogen-associated molecular patterns (PAMPs) or "common elicitors" (Janeway 1989). These receptors are called pattern recognition receptors (PRRs). The best-characterized class of PRRs are the Toll-like receptors (TLRs) (Medzhitov et al. 1997; Akira and Takeda 2004). TLRs are evolutionarily conserved, membrane-bound receptors which act as PRRs for pathogenic compounds containing PAMPs such as bacterial cell wall components (e.g. lipopolysaccharide, Poltorak et al. 1998), unmethylated CpG motifs of bacterial DNA and double stranded RNA of viruses (Cella et al. 1999; Medzhitov and Janeway 2002). These products of microbial metabolism are unique to microorganisms and are not produced by the host. PAMPs thus allow the immune system to distinguish self from microbial non-self (Medzhitov and Janeway 2002).

PAMPs are also recognized by PRRs of the non-TLR type (reviewed by Sansonetti 2006). An example is the PRR family of cytosolic NOD (nucleotide-binding oligomerization domain)-like receptors (NLRs) that seem to function as intracellular PRRs by sensing intracellular muropeptides (Girardin et al. 2001; Inohara et al. 2003; Chamaillard et al. 2003; Girardin et al. 2003a; Girardin et al. 2003b; Mariathasan and Monack 2007). Engagement of either surface or intra-cellular PRRs triggers intracellular signaling cascades that initiate the innate, essentially inflammatory, immune response (Philpott and Girardin 2004). This results in the destruction of pathogens and further in the enhancement of adaptive immune responses, which are required for the specific eradication of microorganisms as well as for the generation of specific memory responses. In addition

Table 1.1 Distinctive features of innate versus adaptive immunity.

	Innate immunity	Adaptive immunity
Receptors	Germline-encoded	Antigen receptors are products of site-specific somatic recombination
Distribution	Subset-specific but non-clonal	Antigen receptors are clonally distributed
Repertoire	Limited	Immense
	Selected in groups of individuals within a given species	Selected in each individual within a given species
Memory	No	Yes

Sources: Modified from Vivier and Malissen (2005)

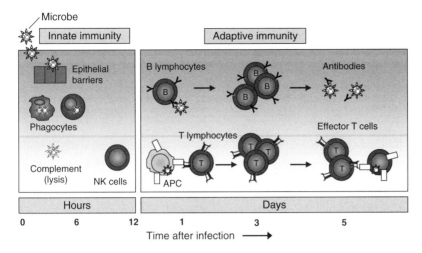

Figure 1.1 Overview of the immune system: Innate versus adaptive immunity.

to the extracellular sensing of pathogens by TLRs and the intracellular sensing by NLRs, other innate sensing systems have been identified suggesting that the innate immune system is composed of a complex and diverse surveillance network with important immune functions that remains yet to be fully characterized (Sansonetti 2006).

Several factors in the formulation of biopharmaceuticals may potentially activate the innate immune system. These include impurities and contaminants that may mimic PAMPs and can thus stimulate immediate innate immune reactions. With the increasing purity of recombinant products such risks are of a diminishing importance. However, repetitive structures, such as protein aggregates present in the formulation of therapeutic proteins, could potentially resemble the repetitive nature of microbial external surfaces and thus function as PAMPs causing activation of immune reactions (Rosenberg 2006). Furthermore, modification of proteins may convert structural epitopes into ligands for PRRs.

For biopharmaceuticals based on nucleic acids, although very few of these are currently marketed, the recognition of PAMPs present on DNA and RNA by PRRs represents a serious concern. It has long been known that viral double stranded RNA and unmethylated CpG motifs of DNA are recognized by TLRs and stimulate innate immune reactions (reviewed in Takeda and Akira 2005). Furthermore, for oligonucleotides, including the promising new class of potential drug molecules based on small interfering RNA (siRNA), a major step prior to the therapeutic use of siRNA is the identification and exclusion of sequence motifs that may act as ligands for TLRs and thereby stimulate unintended immune reactions (reviewed by Marques and Williams 2005).

1.1.2. The Adaptive Immune System

The adaptive immune system constitutes the second line of defense, which initially evolved in jawed vertebrates (reviewed in Pancer and Cooper 2006). The adaptive immune system is capable of mounting highly specific responses against molecular determinants on pathogenic agents that are encountered during the lifetime of a vertebrate. Adaptive immunity is mediated primarily by lymphocytes and has evolved with the ability to generate antibodies against any conceivable pathogenic protein structure by virtue of immunoglobulin gene rearrangements, resulting in the generation of a lymphocyte receptor repertoire of a very high diversity (Gowans 1996). Populations of T and B lymphocytes, each expressing clonally unique receptors, are thus generated by the random rearrangement of V(D)J gene segments, somatic hypermutations in B-cell receptor genes and several other molecular mechanisms that provide for additional diversity to the receptor repertoires.

Antigen-mediated triggering of T and B lymphocytes carrying antigen-specific surface receptors initiates specific cell-mediated and humoral immune responses. Two main lineages of T lymphocytes exist: CD4[+] T helper (Th) cells and CD8[+] cytotoxic T lymphocytes (CTL). Th cells can, among other effector functions, stimulate B-cells to proliferate and differentiate into antibody secreting plasma cells. CTLs exert their most important effector mechanism by antigen-mediated killing of infected cells (Squier and Cohen 1994).

Lymphocytes recirculate between the bloodstream, the lymph and the peripheral lymphoid tissues in a state referred to as naïve cells. To engage in an adaptive immune response, these cells have to become activated in order to proliferate and differentiate into functional effector cells. At least two signals are required to stimulate T-lymphocytes. Specific T-cells recognize peptide fragments bound to the major histocompatibility complex (MHC) class I and class II molecules that display antigenic peptides on the surface of antigen presenting cells (APCs). Such an initial recognition event constitutes the so-called activation signal 1 (Germain 1994). T lymphocytes expressing a diverse repertoire of T-cell receptors (TCR) constitutively "scan" APCs for foreign, MHC-presented antigenic peptides. On B-cells, cell-membrane-bound immunoglobulin recognizes antigen (Reth 1995).

In addition to the signaling initiated by the specific TCR-recognition of peptides displayed on MHC, T-cells need additional stimulation to become fully activated (signal 2), often denoted co-stimulation (Janeway and Bottomly 1994). Receptors on T-cells interact with co-stimulatory molecules on the surface of APCs. Examples of important co-stimulatory molecules on the APC-surface are the B7 family (CD80, CD86), ICOS (*inducible co-s*timulator)-ligand and CD40 that are recognized by CD28, cytotoxic T lymphocyte antigen (CTLA)-4, ICOS and CD40-ligand on T-cells. These additional signals contribute to the priming and differentiation of CTL and Th cells, the latter of which may subsequently deliver help to antigen-specific B-cells. It is believed that in the absence of appropriate co-stimulatory signals, TCR recognition of peptides presented on MHC leads to cell death or anergy, which would constitute a mechanism of tolerance towards self-antigens (Miller and Basten 1996). Thus the presence or the absence of co-stimulation (or signal 2) determines whether naïve antigen-specific T-cells become tolerized or reactive towards the antigen. The differentiation of lymphocytes after an antigen encounter is a process that may proceed over weeks. Moreover, the induction of a robust, adaptive immune response requires repeated exposure to the foreign protein (Ross et al. 2000).

Section 1.2 describes how uptake and processing of antigens occur in APCs and the subsequent loading onto MHC molecules. Section 1.3 deals with the activation of lymphocytes. Immunological tolerance mechanisms are presented in Section 1.4, and Section 1.5 discusses how tolerance can be broken by biopharmaceuticals and presents current views on how the immune system discriminates between self and non-self in relation to the potential immunogenicity of biopharmaceuticals.

1.2. Antigen Uptake, Processing and Presentation by Antigen Presenting Cells

1.2.1. Antigen Presenting Cells

Several different cell types can process and present antigens to T-cells. Certain cell lineages are considered "professional" APCs since they are particularly efficient in presentation of antigenic peptide fragments on MHC class I and MHC class II molecules and in delivering the simultaneous co-stimulatory signals through the expression of molecules such as the B7-family proteins. Such cell types include B-cells, macrophages and DCs (reviewed by Trombetta and Mellman 2005). DCs will be emphasized here due to their documented relative superiority in antigen processing and presentation.

1.2.1.1. B-cells
Antigen presentation by B-cells is linked to their primary function as antibody-producing cells. B-cells are therefore mainly involved in presentation of soluble antigens which the B-cells may bind by their clonally unique surface immunoglobulin receptors. After antigen uptake and processing, peptide fragments are displayed on MHC class II molecules at the B-cell surface (Lanzavecchia 1990). Upon concomitant up-regulation of co-stimulatory activity, induced by for instance microbial constituents, antigen-presenting B-cells may, after an encounter with antigen-specific T-cells, activate the proliferation and differentiation of $CD4^+$ Th cells from which B-cells also receive help (Parker 1993). This reciprocity links the specificity of the humoral antibody- and T-cell mediated responses.

1.2.1.2. Macrophages
Macrophages are specialized in phagocytosis of particulates such as microbes, and they have an extensive capacity for the endocytosis and internalization of a wide range of antigens. They are important cells of the non-specific innate first line of immune defense by their ability to engulf and destruct microorganisms. Macrophages are also able to stimulate adaptive immune responses by presenting antigenic peptides on MHC class I and class II molecules to T-cells and by their expression of co-stimulatory molecules (Pfeifer et al. 1993). MHC and co-stimulatory molecules are upregulated by inflammatory cytokines and bacterial products, but in general, these molecules are expressed in lower levels on macrophages as compared to DCs, and therefore, macrophages are less efficient in antigen presentation and T-cell stimulation than DCs.

1.2.1.3. Dendritic Cells
DCs are nowadays recognized as one of the most potent and important APC-lineages since their ability to stimulate primary immune responses and to

establish immunological memory is superior to that of macrophages (reviewed in Banchereau and Steinman 1998). DCs migrate from peripheral tissues, where antigen uptake can take place, into draining lymph nodes, and thus act as sentinels of the immune system collecting foreign antigens and stimulating effector cells in the lymph nodes, – a capacity characteristic for DCs and not for macrophages (reviewed in Guermonprez et al. 2002). DCs can thus perform functions as different as antigen uptake, antigen processing and T-cell stimulation through a finely regulated developmental program.

DCs are generated from hematopoietic progenitors in the bone marrow that differentiate into precursors circulating in the blood and lymph. In the absence of inflammatory stimuli and foreign antigen exposure, DCs constitutively patrol through the blood, the peripheral tissues, the lymph and the secondary lymphoid organs. DCs also reside in the peripheral tissues, particularly at sites of interface with the environment and thus in areas of potential antigen entry (e.g. the skin epidermis and the mucosa), where they may constitute 1–2% of the total number of cells (Hart 1997; Banchereau and Steinman 1998; Banchereau et al. 2000). This localization allows for an early and efficient uptake of foreign antigens from infectious material by DCs. Administration of a protein biopharmaceutical into sites with a high prevalence of DCs, e.g. by subcutaneous injection, seems to increase the risk of immunogenicity due to prolonged exposure to and uptake by DCs as compared with intravenous administration (Kirchner et al. 1990; Perini et al. 2001).

In the peripheral tissues, DCs exist in a stage called immature DCs characterized by a high sampling of self and non-self antigens (Banchereau and Steinman 1998). In situ, DCs have a unique and characteristic stellate appearance with numerous long dendrites extending from the cell body in many directions, hence the name dendritic cells (Banchereau and Steinman 1998). These dendrites possess high motility and provide the DCs with a large surface area for antigen uptake in the immature stage as well as for T-cell interactions subsequent to DC maturation.

DCs are recruited to sites of antigen deposits where they efficiently take up antigens, process them and load antigen-derived peptides onto MHC class I and class II molecules. Chemokines released by, for instance, infectious tissue damage are responsible for the attraction of DCs that sense chemokine gradients through surface chemokine receptors (CCR) (reviewed in Banchereau et al. 2000). DCs express several CCRs, among them CCR1, CCR2, CCR4, CCR5, CCR6, CXCR1 and CXCR4. These receptors mediate DC migration towards gradients of chemokines such as macrophage inflammatory protein (MIP) 1a, RANTES (short for "regulated upon activation, normal T-cell expressed and secreted"), monophage-derived protein-3, MIP5 and monocyte chemoattractant protein (reviewed in Banchereau et al. 2000). DCs also express adhesion molecules that enable them to enter the peripheral tissues (Tang et al. 1993). Immature DCs are thus specialized in detection and uptake of foreign antigens in the peripheral tissues.

A high degree of heterogeneity exists among DC subsets in situ possibly reflecting the multiple functions of this cell lineage (reviewed in Cella et al. 1997b; Nouri-Shirazi et al. 2000). There is evidence for the existence of at least two different human CD34$^+$ hematopoietic precursors: one of the myeloid lineage, that gives rise to granulocytes/monocytes and myeloid DCs, and the other of the lymphoid lineage giving rise to T-, B-, natural killer

(NK)-cells and lymphoid DCs. The existence of a common human lymphoid precursor is still controversial, but a $CD14^-$ $CD11c^+$ $IL-3R\alpha^+$ precursor may originate from $CD34^+$ lymphoid hematopoietic progenitors (reviewed in Nouri-Shirazi et al. 2000). Thus DCs constitute a heterogeneous lineage with subtypes in different tissues. It is beyond the scope of this chapter to describe these DC subsets further, but the heterogeneity of DCs could be understood in the light of the different functions achieved in multiple anatomical localizations even though the lineage origins and functional differences are not fully clarified yet.

Although DCs continuously sample antigens from the environment, peripheral DCs present antigens quite inefficiently and have been denoted as quiescent (Janeway 1989). So-called "danger signals" from pathogens or inflammatory stimuli activate DCs to undergo the developmental program called maturation. Functions related to antigen acquisition and processing are downregulated during maturation and functions related to antigen presentation and T-cell activation are upregulated turning DCs into potent activators of antigen-specific naïve T-cells (Sallusto and Lanzavecchia 1994). Additionally, maturation induces concomitant migration of DCs from peripheral tissues via the afferent lymphatic vessels into the T-cell areas of the secondary lymphoid organs, where the encounter with naïve antigen-specific T-cells takes place (von Andrian and Mempel 2003). The expression pattern of chemokine receptors and adhesion molecules on the DC surface and the cytoskeleton organization are modified to enable this migration (Banchereau et al. 2000). By this finely coordinated process, only antigens processed by DCs concomitant with the presence of "danger signals" will be able to subsequently activate specific T-cell responses. This ensures that immune responses under normal conditions only are initiated in the presence of additional signals from pathogens and injured tissue, as proposed by P. Matzinger in the "Danger model" (Matzinger 2002).

DCs are activated towards maturation by several signals from pathogens including the direct recognition of PAMPs through specific PRRs and the indirect sensing of infection through inflammatory cytokines or ongoing specific immune responses (Guermonprez et al. 2002). Examples of important groups of receptors on the DC cell surface that are involved by mediating activation of intracellular signal transduction cascades in the induction of DC-maturation include TLRs, cytokine receptors, CD40, Fc receptors (FcR) and sensors for cell death.

Engagement of TLRs thus contributes to the maturation of DCs. DCs can also sense alarm signals through cytokine receptors that bind inflammatory mediators such as tumor necrosis factor (TNF)-α, interleukin (IL)-1β and prostaglandin E2 secreted in response to pathogens (reviewed in Banchereau et al. 2000). $CD4^+$ T-cells can induce DC maturation by triggering of CD40 by CD40 ligand on T-cells (Caux et al. 1994). Immunoglobulin and immunocomplexes can affect DC maturation as well, in a process where FcRs on the DCs are engaged. Finally, maturation of DCs is induced by neighboring cell death. It has been hypothesized that only necrotic and not apoptotic cells induce DC maturation (Gallucci et al. 1999; Sauter et al. 2000), although there are some controversies concerning such distinction in the literature. It has been argued that physiological cell death by apoptosis would not activate immune mechanisms. Apoptotic cells are usually scavenged before they disintegrate, whereas necrotic cells release their content in the extracellular fluid. Several compounds induced by cell death are suggested to induce DC maturation, including nucleotides and heat shock proteins that bind to specific receptors on DCs (Guermonprez et al. 2002).

1.2.2. Antigen Uptake Mechanisms

Antigens are taken up by APCs via several different mechanisms described below, and subsequently delivered to endosomal/lysosomal compartments for further processing (reviewed by Trombetta and Mellman 2005). Endocytosis is usually categorized into four general types based on internalization mechanisms and the size of the antigenic structure: phagocytosis, macropinocytosis, clathrin-dependent receptor-mediated endocytosis and caveolae-mediated endocytosis. These sampling routes have different capacities for the uptake of antigens and cause distinct downstream events.

1.2.2.1. Receptor-Mediated Endocytosis

The capture of antigens by APCs can be facilitated by a broad range of cell surface receptors via receptor-mediated endocytosis (Lanzavecchia 1990). Clathrin-dependent receptor-mediated endocytosis proceeds through specialized regions of the plasma membrane called clathrin-coated pits. Ligand recognition by several different receptors generates a signal in the cytoplasmic tail of the endocytic receptor, which is recognized by a family of adaptor proteins responsible for the recruitment of clathrin lattices and the formation of clathrin-coated endocytosis vesicles of approximately 100 nm (Slepnev and De Camilli 2000). Endocytosis can also, to a lesser extent, proceed via caveolae-mediated endocytosis. Five main types of endocytic receptors with different specificities are present at various levels, depending on the cellular sub-type, on the surface of DCs: FcR specific for the F_C portion of immunoglobulins (Sallusto and Lanzavecchia 1994; Fanger et al. 1996), complement receptors (CR), heat shock protein receptors (Singh-Jasuja et al. 2000), scavenger receptors, receptors of the C-type lectin family such as the macrophage mannose receptor (Sallusto et al. 1995) and DEC-205 (a 205 kDa protein expressed on DCs and thymic epithelium) (Jiang et al. 1995). The fast and efficient acquisition of antigens via receptor-mediated endocytosis enables the immune system to rapidly respond to antigens present in very low concentrations.

1.2.2.2. Macropinocytosis

Immature DCs and probably also macrophages are able to sample large amounts of extracellular fluid and solutes by macropinocytosis in a constitutive, rapid and non-specific way (Steinman and Swanson 1995; Sallusto et al. 1995). The process is actin dependent, requires membrane ruffling, and large pinocytotic vesicles (0.5–3 µm) are formed intracellularly (Amyere et al. 2002). Macropinosomes invaginate from the plasma membrane ruffling domains that fold back against the cell membrane or against each other to enclose a vesicle. The uptake rate of one DC has been estimated to be approximately 1000–1500 μm^3/h corresponding to one cell volume per hour (Jacque et al. 2002). This bulk uptake serves to concentrate antigens in DCs and makes the cells efficient in presenting soluble antigens present in nanomolar to picomolar concentrations in the surroundings. Macropinocytosis is the main mechanism responsible for the uptake by APCs of injected soluble antigens in therapeutic proteins administered by the intravenous, the intraperitoneal or the intradermal route leading to a subsequent transfer of antigens to the lymph nodes (Aderem and Underhill 1999; Delamarre et al. 2005).

1.2.2.3. Phagocytosis

Particulate antigens are taken up primarily by DCs and macrophages via phagocytosis (Reis e Sousa et al. 1993). Phagocytosis includes the uptake of particles too large to be accommodated by clathrin-coated pits. Phagocytosis is in general receptor-mediated, where cross-linking of surface receptors (the same receptors as those used for receptor-mediated endocytosis) by ligands causes avid binding of antigen and triggers signal transduction resulting in cytoskeleton rearrangements, actin polymerization and effective engulfment into phagosomes. Immature DCs phagocytose almost any bacteria (e.g. *Streptococcus aureus*, *Salmonella typhimurium*, *Escherichia coli* and *Mycobacterium tuberculosis*), yeast and parasites like *Leishmania major* (Guermonprez et al. 2002). Immature DCs can also phagocytose apoptotic and necrotic bodies in a process mediated by diverse soluble molecules or receptors (e.g. complement receptors, CD14, integrins and SR-family members) (Rubartelli et al. 1997; Albert et al. 1998). Such sampling of self-antigens from apoptotic cells is believed to play a key role for the maintenance of steady state tolerance (Steinman et al. 2000; Iyoda et al. 2002; Savill et al. 2002).

1.2.3. Antigen Processing and Presentation

Upon uptake, antigens are processed for presentation by MHC molecules via different pathways described below.

1.2.3.1. MHC Class-II-Restricted Antigen Presentation

Antigens present in the extracellular fluids (soluble and particulate) are eventually presented by MHC class II molecules on APCs (Figure 1.2). Proteins are internalized via different mechanisms into the endocytic compartments (as described previously) where a process of acidification of the endocytic vesicles activates proteases that cleave the antigenic proteins into peptides. These peptides are subsequently loaded onto MHC class II molecules (Watts 2001). MHC class II molecules are synthesized in the endoplasmic reticulum (ER) where they bind to the invariant chain molecule (Cresswell 1996). Invariant chain binds to MHC class II with part of its polypeptide chain present in the peptide-binding groove preventing the premature binding of self-peptides or unfolded proteins. Invariant chain targets the delivery of MHC class II molecules from the ER to the low-pH endosomal compartments. Here, invariant chain is cleaved leaving a short peptide fragment CLIP (*cl*ass II-associated *i*nvariant chain *p*eptide) in the peptide-binding groove (Villadangos et al. 1999). Removal of CLIP and binding of endocytosed antigenic peptides is catalyzed by human leukocyte antigen (HLA) DM (Kropshofer et al. 1999). The MHC class II-peptide-complexes are then transported to the cell surface, where they may interact with antigen-specific TcRs of CD4+ T-cells.

1.2.3.2. MHC Class I-Restricted Antigen Presentation

MHC class I molecules display peptides from foreign proteins expressed in the cytosol of cells (Cresswell et al. 1999) and are thus of less importance (if cross-presentation is not involved, see below) for the induction of immunogenicity

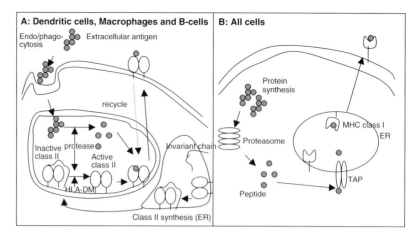

Figure 1.2 Antigen-presenting pathways. (A) In the endoplasmic reticulum (ER), MHC class II molecules, heterodimers composed of an α- and β-chain, associate with the invariant chain, which prevents them from binding peptides. This complex is transported to endocytic vesicles where the invariant chain is hydrolyzed and its bound fragments removed by HLA-DM molecules. MHC class II molecules then bind peptides that are generated by proteolysis of proteins that are present in endocytic compartments (e.g. from internalized proteins). The class II molecules transport the bound peptides for display at the cell surface and may recycle back into endosomes to acquire new peptides. This pathway is operative in DCs, macrophages and B lymphocytes. (B) In all cells, viral and cellular proteins are cleaved into oligopeptides by proteasomes in the cytoplasm, a fraction of which are transported into the ER by TAP. Newly synthesized MHC class I molecules bind these peptides and transport them to the cell surface. Modified from Raychaudhuri and Rock (1998).

towards biopharmaceuticals than MHC class II molecules (Figure 1.2). The cytosolic proteins can be viral or bacterial proteins or endogenous proteins expressed by cells. The majority of the MHC class I-restricted peptides are generated in the cytoplasm by proteolytic degradation of the proteins into peptides catalyzed by the proteasome (Shastri et al. 2002). The proteasome is a large, multicatalytical protease complex with a hollow core wherein proteins are broken down into peptide fragments. Cytosolic chaperones are thought to protect peptides from exhaustive degradation in the cytosol (Kunisawa and Shastri 2003). The peptide fragments are then transported into the lumen of the ER via the transporters associated with antigen processing (TAP), where final trimming of peptides is thought to occur, and the peptide fragments are then loaded onto newly synthesized MHC class I molecules (Bouvier 2003). Peptide-loaded MHC class I molecules are transported through the Golgi apparatus to the cell surface for presentation to CD8+ T-cells.

1.2.3.3. Cross-Presentation

Most antigens present in the extracellular fluid are presented by the MHC class II presentation pathway but not the MHC class I pathway (Raychaudhuri and Rock 1998). However, recent findings suggest that there is a cross-talk between the two pathways, since certain types of exogenous antigens can also be presented by MHC class I molecules on DCs in particular, and to a lesser extent also on macrophages, a process referred to as cross-presentation (Yewdell et al. 1999; Ackerman and Cresswell 2004). Several models for cross-presentation have been proposed, and these may be classified according to their dependency of TAP, since both a TAP-dependent and a TAP-independent mechanism exist (Yewdell et al. 1999).

For the TAP-independent mechanism, uptake of antigens by phagocytosis proceeds via vacuolar pathways whereby peptides derived from exogenous antigens bind to MHC class I molecules within the post-Golgi vacuolar compartment or on the cell surface (Pfeifer et al. 1993). The model of TAP-dependent cross-presentation suggests that whole organisms or antigens escape from vacuolar compartments after phagocytosis into the cytosol, undergo cytosolic processing and subsequently bind to MHC class I molecules in the ER (Kovacsovics-Bankowski et al. 1993; Norbury et al. 1997; Rodriguez et al. 1999; Regnault et al. 1999). There is evidence for a membrane transport pathway, linking the lumen of endocytic compartments and the cytosol in DCs (Rodriguez et al. 1999) and macrophages (Kovacsovics-Bankowski and Rock 1995) that participates in the TAP-dependent cross-priming.

Several uptake mechanisms in DCs may participate in the delivery of antigens for cross-presentation. These includes macropinocytosis (Norbury et al. 1997), phagocytosis (Kovacsovics-Bankowski et al. 1993; Albert et al. 1998; Wick and Ljunggren 1999) and receptor-mediated endocytosis (reviewed in (Guermonprez et al. 2002)).

1.3. Lymphocyte Activation

Upon antigen uptake, processing and MHC loading, APCs present antigen to T lymphocytes. Below is presented how one type of APC, the DCs, stimulates lymphocytes to proliferate and differentiate into functional effector cells. Activation of B lymphocytes by thymus-independent antigens is described in Section 1.3.3.

1.3.1. Regulation of MHC upon DC Maturation

Maturation of DCs induces changes in antigen presentation. Antigen uptake is downregulated during the process of maturation due to loss of endocytotic/phagocytotic receptors and decreased macropinocytosis. Soluble and particulate antigens after uptake are directed to MHC class II compartments in the DCs (Sallusto and Lanzavecchia 1994; Inaba et al. 1998). The antigens are degraded into peptide fragments due to the lysosomal-like environment in the MHC class II compartments that causes weak proteolytic degradation. In immature DCs, MHC class II molecules are continuously synthesized and have a fast turnover rate in MHC class II compartments (Kleijmeer et al. 1995). Upon maturation the turnover decreases, there is a transient burst in MHC class II synthesis, peptide fragments are loaded on the molecules after removal of invariant chain, and the complexes are translocated to the cell surface and assembled into clusters of molecules involved in T-cell stimulation (Turley et al. 2000). MHC class I synthesis and half-life are increased upon induction of maturation (Rescigno et al. 1998), although to a lower extent than those of MHC class II (Cella et al. 1997a). The decreased turnover rate of MHC molecules upon DC maturation leads to an increased duration of the surface peptide presentation, enhancing the probability of encounter with and activation of specific T-cells (Steinman et al. 1999). MHC class I presentation is also altered upon DC maturation.

1.3.2. Priming of Lymphocytes by DC

T-cell priming is achieved in the T-cell areas of the secondary lymphoid organs into which DCs rapidly migrate upon maturation (Randolph 2001; Mempel et al. 2004). DC and T-cell clustering in lymph nodes is mediated by adhesion molecules such as integrin $\beta 1$, CD2, CD50, CD54 and CD58. Morphological changes, including cytoskeleton rearrangements and increased cellular motility, result in the formation of cytoplasmic projections, so-called veils, that create a large surface area for interaction with up to 3000 T-cells per DC (Mellman and Steinman 2001). Antigen-specific interactions occur between peptide-loaded MHC complexes on DCs and antigen-specific TCRs on T-cells. The second activation signal is mediated by co-stimulatory molecules on DCs (e.g. ICOS, CD40, CD80) and their respective ligand or receptor on T-cells thus sustaining and amplifying the activation signaling. T-cells and APCs establish contact by forming an "immunological synapse", where TCRs and co-stimulatory molecules are congregated in a central area surrounded by a ring of adhesion molecules (Dustin and Cooper 2000). Naïve T-cells that have received signal 1 and 2 from APCs become activated and both secrete and respond to IL-2, which induces proliferation and differentiation into functional effector T-cells (Janeway and Bottomly 1994).

Naïve antigen-specific $CD4^+$ T-cells are primed by antigen-presenting DCs, and these Th-cells can interact with B-cells and stimulate antigen-specific antibody production (a Th-dependent response). DCs can also prime naïve $CD8^+$ T-cells in the absence of $CD4^+$ T-cells, but in general, the induction of an antigen-specific T-cell response requires $CD4^+$ T-cell help (Banchereau and Steinman 1998).

After activation, naïve $CD4^+$ T-cells differentiate into functional sub-lineages, including Th1 cells and Th2 cells (reviewed in Mosmann and Coffman 1989). The division into Th-subsets is largely based on their secretion of different cytokines, and since the identification of Th1/Th2 cells, additional Th lineages have been identified such as Th3 and Th17 (Weaver et al. 2006). Th1 cells are characterized mainly by the secretion of interferon (IFN)-γ, and they promote cell-mediated immune responses to intracellular pathogens. Th1 activity is dependent on IL-12-production from APCs following exposure to pathogens. Th2 cells are characterized by the secretion of cytokines, such as IL-4, IL-5, IL-10 and IL13. Th2 cells support the production of circulating antibodies and participate in immune responses against extracellular pathogens. IL-4 production by APCs tends to favor a Th2 type of response.

The differentiation into either Th1 or Th2 cells is mutually antagonistic since up-regulation of one subset leads to down-regulation of the other subset. Different DC subsets have been shown to posses diverse capacities to polarize Th-cell responses, but other factors are also important for polarization, such as the local cytokine environment, the presence of pathogenic signals, tissue-specific environmental factors, the DC/T-cell ratio and the duration of DC stimulation (Guermonprez et al. 2002).

$CD8^+$ T-cells mediate their effector function through the production of cytokines such as IFN-γ and TNF-α and through direct cytolytic effects

(Squier and Cohen 1994). The cytotoxicity is mediated by the release of granule contents, such as perforin and granzyme that lyse target cells by creating pores in the cell membrane. In addition, $CD8^+$ CTL can kill target cells by a process of Fas-mediated apoptosis (Fisher et al. 1995).

1.3.3. T-cell-Independent Activation of B-lymphocytes

B-cell responses to most protein antigens require $CD4^+$ T-cell mediated help. However, polymeric antigens with multiple repeating antigenic epitopes are able to directly activate B-cells by cross-linking of the immunoglobulin receptors (Fluckiger et al. 1998). These antigens, referred to as thymus-independent antigens, include bacterial cell wall components, for example, lipopolysaccharide. B-cell activation by such thymus-independent antigens are important for the rapid production of antibodies towards microbial antigens consisting of repeated determinants (Vos et al. 2000) but may also be involved in the immune reactions towards biopharmaceuticals with highly repetitive structures, where the co-stimulatory signal can be mediated via alternative signaling pathways (e.g. TLR engagement) (Rosenberg 2006).

1.4. Immunological Tolerance

B-cell receptors (BCRs) and TCRs, randomly generated by gene rearrangements in developing lymphocytes, as previously mentioned, ensure a highly diverse B- and T-cell repertoire providing for a potential recognition of a vast array of antigens. A subset of these lymphocytes will express self-reactive receptors and hence must be regulated in order to prevent autoimmune responses. It has been estimated that up to 75% of newly generated immature B-cells in the bone marrow of healthy individuals are polyreactive and capable of binding self-antigens (De Boer and Perelson 1993; Nemazee 1996; Wardemann et al. 2003), whereas up to 30% of the naïve T-cells exiting from the thymus may be autoreactive (Zerrahn et al. 1997). A proportion of autoreactive cells enter the mature B- and T-cell pool and may in rare cases contribute to the generation of autoimmune diseases. A series of "checkpoints" in the pathway of lymphocyte differentiation have evolved that ensures that autoreactive T- and B-cells are regulated through what is called central and peripheral tolerance mechanisms, which are described below (Figure 1.3).

1.4.1. Central Tolerance

The initial mechanism in order to achieve immunological tolerance engages the populations of immature T-cells in the thymus and immature B-cells developing in the bone marrow. By a negative selection procedure, also referred to as a central tolerance mechanism, any newly generated lymphocyte expressing a receptor that binds a self-antigen with sufficiently high affinity may be deleted (induced cell death) in a clonally specific fashion (Surh and Sprent 1994; Cornall et al. 1995).

T-cell development requires TCR gene rearrangements (variable α-, β-gene segments) in the thymic cortex followed by a halt of recombination. Following positive selection of single-positive ($CD4^+$ or $CD8^+$) T-cells, clonal deletion (negative selection) may be ensured in the thymic medulla

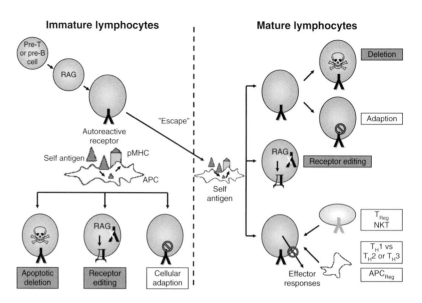

Figure 1.3 Mechanisms that regulate lymphocytes expressing autoreactive receptors. Some of the T-cell- and B-cell-receptors generated by random recombination in developing lymphocytes possess the ability to bind to a self-antigen. These autoreactive immature lymphocytes may either be deleted (cell death by apoptosis) or a receptor re-editing mechanism, initiated when the receptor engages a self-antigen, may lead to an altered specificity (dark grey labels). Alternatively, the cells may undergo functional alterations (white labels). In the case of T-cell recognition, the specific antigen has to be processed and presented on self-MHC molecules, (pMHC) while B-cells can recognize intact soluble or membrane-bound antigens. Autoreactive lymphocytes may alternatively be regulated by the induction of negative intracellular signaling (down-regulation leading to anergy) which prevents specific responses to self-antigens. Autoreactive lymphocytes that escape these processes and join the peripheral pool of mature lymphocytes may be deleted or down-regulated in the periphery which is for the T-cells dependent on the encounter of autoantigen-presenting cells. Finally, the ability of potentially autoreactive lymphocytes to induce pathology can be controlled by interactions with peripheral regulatory cells (including regulatory T-cells, NK cells, regulatory APCs). Modified from Singh and Schwartz (2006).

(Surh and Sprent 1994). The thymus is a unique organ also in the sense that certain cells within the thymus not only express thymus-specific antigens but also non-thymic, tissue-specific gene products. The thymus thus "mirrors" other tissues in the body (Kyewski and Klein 2006). Presentation of these ectopically expressed antigens in the context of MHC molecules by thymic APCs leads to the deletion of tissue-specific autoreactive T-cells (Gotter et al. 2004). Depending on high-affinity recognition, potentially autoreactive cells are deleted and thus eliminated already at their site of differentiation. Autoreactive lymphocytes may escape this clonal deletion fate, for instance, by virtue of secondary recombination ("re-editing") to a non-self reactive receptor specificity (Nemazee and Hogquist 2003), though there are some controversies concerning the importance of such a mechanism.

For the autoreactive immature B-cells, the mechanisms of deletion and possibly receptor re-editing are believed to be initiated by the encounter with high-avidity antigens that mediate signaling through the BCR, leading to a developmental arrest (Nemazee and Burki 1989; Hartley et al. 1991; Hartley et al. 1993; Lang et al. 1996). Deletion of autoreactive B-cells thus does not require APCs. The cells can escape death by re-editing of the BCR (Erikson et al. 1991; Tiegs et al. 1993). If such receptor DNA recombination towards a non-autoreactive BCR fails, the cell dies within 1–2 days.

1.4.2. Peripheral Tolerance

In spite of the central tolerance mechanisms in the bone marrow and in the thymus, many autoreactive lymphocytes exit into the peripheral pool of circulating lymphocytes. Additional mechanisms, collectively referred to as peripheral tolerance mechanisms, ensure the low incidence of autoimmune reactions towards self-antigens. In general, peripheral autoreactive lymphocytes are thought to be either eliminated or regulated upon recognition of specific self-antigens, or alternatively existing in different stages of anergy, the latter of which may represent a reversible state of tolerance (reviewed by Singh and Schwartz 2006).

1.4.2.1. Peripheral B-cell Tolerance

The majority of autoreactive B-cells dies after a short lifespan in the spleen and other in secondary lymphoid organs (MacLennan and Gray 1986; Chan and MacLennan 1993). Engagement of the BCR via low-avidity binding to auto-antigens can induce a state of anergy or resistance to activation (Healy and Goodnow 1998; Hippen et al. 2005). Anergy is characterized by a developmental arrest and an increased threshold for activation by antigens (Cooke et al. 1994). Anergic B-cells may interact with CD4$^+$ T-cells, but in the absence of BCR signaling, no activation occurs. Instead, the B-cells may be killed in a CD40-ligand Fas-dependent manner (Rathmell et al. 1995; Rathmell et al. 1996).

Some anergic B-cells can escape cell death and survive for longer periods after chronic self-antigen engagement. Negative signaling molecules, such as intracellular phosphatases, can balance the activating signal from BCR engagement resulting in anergy (Cannons and Schwartzberg 2004). Higher avidity antigens may overcome BCR signaling blockade, and anergic B-cells can be recruited into an immune response (Cooke et al. 1994). Such antigens include structurally organized antigens from pathogens or aggregates of biopharmaceutical proteins. T-cell help is probably needed for such B-cell activation to occur, thus requiring both breaking of B-cell and T-cell tolerance (Rathmell et al. 1998). B-cells directed against rare, low-affinity, tissue-specific or highly sequestered intracellular antigens may not be initially tolerized.

1.4.2.2. Peripheral T-cell Tolerance

T-cells are only activated into an efficient immune response if the antigen recognition takes place in the presence of co-stimulatory signals from APCs. This mechanism ensures that T-cells are specifically activated in the periphery upon encounter with pathogens or "tissue danger" as sensed by the APCs, as described above. Furthermore, self-reactive T-cells can adapt towards an un-reactive phenotype in the periphery. Block of TCR signaling causes the inhibition of production of cytokines as well as the inhibition of a clonal expansion in response to TCR engagement (Schwartz 2003).

Regulation of peripheral autoreactive T-cells may also be achieved by the upregulation of co-inhibitory molecules expressed by lymphocytes (reviewed in Leibson 2004). Examples of such molecules are CTLA-4, programmed cell death 1 (PD1) and CD22 (Probst et al. 2005). Finally, certain types of lymphocytes have been shown to regulate the autoreactivity of autologous lymphocytes. An example is the $CD25^+$ regulatory T-cells that represent 5–7% of the normal peripheral $CD4^+$ T-cell population (Sakaguchi et al. 1995). $CD25^+$ $Foxp3^+$regulatory T-cells can inhibit the activation of autoreactive T-cells. Other examples of cells with regulatory functions are NKT-cells and certain APCs (Taniguchi et al. 2003; Smits et al. 2005; Lund et al. 2005).

1.5. Self Versus Non-self, the Danger Model and Biopharmaceuticals

Over the years, different theories have aimed at explaining how the immune system is able to discriminate between self and foreign antigens. Early observations suggested that signaling through antigen-specific receptors initiates an immune response exclusively towards non-self antigens, since self-reactive lymphocytes are deleted early in life as described in previous section. The theory was later modified upon the discovery of the need for co-stimulation in the activation of T-cells (as described in Section 1.1.2; Jenkins and Schwartz 1987), and further modified by Janeway in 1989 into an "infectious non-self" and "non-infectious self" model upon the discovery of activation of APCs by PAMPs via PRRs (Janeway 1989). More recently, Matzinger proposed in the "danger model" that it is alarm signals in response to damage that initially activate the immune system and not merely the recognition of non-self antigens (Matzinger 1994). According to this theory, APCs are activated by danger/alarm signals from injured cells, such as cells exposed to pathogens, toxins and mechanical damage. These alarm signals are of a diverse nature and can be intracellular, secreted or part of the extracellular matrix.

Concerning potential immune reactions towards biopharmaceuticals upon administration to patients, these theories imply that the immune system is mainly activated if the administered drug formulation elicits APC-activating alarm signals. Such signals may be related to the drug molecule itself (e.g. double stranded RNA or CpG motif on DNA), the formulation of the drug (e.g. protein aggregates, impurities or improper choice of exipients), the administration of the drug (e.g. necrosis at an injection site) and the general immune status of the patient. An example of the requirements for additional stimulation of an antigen-specific immune response is provided by the field of vaccinology, where it is well known that adjuvants are necessary in order to induce efficient and robust adaptive immune responses towards therapeutics based on certain xenogeneic proteins, i.e. the foreignness of the protein itself may be an insufficient immune stimulator.

However, it is generally accepted that the immunogenicity of therapeutic proteins is influenced by the degree of difference in amino acid sequence between the therapeutic protein and the endogenous counterpart. Protein therapeutics based on human endogenous proteins should obviously be the least immunogenic, for example, products purified from human blood or recombinant cytokines and growth factors (Schellekens 2002). Still, many of the conserved human proteins contain a degree of allogeneic variability that may cause immunological and clinical consequences. An example that illustrates the clinical importance of genetic (and protein) matching is provided by the medical issues which may be encountered after allogeneic tissue transplantations.

Protein therapeutics of a xenogeneic origin imply the highest risk of immunogenicity due to the presence of foreign epitopes (e.g. expressed on murine antibodies produced for clinical therapy). Such products can, after uptake by APCs, in addition to a possible direct stimulation of B-cells and macrophages, result in a specific B- and Th-cell stimulation and the production of specific antibodies as well as the induction of memory cells. Such responses tend to decrease the treatment efficacy via neutralization and increased elimination of the administered foreign antibody or protein. An additional important effect due to such production of antibodies may be a neutralization of the endogenous counterpart molecule. Furthermore, there may be an induction of inflammatory and allergic reactions of potential clinical importance. Over the past years, research has aimed at overcoming such obstacles as exemplified by the development of, in the case of antibody treatments, chimeric or "humanized" monoclonal antibodies.

In addition, as previously mentioned, factors related to the product manufacture may also influence the immunogenicity of the administered product, such as contamination of the product by material of non-self origin. Protein purification is a complex process and even minor changes in the manufacturing procedures can result in markedly different immunogenicity due to structural alterations that create new epitopes recognized as non-self (Ryff 1997). Chemical instability (oxidation, deamidation) can also lead to structural changes and formation of non-self epitopes. Upon repeated administration such non-self epitopes could, together with "activators" of the innate immune system (adjuvants), function as "vaccines" enhancing the immunogenicity of a particular therapeutic protein leading to increased immune reactions ("secondary immune response").

Some protein therapeutics have been observed to break immunological tolerance and may induce specific immune responses. These therapeutics include recombinant human self-proteins such as insulin and granulocyte macrophage colony stimulating factor (GM-CSF), which is further described in later chapters of this book. The disruption of tolerance may be a slow process developing over months or longer. However, it does not necessarily imply obvious immediate consequences for the patient.

As described in Section 1.4, multiple mechanisms ensure that the lymphocyte repertoire is tolerized towards self-antigens. However, since both autoreactive T-cells and B-cells in the periphery may become activated, the latter by Th-cells in CD40-ligand-CD40-dependent ways, or in a T-cell-independent fashion, tolerance can be broken (Melchers and Rolink 2006). Microbial infectious agents and impurities or aggregates of therapeutic proteins may cause an activation of auto-reactive lymphocytes through (1) the release of sequestered autoantigens in the context of alarm signals as exemplified above; (2) activation of autoreactive lymphocytes due to molecular mimicry of autoantigens; or (3) polyclonal activation of T- and/or B-cells (Rosenberg 2006), etc. The result of an autoantigen-driven immune response may be the generation of autoantibodies and the expansion of long-lived memory B and plasma cells. High-avidity autoantigen-specific B-cells can interact efficiently with Th cells in response to very low concentrations of autoantigens (Coutinho et al. 1975; Lanzavecchia 1987), mechanisms which imply a potential risk of pathological consequences for the individual.

1.6. Concluding Remarks

Our immune system, composed of innate and adaptive defense mechanisms, has evolved towards the specific recognition of non-self and the tolerance to self-molecules. Biopharmaceuticals, with the exception of vaccines, should optimally consist exclusively of homologous "self-like" molecules, but can under certain circumstances contain non-self epitopes that activate innate and/or adaptive immune reactions thereby breaking immunological tolerance. Examples of such unfortunate events induced by biopharmaceuticals are presented in this book. An increased understanding of basic mechanisms underlying the activation and especially the regulation of specific and non-specific immune responses will help us to design formulations of future biopharmaceuticals with a reduced risk of inducing unwanted immunoreactivity.

Acknowledgements. We gratefully acknowledge the Danish Research Council for Technology and Production Sciences for financial support (CF).

References

Ackerman, A.L. and Cresswell, P. 2004. Cellular mechanisms governing cross-presentation of exogenous antigens. Nat. Immunol. 5:678–684

Aderem, A. and Underhill, D.M. 1999. Mechanisms of phagocytosis in macrophages. Annu. Rev. Immunol. 17:593–623

Akira, S. and Takeda, K. 2004. Toll-like receptor signalling. Nat. Rev. Immunol. 4:499–511

Albert, M.L., Pearce, S.F., Francisco, L.M., Sauter, B., Roy, P., Silverstein, R.L., and Bhardwaj, N. 1998. Immature dendritic cells phagocytose apoptotic cells via alphavbeta5 and CD36, and cross-present antigens to cytotoxic T lymphocytes. J. Exp. Med. 188:1359–1368

Amyere, M., Mettlen, M., Van, D., Platek, A., Payrastre, B., Veithen, A., and Courtoy, P.J. 2002. Origin, originality, functions, subversions and molecular signalling of macropinocytosis. Int. J. Med. Microbiol. 291:487–494

Banchereau, J., Briere, F., Caux, C., Davoust, J., Lebecque, S., Liu, Y.J., Pulendran, B., and Palucka, K. 2000. Immunobiology of dendritic cells. Annu. Rev. Immunol. 18:767–811

Banchereau, J. and Steinman, R.M. 1998. Dendritic cells and the control of immunity. Nature 392:245–252

Bouvier, M. 2003. Accessory proteins and the assembly of human class I MHC molecules: a molecular and structural perspective. Mol. Immunol. 39:697–706

Cannons, J.L. and Schwartzberg, P.L. 2004. Fine-tuning lymphocyte regulation: what's new with tyrosine kinases and phosphatases? Curr. Opin. Immunol. 16:296–303

Caux, C., Massacrier, C., Vanbervliet, B., Dubois, B., Van Kooten, C., Durand, I., and Banchereau, J. 1994. Activation of human dendritic cells through CD40 cross-linking. J. Exp. Med. 180:1263–1272

Cella, M., Engering, A., Pinet, V., Pieters, J., and Lanzavecchia, A. 1997a. Inflammatory stimuli induce accumulation of MHC class II complexes on dendritic cells. Nature 388:782–787

Cella, M., Salio, M., Sakakibara, Y., Langen, H., Julkunen, I., and Lanzavecchia, A. 1999. Maturation, activation, and protection of dendritic cells induced by double-stranded RNA. J. Exp. Med. 189:821–829

Cella, M., Sallusto, F., and Lanzavecchia, A. 1997b. Origin, maturation and antigen presenting function of dendritic cells. Curr. Opin. Immunol. 9:10–16

Chamaillard, M., Hashimoto, M., Horie, Y., Masumoto, J., Qiu, S., Saab, L., Ogura, Y., Kawasaki, A., Fukase, K., Kusumoto, S., Valvano, M.A., Foster, S.J., Mak, T.W., Nunez, G., and Inohara, N. 2003. An essential role for NOD1 in host recognition of bacterial peptidoglycan containing diaminopimelic acid. Nat. Immunol. 4:702–707

Chan, E.Y. and MacLennan, I.C. 1993. Only a small proportion of splenic B cells in adults are short-lived virgin cells. Eur. J. Immunol. 23:357–363

Cooke, M.P., Heath, A.W., Shokat, K.M., Zeng, Y., Finkelman, F.D., Linsley, P.S., Howard, M., and Goodnow, C.C. 1994. Immunoglobulin signal transduction guides the specificity of B cell-T cell interactions and is blocked in tolerant self-reactive B cells. J. Exp. Med. 179:425–438

Cornall, R.J., Goodnow, C.C., and Cyster, J.G. 1995. The regulation of self-reactive B cells. Curr. Opin. Immunol. 7:804–811

Coutinho, A., Gronowicz, E., and Moller, G. 1975. Mechanism of B-Cell Activation and Paralysis by Thymus-Independent Antigens – Additive Effects Between Nnp-Lps and Lps in Specific Response to Hapten. Scand. J. Immunol. 4:89–94

Cresswell, P. 1996. Invariant chain structure and MHC class II function. Cell 84: 505–507

Cresswell, P., Bangia, N., Dick, T., and Diedrich, G. 1999. The nature of the MHC class I peptide loading complex. Immunol. Rev. 172:21–28

De Boer, R.J. and Perelson, A.S. 1993. How diverse should the immune system be? Proc. Biol. Sci. 252:171–175

Delamarre, L., Pack, M., Chang, H., Mellman, I., and Trombetta, E.S. 2005. Differential lysosomal proteolysis in antigen-presenting cells determines antigen fate. Science 307:1630–1634

Dustin, M.L. and Cooper, J.A. 2000. The immunological synapse and the actin cytoskeleton: molecular hardware for T cell signaling. Nat. Immunol. 1:23–29

Erikson, J., Radic, M.Z., Camper, S.A., Hardy, R.R., Carmack, C., and Weigert, M. 1991. Expression of anti-DNA immunoglobulin transgenes in non-autoimmune mice. Nature 349:331–334

Fanger, N.A., Wardwell, K., Shen, L., Tedder, T.F., and Guyre, P.M. 1996. Type I (CD64) and type II (CD32) Fc gamma receptor-mediated phagocytosis by human blood dendritic cells. J. Immunol. 157:541–548

Fisher, G.H., Rosenberg, F.J., Straus, S.E., Dale, J.K., Middleton, L.A., Lin, A.Y., Strober, W., Lenardo, M.J., and Puck, J.M. 1995. Dominant interfering Fas gene mutations impair apoptosis in a human autoimmune lymphoproliferative syndrome. Cell 81:935–946

Fluckiger, A.C., Li, Z.M., Kato, R.M., Wahl, M.I., Ochs, H.D., Longnecker, R., Kinet, J.P., Witte, O.N., Scharenberg, A.M., and Rawlings, D.J. 1998. Btk/Tec kinases regulate sustained increases in intracellular Ca2+ following B-cell receptor activation. EMBO J. 17:1973–1985

Gallucci, S., Lolkema, M., and Matzinger, P. 1999. Natural adjuvants: endogenous activators of dendritic cells. Nat. Med. 5:1249–1255

Germain, R.N. 1994. MHC-dependent antigen processing and peptide presentation: providing ligands for T lymphocyte activation. Cell 76:287–299

Girardin, S.E., Boneca, I.G., Carneiro, L.A.M., Antignac, A., Jehanno, M., Viala, J., Tedin, K., Taha, M.K., Labigne, A., Zahringer, U., Coyle, A.J., Bertin, J., Sansonetti, P.J., and Philpott, D.J. 2003a. Nod1 detects a unique muropeptide from Gram-negative bacterial peptidoglycan. Science 300:1584–1587

Girardin, S.E., Boneca, I.G., Viala, J., Chamaillard, M., Labigne, A., Thomas, G., Philpott, D.J., and Sansonetti, P.J. 2003b. Nod2 is a general sensor of peptidoglycan through muramyl dipeptide (MDP) detection. J. Biol. Chem. 278:8869–8872

Girardin, S.E., Tournebize, R., Mavris, M., Page, A.L., Li, X., Stark, G.R., Bertin, J., DiStefano, P.S., Yaniv, M., Sansonetti, P.J., and Philpott, D.J. 2001. CARD4/Nod1 mediates NF-kappaB and JNK activation by invasive Shigella flexneri. EMBO Rep. 2:736–742

Gotter, J., Brors, B., Hergenhahn, M., and Kyewski, B. 2004. Medullary epithelial cells of the human thymus express a highly diverse selection of tissue-specific genes colocalized in chromosomal clusters. J. Exp. Med. 199:155–166

Gowans, J.L. 1996. The lymphocyte–a disgraceful gap in medical knowledge. Immunol. Today 17:288–291

Guermonprez, P., Valladeau, J., Zitvogel, L., Thery, C., and Amigorena, S. 2002. Antigen presentation and T cell stimulation by dendritic cells. Annu. Rev. Immunol. 20:621–667

Hart, D.N. 1997. Dendritic cells: unique leukocyte populations which control the primary immune response. Blood 90:3245–3287

Hartley, S.B., Cooke, M.P., Fulcher, D.A., Harris, A.W., Cory, S., Basten, A., and Goodnow, C.C. 1993. Elimination of self-reactive B lymphocytes proceeds in two stages: arrested development and cell death. Cell 72:325–335

Hartley, S.B., Crosbie, J., Brink, R., Kantor, A.B., Basten, A., and Goodnow, C.C. 1991. Elimination from peripheral lymphoid tissues of self-reactive B lymphocytes recognizing membrane-bound antigens. Nature 353:765–769

Healy, J.I. and Goodnow, C.C. 1998. Positive versus negative signaling by lymphocyte antigen receptors. Annu. Rev. Immunol. 16:645–670

Hippen, K.L., Schram, B.R., Tze, L.E., Pape, K.A., Jenkins, M.K., and Behrens, T.W. 2005. In vivo assessment of the relative contributions of deletion, anergy, and editing to B cell self-tolerance. J. Immunol. 175:909–916

Inaba, K., Turley, S., Yamaide, F., Iyoda, T., Mahnke, K., Inaba, M., Pack, M., Subklewe, M., Sauter, B., Sheff, D., Albert, M., Bhardwaj, N., Mellman, I., and Steinman, R.M. 1998. Efficient presentation of phagocytosed cellular fragments on the major histocompatibility complex class II products of dendritic cells. J. Exp. Med. 188:2163–2173

Inohara, N., Ogura, Y., Fontalba, A., Gutierrez, O., Pons, F., Crespo, J., Fukase, K., Inamura, S., Kusumoto, S., Hashimoto, M., Foster, S.J., Moran, A.P., Fernandez-Luna, J.L., and Nunez, G. 2003. Host recognition of bacterial muramyl dipeptide mediated through NOD2. J. Biol. Chem. 278:5509–5512

Iyoda, T., Shimoyama, S., Liu, K., Omatsu, Y., Akiyama, Y., Maeda, Y., Takahara, K., Steinman, R.M., and Inaba, K. 2002. The CD8+ dendritic cell subset selectively endocytoses dying cells in culture and in vivo. J. Exp. Med. 195:1289–1302

Jacque, J. M., Triques, K., and Stevenson, M. 2002. Modulation of HIV-1 replication by RNA interference. Nature 418:435–438

Janeway, C.A. Jr. 1989. Approaching the asymptote? Evolution and revolution in immunology. Cold Spring Harb. Symp. Quant. Biol. 54 Pt 1:1–13

Janeway, C.A. Jr. and Bottomly, K. 1994. Signals and signs for lymphocyte responses. Cell 76:275–285

Jenkins, M.K. and Schwartz, R.H. 1987. Antigen presentation by chemically modified splenocytes induces antigen-specific T-cell unresponsiveness in vitro and in vivo. J. Exp. Med. 165:302–319

Jiang, W., Swiggard, W.J., Heufler, C., Peng, M., Mirza, A., Steinman, R.M., and Nussenzweig, M.C. 1995. The receptor DEC-205 expressed by dendritic cells and thymic epithelial cells is involved in antigen processing. Nature 375:151–155

Kirchner, H., Korfer, A., Palmer, P.A., Evers, P., De Riese, W., Knuver-Hopf, J., Hadam, M., Goldman, U., Franks, C.R., and Poliwoda, H. 1990. Subcutaneous interleukin-2 and interferon-alpha 2b in patients with metastatic renal cell cancer: the German outpatient experience. Mol. Biother. 2:145–154

Kleijmeer, M.J., Ossevoort, M.A., van Veen, C.J., van Hellemond, J.J., Neefjes, J.J., Kast, W.M., Melief, C.J., and Geuze, H.J. 1995. MHC class II compartments and the kinetics of antigen presentation in activated mouse spleen dendritic cells. J. Immunol. 154:5715–5724

Kovacsovics-Bankowski, M., Clark, K., Benacerraf, B., and Rock, K.L. 1993. Efficient major histocompatibility complex class I presentation of exogenous antigen upon phagocytosis by macrophages. Proc. Natl. Acad. Sci. USA 90:4942–4946

Kovacsovics-Bankowski, M. and Rock, K.L. 1995. A phagosome-to-cytosol pathway for exogenous antigens presented on MHC class I molecules. Science 267:243–246

Kropshofer, H., Hammerling, G.J., and Vogt, A.B. 1999. The impact of the non-classical MHC proteins HLA-DM and HLA-DO on loading of MHC class II molecules. Immunol. Rev. 172:267–278

Kunisawa, J. and Shastri, N. 2003. The group II chaperonin TRiC protects proteolytic intermediates from degradation in the MHC class I antigen processing pathway. Mol. Cell 12:565–576

Kyewski, B. and Klein, L. 2006. A central role for central tolerance. Annu. Rev. Immunol. 24:571–606

Lang, J., Jackson, M., Teyton, L., Brunmark, A., Kane, K., and Nemazee, D. 1996. B cells are exquisitely sensitive to central tolerance and receptor editing induced by ultralow affinity, membrane-bound antigen. J. Exp. Med. 184:1685–1697

Lanzavecchia, A. 1987. Antigen uptake and accumulation in antigen-specific B-cells. Immunol. Rev. 99:39–51

Lanzavecchia, A. 1990. Receptor-mediated antigen uptake and its effect on antigen presentation to class II-restricted T lymphocytes. Annu. Rev. Immunol. 8:773–793

Leibson, P.J. 2004. The regulation of lymphocyte activation by inhibitory receptors. Curr. Opin. Immunol. 16:328–336

Lund, F.E., Garvy, B.A., Randall, T.D., and Harris, D.P. 2005. Regulatory roles for cytokine-producing B cells in infection and autoimmune disease. Curr. Dir. Autoimmun. 8:25–54

MacLennan, I.C. and Gray, D. 1986. Antigen-driven selection of virgin and memory B cells. Immunol. Rev. 91:61–85

Mariathasan, S. and Monack, D.M. 2007. Inflammasome adaptors and sensors: intra-cellular regulators of infection and inflammation. Nat. Rev. Immunol. 7:31–40

Marques, J.T. and Williams, B.R.G. 2005. Activation of the mammalian immune system by siRNAs. Nat. Biotechnol. 23:1399–1405

Matzinger, P. 1994. Tolerance, danger, and the extended family. Annu. Rev. Immunol. 12:991–1045

Matzinger, P. 2002. The danger model: a renewed sense of self. Science 296:301–305

Medzhitov, R. and Janeway, C.A. Jr. 2002. Decoding the patterns of self and nonself by the innate immune system. Science 296:298–300

Medzhitov, R., Preston-Hurlburt, P., and Janeway, C.A. 1997. A human homologue of the Drosophila Toll protein signals activation of adaptive immunity. Nature 388:394–397

Melchers, F. and Rolink, A.R. 2006. B cell tolerance – How to make it and how to break it. Curr. Concepts Autoimmun. Chron. Inflam. 305:1–23

Mellman, I. and Steinman, R.M. 2001. Dendritic cells: specialized and regulated antigen processing machines. Cell 106:255–258

Mempel, T.R., Henrickson, S.E., and von Andrian, U.H. 2004. T-cell priming by dendritic cells in lymph nodes occurs in three distinct phases. Nature 427:154–159

Miller, J.F. and Basten, A. 1996. Mechanisms of tolerance to self. Curr. Opin. Immunol. 8:815–821

Mosmann, T.R. and Coffman, R.L. 1989. TH1 and TH2 cells: different patterns of lymphokine secretion lead to different functional properties. Annu. Rev. Immunol. 7:145–173

Nemazee, D. 1996. Antigen receptor 'capacity' and the sensitivity of self-tolerance. Immunol. Today 17:25–29

Nemazee, D. and Hogquist, K.A. 2003. Antigen receptor selection by editing or downregulation of V(D)J recombination. Curr. Opin. Immunol. 15:182–189

Nemazee, D.A. and Burki, K. 1989. Clonal deletion of B lymphocytes in a transgenic mouse bearing anti-MHC class I antibody genes. Nature 337:562–566

Norbury, C.C., Chambers, B.J., Prescott, A.R., Ljunggren, H.G., and Watts, C. 1997. Constitutive macropinocytosis allows TAP-dependent major histocompatibility complex class I presentation of exogenous soluble antigen by bone marrow-derived dendritic cells. Eur. J. Immunol. 27:280–288

Nouri-Shirazi, M., Banchereau, J., Fay, J., and Palucka, K. 2000. Dendritic cell based tumor vaccines. Immunol. Lett. 74:5–10

Pancer, Z. and Cooper, M.D. 2006. The evolution of adaptive immunity. Annu. Rev. Immunol. 24:497–518

Parker, D.C. 1993. T-Cell - Dependent B-Cell Activation. Annu. Rev. Immunol. 11:331–360

Perini, P., Facchinetti, A., Bulian, P., Massaro, A.R., De Pascalis, D., Bertolotto, A., Biasi, G., and Gallo, P. 2001. Interferon-beta (IFN-beta) antibodies in interferon-beta 1a-and interferon-beta 1b-treated multiple sclerosis patients. Prevalence, kinetics, cross-reactivity, and factors enhancing interferon-beta immunogenicity in vivo. Eur. Cytokine Network 12:56–61

Pfeifer, J.D., Wick, M.J., Roberts, R.L., Findlay, K., Normark, S.J., and Harding, C.V. 1993. Phagocytic processing of bacterial antigens for class I MHC presentation to T cells. Nature 361:359–362

Philpott, D.J. and Girardin, S.E. 2004. The role of Toll-like receptors and Nod proteins in bacterial infection. Mol. Immunol. 41:1099–1108

Poltorak, A., He, X., Smirnova, I., Liu, M.Y., Van Huffel, C., Du, X., Birdwell, D., Alejos, E., Silva, M., Galanos, C., Freudenberg, M., Ricciardi-Castagnoli, P., Layton, B., and Beutler, B. 1998. Defective LPS signaling in C3H/HeJ and C57BL/10ScCr mice: mutations in Tlr4 gene. Science 282:2085–2088

Probst, H.C., McCoy, K., Okazaki, T., Honjo, T., and Van Den, B.M. 2005. Resting dendritic cells induce peripheral CD8+ T cell tolerance through PD-1 and CTLA-4. Nat. Immunol. 6:280–286

Randolph, G.J. 2001. Dendritic cell migration to lymph nodes: cytokines, chemokines, and lipid mediators. Semin. Immunol. 13:267–274

Rathmell, J.C., Cooke, M.P., Ho, W.Y., Grein, J., Townsend, S.E., Davis, M.M., and Goodnow, C.C. 1995. CD95 (Fas)-dependent elimination of self-reactive B cells upon interaction with CD4+ T cells. Nature 376:181–184

Rathmell, J.C., Fournier, S., Weintraub, B.C., Allison, J.P., and Goodnow, C.C. 1998. Repression of B7.2 on self-reactive B cells is essential to prevent proliferation and allow Fas-mediated deletion by CD4(+) T cells. J. Exp. Med. 188:651–659

Rathmell, J.C., Townsend, S.E., Xu, J.C., Flavell, R.A., and Goodnow, C.C. 1996. Expansion or elimination of B cells in vivo: dual roles for. Cell 87:319–329

Raychaudhuri, S. and Rock, K.L. 1998. Fully mobilizing host defense: building better vaccines. Nat. Biotechnol. 16:1025–1031

Regnault, A., Lankar, D., Lacabanne, V., Rodriguez, A., Thery, C., Rescigno, M., Saito, T., Verbeek, S., Bonnerot, C., Ricciardi-Castagnoli, P., and Amigorena, S. 1999. Fcgamma receptor-mediated induction of dendritic cell maturation and major histocompatibility complex class I-restricted antigen presentation after immune complex internalization. J. Exp. Med. 189:371–380

Reis e Sousa, C., Stahl, P.D., and Austyn, J.M. 1993. Phagocytosis of antigens by Langerhans cells in vitro. J. Exp. Med. 178:509–519

Rescigno, M., Citterio, S., Thery, C., Rittig, M., Medaglini, D., Pozzi, G., Amigorena, S., and Ricciardi-Castagnoli, P. 1998. Bacteria-induced neo-biosynthesis, stabilization, and surface expression of functional class I molecules in mouse dendritic cells. Proc. Natl. Acad. Sci. USA 95:5229–5234

Reth, M. 1995. The B-cell antigen receptor complex and co-receptors. Immunol. Today 16:310–313

Rodriguez, A., Regnault, A., Kleijmeer, M., Ricciardi-Castagnoli, P., and Amigorena, S. 1999. Selective transport of internalized antigens to the cytosol for MHC class I presentation in dendritic cells. Nat. Cell. Biol. 1:362–368

Rosenberg, A.S. 2006. Effects of protein aggregates: an immunologic perspective. AAPS J 8:E501–E507

Ross, C., Clemmesen, K.M., Svenson, M., Sorensen, P.S., Koch-Henriksen, N., Skovgaard, G.L., and Bendtzen, K. 2000. Immunogenicity of interferon-beta in multiple sclerosis patients: Influence of preparation, dosage, dose frequency, and route of administration. Ann. Neurol. 48:706–712

Rubartelli, A., Poggi, A., and Zocchi, M.R. 1997. The selective engulfment of apoptotic bodies by dendritic cells is mediated by the alpha(v)beta3 integrin and requires intracellular and extracellular calcium. Eur. J. Immunol. 27:1893–1900

Ryff, J.C. 1997. Clinical investigation of the immunogenicity of interferon-alpha 2a. J. Interferon Cytokine Res. 17 Suppl 1:S29–S33

Sakaguchi, S., Sakaguchi, N., Asano, M., Itoh, M., and Toda, M. 1995. Immunological self-tolerance maintained by activated T-cells expressing Il-2 receptor alpha-chains (Cd25) – breakdown of a single mechanism of self-tolerance causes various autoimmune-diseases. J. Immunol. 155:1151–1164

Sallusto, F., Cella, M., Danieli, C., and Lanzavecchia, A. 1995. Dendritic cells use macropinocytosis and the mannose receptor to concentrate macromolecules in the major histocompatibility complex class II compartment: downregulation by cytokines and bacterial products. J. Exp. Med. 182:389–400

Sallusto, F. and Lanzavecchia, A. 1994. Efficient presentation of soluble antigen by cultured human dendritic cells is maintained by granulocyte/macrophage colony-stimulating factor plus interleukin 4 and downregulated by tumor necrosis factor alpha. J. Exp. Med. 179:1109–1118

Sansonetti, P.J. 2006. The innate signaling of dangers and the dangers of innate signaling. Nat. Immunol. 7:1237–1242

Sauter, B., Albert, M.L., Francisco, L., Larsson, M., Somersan, S., and Bhardwaj, N. 2000. Consequences of cell death: exposure to necrotic tumor cells, but not primary tissue cells or apoptotic cells, induces the maturation of immunostimulatory dendritic cells. J. Exp. Med. 191:423–434

Savill, J., Dransfield, I., Gregory, C., and Haslett, C. 2002. A blast from the past: clearance of apoptotic cells regulates immune responses. Nat. Rev. Immunol. 2: 965–975

Schellekens, H. 2002. Immunogenicity of therapeutic proteins: clinical implications and future prospects. Clin. Ther. 24:1720–1740

Schellekens, H. 2005. Factors influencing the immunogenicity of therapeutic proteins. Nephrol. Dial. Transpl. 20:3–9

Schwartz, R.H. 2003. T cell anergy. Annu. Rev. Immunol. 21:305–334

Shastri, N., Schwab, S., and Serwold, T. 2002. Producing nature's gene-chips: The generation of peptides for display by MHC class I molecules. Annu. Rev. Immunol. 20:463–493

Singh, N.J. and Schwartz, R.H. 2006. Primer: mechanisms of immunologic tolerance. Nat. Clin. Pract. Rheumatol. 2:44–52

Singh-Jasuja, H., Scherer, H.U., Hilf, N., Arnold-Schild, D., Rammensee, H.G., Toes, R.E., and Schild, H. 2000. The heat shock protein gp96 induces maturation of dendritic cells and down-regulation of its receptor. Eur. J. Immunol. 30:2211–2215

Slepnev, V.I. and De Camilli, P. 2000. Accessory factors in clathrin-dependent synaptic vesicle endocytosis. Nat. Rev. Neurosci. 1:161–172

Smits, H.H., de Jong, E.C., Wierenga, E.A., and Kapsenberg, M.L. 2005. Different faces of regulatory DCs in homeostasis and immunity. Trends Immunol. 26:123–129

Squier, M.K. and Cohen, J.J. 1994. Cell-mediated cytotoxic mechanisms. Curr. Opin. Immunol. 6:447–452

Steinman, R.M., Inaba, K., Turley, S., Pierre, P., and Mellman, I. 1999. Antigen capture, processing, and presentation by dendritic cells: recent cell biological studies. Hum. Immunol. 60:562–567

Steinman, R.M. and Swanson, J. 1995. The endocytic activity of dendritic cells. J. Exp. Med. 182:283–288

Steinman, R.M., Turley, S., Mellman, I., and Inaba, K. 2000. The induction of tolerance by dendritic cells that have captured apoptotic cells. J. Exp. Med. 191:411–416

Surh, C.D. and Sprent, J. 1994. T-cell apoptosis detected in situ during positive and negative selection in the thymus. Nature 372:100–103

Takeda, K. and Akira, S. 2005. Toll-like receptors in innate immunity. Int. Immunol. 17:1–14

Tang, A., Amagai, M., Granger, L.G., Stanley, J.R., and Udey, M.C. 1993. Adhesion of epidermal Langerhans cells to keratinocytes mediated by E- cadherin. Nature 361:82–85

Taniguchi, M., Harada, M., Kojo, S., Nakayama, T., and Wakao, H. 2003. The regulatory role of V alpha 14 NKT cells in innate and acquired immune response. Annu. Rev. Immunol. 21:483–513

Tiegs, S.L., Russell, D.M., and Nemazee, D. 1993. Receptor editing in self-reactive bone marrow B cells. J. Exp. Med. 177:1009–1020

Trombetta, E.S. and Mellman, I. 2005. Cell biology of antigen processing in vitro and in vivo. Annu. Rev. Immunol. 23:975–1028

Turley, S.J., Inaba, K., Garrett, W.S., Ebersold, M., Unternaehrer, J., Steinman, R.M., and Mellman, I. 2000. Transport of peptide-MHC class II complexes in developing dendritic cells. Science 288:522–527

Villadangos, J.A., Bryant, R.A., Deussing, J., Driessen, C., Lennon-Dumenil, A.M., Riese, R.J., Roth, W., Saftig, P., Shi, G.P., Chapman, H.A., Peters, C., and Ploegh, H.L. 1999. Proteases involved in MHC class II antigen presentation. Immunol. Rev. 172:109–120

Vivier, E. and Malissen, B. 2005. Innate and adaptive immunity: specificities and signaling hierarchies revisited. Nat. Rev. Immunol. 6:17–21

von Andrian, U.H. and Mempel, T.R. 2003. Homing and cellular traffic in lymph nodes. Nat. Rev. Immunol. 3:867–878

Vos, Q., Lees, A., Wu, Z.Q., Snapper, C.M., and Mond, J.J. 2000. B-cell activation by T-cell-independent type 2 antigens as an integral part of the humoral immune response to pathogenic microorganisms. Immunol. Rev. 176:154–170

Wardemann, H., Yurasov, S., Schaefer, A., Young, J.W., Meffre, E., and Nussenzweig, M.C. 2003. Predominant autoantibody production by early human B cell precursors. Science 301:1374–1377

Watts, C. 2001. Antigen processing in the endocytic compartment. Curr. Opin. Immunol. 13:26–31

Weaver, C.T., Harrington, L.E., Mangan, P.R., Gavrieli, M., and Murphy, K.M. 2006. Th17: an effector CD4 T cell lineage with regulatory T cell ties. Immunity 24: 677–688

Wick, M.J. and Ljunggren, H.G. 1999. Processing of bacterial antigens for peptide presentation on MHC class I molecules. Immunol. Rev. 172:153–162

Yewdell, J.W., Norbury, C.C., and Bennink, J.R. 1999. Mechanisms of exogenous antigen presentation by MHC class I molecules in vitro and in vivo: implications for generating CD8+ T cell responses to infectious agents, tumors, transplants, and vaccines. Adv. Immunol. 73:1–77

Zerrahn, J., Held, W., and Raulet, D.H. 1997. The MHC reactivity of the T cell repertoire prior to positive and negative selection. Cell 88:627–636

Zinkernagel, R.M. 2000. What is missing in immunology to understand immunity? Nat. Immunol. 1:181–185

Clinical Aspects of Immunogenicity to Biopharmaceuticals

Simona Malucchi and Antonio Bertolotto

2.1. Introduction

The range of biopharmaceuticals available is steadily increasing. The first generation of products were copies of naturally occurring growth factors, or hormones or cytokines. With the development of new techniques, such as pegylation and glycosylation, second-generation biopharmaceuticals with increased bioavailability and higher therapeutic index are available.

Most biopharmaceuticals induce immune responses. The theoretical basis for immunogenicity to biopharmaceuticals is based either on their foreign nature, being of exogenous origin (neo-antigens or non-self-antigens), or on their similarity to self-molecules (self-antigens). In both cases, clinical manifestation of immunogenicity depends on the activation of antibody-secreting B cells. Besides this, many factors contribute to immunogenicity, such as product-related factors and host-related factors. These are discussed in more detail in Chapter 5.

Immunogenicity can cause a range of consequences, as summarized in Table 2.1. In many cases, antibodies against biopharmaceuticals have little or no consequences. In some cases, they can cause a loss of efficacy of the therapeutic proteins, but the most dangerous effect occurs when autoimmunity is directed against the endogenous molecule (Kromminga and Schellekens 2005). On the next pages, the different effects of antigenicity and immunogenicity will be discussed, and each type of effect will be illustrated by examples.

2.2. Clinical Aspects of Immunogenicity

2.2.1. No Apparent Effect of Antibody Formation: Growth Hormone

Since the 1980s, recombinant forms of human growth hormone (rhGH, *Escherichia coli* derived) have been used as therapy for deficiencies in GH production or response. Most studies have not shown any effect of anti-GH antibodies on growth rate. In a study by Albertsson-Wikland (1987), anti-GH antibodies were found in 1 out of 47 (2.1%) children treated for up to

Table 2.1 Consequences of immunogenicity.

Biopharmaceutical	Clinical use	Consequences of immunogenicity	References
rh-GH	GH deficiency	No evidence of any effect on clinical efficacy	Albertsson-Wikland 1987; Takano et al. 1989
rh-Insulin	Diabetes mellitus	Alteration of the drug pharmacokinetics	Walford et al. 1982; Ishibashi et al. 1986; Van Haeften 1989
GM-CSF	Some cancers	Reduction in drug efficacy	Ragnhammar et al. 1994; Rini et al. 2005
IFNα	Hepatitis C, some cancers	Reduction in drug efficacy	Figlin and Itri 1988; Lok, Lai and Leung 1990; Douglas et al. 1993; Bonetti et al. 1994
IFNβ	Multiple sclerosis	Reduction/loss in drug efficacy	See Table 2.6
Factors VIII and IX	Haemophilia A and B	Cross-reaction with endogenous protein	Lacroix-Desmazes et al. 2002; Lusher 2000; Schellekens and Casadevall 2004.
rh-MDGF		Cross-reaction with endogenous protein	Kuter 2000; Li et al. 2001
rh-EPO	Anaemia	Cross-reaction with endogenous protein	Casadevall 2002; Locatelli et al. 2004
Natalizumab	Multiple sclerosis	Adverse drug reactions and loss of clinical efficacy	AFFIRM study 2006; SENTINEL study 2006
GA	Multiple sclerosis	Unknown effect	Teitelbaum et al. 1996; Brenner et al. 2001; Salama et al. 2003; Farina et al. 2005

Note: rh= recombinant human; GH= growth hormone; GM-CSF= granulocyte-macrophage colony-stimulating factor; IFN= interferon; MDGF= megakaryocyte differentiation and growth factor; GA= glatiramer acetate six months with recombinant somatotrophin, without observing any adverse effect on growth rate. In another study by Takano (1989), three different kinds of rhGH preparations were administered to 203 patients affected by Turner's syndrome and antibodies were detected in 71.4% and 10.8% of the methionyl-rhGH and methionine-free-rhGH treated patients, respectively; no inhibition of growth rate was observed in these patients.

However, some authors have described a reduction in clinical response in a few patients with high titres of anti-GH antibodies. Kaplan et al. (1986) evaluated the development of antibodies against GH in 36 children who had been treated with methionyl-rhGH intramuscularly for up to four years, finding that the incidence of antibodies was higher than in subjects treated with GH derived from bovine pituitaries. No allergic manifestation or systemic side effects were demonstrable in patients who developed antibodies, but a poor growth was observed in one patient who acquired high-titre, high-binding-capacity antibodies to hGH.

A similar finding has been described in a Japanese study by Okada et al. (1987), in which the authors reported a case of a 10-year-old child treated with methionyl-rhGH for an idiopathic growth hormone deficiency. The child had a decrease in growth rate by the ninth month of therapy, and anti-GH had been detected at two months of treatment, with maximum titre at nine months. A switch from methionyl-rhGH to pituitary-extracted hGH was able to produce a new increase in growth rate, and the cause of growth attenuation was attributed to the high titre of anti-GH antibodies.

It has been observed that antibody titres are inversely related to the purity of the methionyl-rhGH preparation (Takano, Shizume and Hibi 1989). Subsequent studies based on subcutaneous administration and on the use of *N*-methionine-free rhGH were associated with a lower incidence of antibodies.

More recent preparations of rhGH are less immunogenic (antibody incidence of 1.1%) after one year of treatment (Lundin et al. 1991). Massa and co-workers (1993) studied anti-GH antibodies induced by treatment with methionyl-rhGH, finding that antibodies developed in 3 out of 26 patients (12%) who were previously treated with pituitary-extracted hGH, and in 15 out of 20 patients (75%) who were previously untreated. The majority of antibodies positive patients, 15 out of 18, developed antibodies during the first year of treatment, whereas in 3 out of 18 patients, antibodies developed during the second year; they disappeared after the discontinuation of treatment and no effect on growth rate was observed.

It has been suggested that antibodies and GH receptor bind to different epitopes on the GH molecule, which can explain the fact that anti-rhGH antibodies generally do not influence growth (Schellekens and Casadevall 2004).

2.2.2. Change in Drug Pharmacokinetics: Insulin

Insulin replacement therapy is the mainstay pharmacological treatment for patients with type 1 and with advanced type 2 diabetes (DeWitt and Hirsch 2003). Insulin is a 51-amino acid peptide hormone and consists of a 21-amino acid alpha-chain linked by disulphide bonds to a 30-residue beta-chain (Figure 2.1).

At physiological concentrations, insulin molecules exist in monomeric form, but when stored at commercial therapeutic dose concentrations,

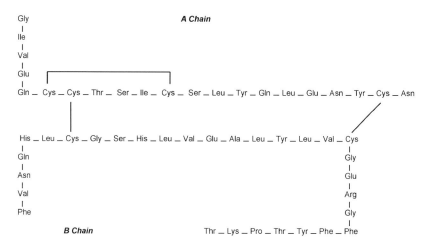

Figure 2.1 Amino acid sequence of human insulin.

individual insulin molecules interact with one another, forming dimers and hexamers (Bristol 1993). Upon subcutaneous administration, an insulin depot is formed, and individual molecules must dissociate before entering the blood-stream. This causes a delayed entry into the blood, and consequently, insulin plasma levels peak 90–120 min after injection. This is why insulin has to be injected up to one hour before food consumption (Walsh 2004).

2.2.2.1. Bovine and Porcine Insulins

In the 1920s, insulin was introduced in the treatment for diabetes; the first insulins were either single species or mixtures of bovine and porcine insulins isolated from pancreata. Bovine, porcine and human insulins differ in their primary structure. Porcine and human insulins have a different amino acid in the beta-chain, whereas bovine insulin differs from porcine and human insulins in two amino acids in the alpha-chain (Smith 1966).

In the 1950s, the in vitro use of radioactive insulin showed that 100% of patients treated with animal insulins produced high levels of circulating anti-insulin antibodies (Berson et al. 1956). Several studies described cutaneous and systemic allergic reactions linked to insulin antibodies (Hanauer and Batson 1961, deShazo et al. 1977, Velcovsky, Beringhoff and Federlin 1978, Deleeuw, Delvigne and Beckaert 1982, Carveth-Johnson, Mylvaganam and Child 1982, Blandford et al. 1982, Altman et al. 1983, Garcia-Ortega, Knobel and Miranda 1984, Gossain, Rouner and Homak 1985, Kumar 1997, Frigerio, Aubry and Gomez 1997) and insulin resistance (Andersen 1973, Witters et al. 1977, Davidson and DeBra 1978, Grammer et al. 1987, Lahtela et al. 1997). In one study by Deckert (1985), hypersensitivity reactions and IgE-mediated responses were described in up to 30% of patients and severe systemic immunological reactions in less than 0.1% of patients treated with insulin of animal origin.

In patients treated with animal insulin, it seems that the development of insulin antibodies correlates with increased insulin requirements. In a study by Walford and co-workers (1982), 40 diabetic patients were switched from bovine to highly purified porcine insulin for a period of six months, and the patients underwent sequential determination of anti-insulin IgG. The authors observed a positive correlation between percentage change in insulin dose and change in insulin-binding capacity and concluded that the level of circulating antibodies affected the dose of insulin required to maintain stable diabetic control.

Another problem associated with the first animal insulins was that they were contaminated with several other islet cell peptides such as proinsulin, C-peptide and glucagons (Chance, Root and Galloway 1976), which enhanced immunogenicity. The later version of more purified porcine insulin gave a 60% incidence; however, human insulin was lower still at 40–50% incidence (Fireman, Fineberg and Galloway 1982, Fineberg et al. 1983).

2.2.2.2. *Human Insulin*

During human insulin treatment, both IgG and IgE antibodies have been detected. However, the titres were low and the incidence decreased in patients treated exclusively with human insulin (Velcovsky and Federlin 1982). Antibodies were initially detected 1–2 months after the beginning of therapy and were described at two years in some long-term studies (Schernthaner 1993, Velcovsky and Federlin 1982). They appear not to be specific for variant residues, but rather react with determinants shared by the human protein (Reeves and Kelly 1982, Marshall et al. 1988).

Even though human insulin is less immunogenic than the animal ones, high titres of IgG insulin antibodies were shown to bind and neutralize insulin, leading to insulin resistance by interfering with receptor binding (Van Haeften 1989). It has been described that antibodies alter insulin pharmacokinetics, causing an increase in daily insulin requirements (Ishibashi et al. 1986, Peters et al. 1995). However, in some large-scale trials, the presence of antibodies has not been shown to alter long-term glycaemic control directly (Van Haeften 1989, Chen et al. 2005).

In the last three decades, the prevalence of anti-insulin antibodies has decreased, thanks to the improvements in the purification of insulin preparations and to the development of monocomponent insulins (Fineberg et al. 1983, Van Haeften 1989, Walford, Allison and Reeves 1982). Moreover, the availability of recombinant human forms of insulin contributed to a further decrease of the immunogenicity (Fineberg et al. 2003). However, also recombinant human insulin is immunogenic (Fineberg et al. 1983, Fireman, Fineberg and Galloway 1982), but allergic phenomena are unusual and insulin antibody-mediated insulin resistance is an extremely rare complication of therapy (Fineberg 1994).

In most countries, the use of animal insulins has been largely replaced with recombinant human insulins. Recombinant insulin was the first product of recombinant DNA technology to gain approval in 1982. In the case of insulin, the main focus of engineering was to develop "fast-acting" insulin analogues, which could be administered with meals. These fast-acting analogues were obtained by making amino acid substitutions that increased steric hindrance between individual insulin molecules (Walsh 2005). In addition, various "long-acting" insulin analogues, which have a retarded entry into the bloodstream, have recently been engineered. The immunogenicity of insulin and these novel analogues is discussed in more detail in Chapter 8.

2.2.3. Reduction in Drug Efficacy

The formation of antibodies may reduce the drug efficacy, without these antibodies having any distinct (or known) effects on the pharmacokinetics.

This is exemplified below using granulocyte-macrophage colony-stimulating factor and type I interferons.

2.2.3.1. *Granulocyte-Macrophage Colony-Stimulating Factor*

Granulocyte-macrophage colony-stimulating factor (GM-CSF) is a cytokine which is able to stimulate the production of neutrophilic granulocytes, macrophages and mixed granulocyte-macrophage colonies from bone marrow cells. It can also stimulate some functional activities in mature granulocytes and macrophages. GM-CSF binds to a specific receptor which has significant homologies with other receptors for haematopoietic growth factors, such as interleukin-2b, interleukin-3, interleukin-6, interleukin-7 and erythropoietin. GM-CSF receptors are present in tissues derived from haematopoietic cells as well as in other cell types including those in the nervous system (Antignani and Youle 2007).

GM-CSF is mostly used to accelerate marrow recovery after cancer chemotherapy. Moreover, GM-CSF may enhance the immunogenicity of tumour cells by facilitating tumour antigen presentation (Hill et al. 1993, Charak, Agah and Mazumder 1993, Hooijberg et al. 1995). Studies made in animal models (Hill et al. 1993, Charak, Agah and Mazumder 1993) showed that GM-CSF, either alone or in combination with other therapeutic agents, is able to reduce the growth of tumour cells by the activation of macrophages. These data, together with results obtained in vitro (Masucci et al. 1989, Ragnhammar et al. 1994a), support the use of GM-CSF alone (as has been used widely for therapy of malignant diseases) or in combination with tumour-specific antibodies or immunomodulatory cytokines (e.g. interleukin-2) as an immunotherapeutic approach in patients with cancer.

Recombinant human GM-CSF produced in *E. coli* is a single, non-glycosylated, polypeptide chain containing 127 amino acids and with a molecular mass of 14477 dalton. The therapeutic administration of GM-CSF causes the development of antibodies in patients (Ragnhammar et al. 1994a). There are few data about the induction of antibodies in patients treated with GM-CSF because this cytokine is especially used in patients who are immuno-suppressed.

Antibodies against yeast-derived recombinant human GM-CSF as well as *E. coli*-derived rhGM-CSF have been described. Gribben et al. (1990) observed antibodies in 31% of patients affected by chemotherapy-resistant solid tumours treated with yeast-derived rhGM-CSF. In another study by Ragnhammar et al. (1994b), 95% of cancer patients treated with *E. coli*-derived rhGM-CSF subcutaneously, at $250 \ \mu g/m^2/day$ for 10 days every month for four months, developed binding antibodies after the second cycle. The same percentage of antibody-positive patients has been reported in a study by Wadhwa et al. (1996) on 20 colon carcinoma affected patients treated with a combination therapy (GM-CSF plus a colon carcinoma reactive antibody); in 40% of patients, these antibodies had neutralizing activity in an in vitro bioassay.

Results from a study by Rini and co-workers (2005) conducted on 15 prostate cancer patients demonstrated that antibodies against GM-CSF developed in all patients. In 87% of the patients they developed within three months, while in the other patients antibodies developed after additional cycles of GM-CSF. Sixty percent of the patients developed GM-CSF antibodies which neutralized the biological activity of GM-CSF in vitro in a cell-based bioassay. These antibodies also recognized GM-CSF from different expression systems, indicating that they are directed towards the amino acid backbone of the protein. In fact, it has been suggested that antibodies recognize an epitope of the protein backbone, which in the native protein is normally masked by a carbohydrate residue, whereas it is exposed in the *E. coli*-derived as well as in the yeast-derived rhGM-CSF (Gribben et al. 1990, Mellstedt 1994).

Antibodies appear to modify GM-CSF pharmacokinetics, but this phenomenon is not clear. It is suggested that the mitogenic activity of the drug leads to an increase in target cells and their mitogen receptors. This phenomenon has led to observation of an inverse relationship between neutrophil count and serum levels of GM-CSF (Petros et al. 1992). Thus, changes in pharmacokinetics may not be directly attributed to circulating antibodies.

2.2.3.2. Type I Interferons

Interferons (IFNs) are a family of regulatory proteins, the majority of which are composed by 166 amino acid residues with molecular weight of 16–26 kilodalton. Based on the homology in their sequences, IFNs are classified into two groups: type I and type II.

Type I IFNs include seven families with different antigenic characteristics: alpha (α), beta (β), delta (δ), kappa (κ), epsilon (ϵ), omega (ω) and tau (τ) (Pestka et al. 2004). They are encoded by a cluster of genes located on chromosome 9, are produced in response to a viral stimulation and recognize the same membrane receptor, IFNAR (Pestka, Krause and Walter 2004; Bekisz et al. 2004).

Currently, only one member of type II IFNs is known: IFNγ, which is encoded by a gene located on chromosome 12 and which is produced by T lymphocytes and natural killer cells in response to non-self-antigen presentation. Its receptor is different from IFNAR. Here, attention is focused on type I IFNs, in particular to IFNα and IFNβ.

2.2.3.2.1. Interferon-Alfa: Interferon alfa (IFNα) is a protein, composed of 166 amino acids. Several genes of IFNα have been identified which share a high degree of homology. These proteins have antiviral activity, inhibit viral replication, increase class I MHC, stimulate Th1 cells and inhibit proliferation of many cell types.

IFNα is used for the treatment of many malignant diseases and for chronic hepatitis C and B. Several different recombinant preparations of IFNα exist. The most commonly used include IFNα-2a and IFNα-2b, which differ in the amino acid in position 23 (lysine in IFNα-2a and arginine in IFNα-2b); both preparations are glycosylated. Many studies have reported the development of antibodies in patients chronically treated with the two preparations, with different percentages, ranging from 19 to 61% and with a higher incidence in patients treated with IFNα-2a compared with patients treated with IFNα-2b (Quesada et al. 1985, von Wussow et al. 1987, Steis et al. 1988, Spiegel, Jacobs and Treuhaft 1989, Freund et al. 1989; Berman et al. 1990). As the gene for IFNα-2a is not present in the population, it is possible that this type of IFN carries a neo-antigen, but extensive studies have shown that the structural differences between the two products may not be the reason for the difference in immunogenicity (Kromminga and Schellekens 2005).

Discordant data exist about the role of anti-interferon antibodies on the drug clinical efficacy. In the study by Berman et al. (1990) on hairy cell leukaemia-affected subjects, 19% of patients with antibodies showed a resistance to treatment. In another study of IFNα-treated patients affected by hairy cell leukaemia (Steis et al. 1988), antibodies were reported in 16 out of 51 (31%) subjects, but a clinical resistance was observed in 6 out of 16 (38%) of these antibody-positive patients. Freund et al. (1989) evaluated IFNα-2b-treated patients affected by myelogenous leukaemia, finding antibodies in 8 out of 27 (30%) subjects and observing a resistance to therapy in all the antibody-positive patients.

Different data arise from other studies: Figlin and Itri (1988) described anti-interferon antibodies in 12 out of 19 renal carcinoma patients treated with IFNα-2a intramuscularly, reporting that 6 out of these 12 patients developed neutralizing antibodies, but no correlation between antibody presence and clinical response to therapy nor clinical toxicity was found. A review by Jones and Itri (1986) evaluated more than 1300 cancer patients who had received IFNα-2a treatment. The authors reported that about 27% of patients developed antibodies, but they did not find any adverse clinical manifestation associated with them.

The kinetics of antibody development seems to be linked to the type of disease. For example, in patients affected by renal cell carcinoma, antibodies have been described after a median time of eight weeks, while in patients affected by hairy cell leukaemia they have been reported to arise after an average of seven months (Figlin and Itri 1988).

IFNα-2a is also widely used for the treatment of chronic hepatitis C. A study by Bonetti et al. (1994) evaluated antibodies against therapeutic IFNα-2a in 60 patients affected by chronic hepatitis C and observing 61% of antibody-positive patients within six months of treatment. Interestingly, they found that 75% of patients who showed no therapeutic response to IFN had detectable antibodies. Similarly, in one study by Douglas (Douglas et al. 1993) on IFNα-2a for hepatitis C, antibodies were present in 32% of treated patients, and when comparing responder and non-responder patients, a higher percentage of antibodies positive subjects were found in the group of non-responders (40% versus 14%, respectively). In an Italian study by the group of Dianzani et al. (1989), the authors analysed 175 patients treated with recombinant IFNα-2b, trying to correlate the presence of antibodies with a reduction in clinical response, but antibodies were found in only one patient. A Chinese trial of IFNα-2a in hepatitis B-affected patients reported that 39% of patients developed antibodies. They were more likely to develop in the group of patients treated with a low dose than in the group treated with a high dose of drug. A high antibody titre correlated with a failure in treatment response (Lok, Lai and Leung 1990).

With the introduction of pegylated-IFNα, the prevalence of neutralizing antibodies is about 1–2% (Frost 2005). This corresponds well with the hypothesis that the backbone is the antigenic epitope and that shielding thereof by glycosylation or PEGylation reduces unwanted antibody formation.

2.2.3.3. Interferon Beta

Interferon beta (IFNβ) is used in the treatment of multiple sclerosis. Clinical aspects of the formation of neutralizing antibodies against IFNβ will be discussed further below in Section 2.5, and immune responses to IFNβ are discussed in great detail in Chapter 7.

2.2.4. Cross-Reaction with Endogenous Protein

2.2.4.1. Megakaryocyte Differentiation and Growth Factor

The most dangerous consequence of the development of antibodies occurs when the endogenous protein is neutralized. This effect has been described for megakaryocyte differentiation and growth factor (MDGF) and for erythropoietin (EPO). The development of first-generation thrombopoietic growth factor (human recombinant thrombopoietin, TPO, and pegylated recombinant human MDGF) has been stopped due to the development of antibodies against endogenous TPO, causing severe thrombocytopenia in 13 out of 325 healthy volunteers and in 4 out of 650 cancer patients (Kuter 2000). In a study by Li and co-workers (Li et al. 2001), the authors evaluated three of these thrombocytopenic subjects (two volunteers and one cancer patient). They found that that in all of the patients thrombocytopenia was due to the development of antibodies which cross-reacted with endogenous TPO, neutralizing its biological activity. All the subjects underwent bone marrow examination that showed a marked reduction in megakaryocytes. All anti-TPO antibodies were IgG and most of the anti-TPO were IgG4. The biological activity of endogenous TPO was inhibited by the binding of anti-TPO to the first 163 amino acids of TPO, preventing TPO from binding to its receptor. In two subjects endogenous TPO level were elevated, but biologically inactive, as it formed an immune complex with IgG. A study of the time course of anti-TPO development was performed in all the three subjects, showing that no subject had antibodies before the first injection of PEG-rhMDGF and that there was no IgM response. In one subject, IgG appeared on day 56 after the drug injection, when the platelet count had already begun to fall and was maximal on day 147; these antibodies progressively decreased and disappeared. In another subject, anti-TPO rapidly disappeared after treatment with cyclosporine, and in the third subject (the oncologic patient), antibodies persisted at high titre despite plasmapheresis.

New non-immunogenic second-generation thrombopoietic growth factors have been developed; they have been tested in healthy humans, producing a dose-dependent rise in platelet count, without adverse effects (Kuter 2007).

2.2.4.2. Erythropoietin

Recombinant human erythropoietin (rhEPO) has been successfully used for the treatment of anaemia due to chronic renal failure. Several patients affected by chronic kidney disease and treated with recombinant epoetin-α developed pure red cell aplasia (PRCA), due to the production of antibodies directed against recombinant EPO as well as against the endogenous EPO (Locatelli et al. 2004). The immune response to EPO is discussed in detail in Chapter 6.

PRCA is a rare disorder, which can arise either spontaneously or in association with thymoma, lymphoid proliferation or an immune-related disorder, such as lupus erythematosus or rheumatoid arthritis. It can also occur secondary to viral infections or to drugs. In adults it is usually an autoimmune disorder, in which antibodies of cytotoxic T lymphocytes are directed against erythroid progenitors (Casadevall 2002).

The use of recombinant EPO started in 1988, initially by the intravenous route, and since 1990, by the subcutaneous route. The molecular mass of the peptidic part of both endogenous EPO and rhEPO is 18 kilodalton. The erythropoietin molecule folds into four alpha helices stabilized by two disulphide bonds, which are essential for biological activity. EPO is a glycosylated molecule, causing an increase in the molecular mass to about 30 kilodalton, and the glycosylation is essential to the biological activity of the molecule. Therefore, rhEPO is produced in mammalian cell lines, as bacterial cell lines are not able to produce this post-translational modification. Endogenous EPO and most rhEPO variants have minor differences in glycosylation, with variation in the sialic acid composition of the oligosaccharide groups (Sasaki et al. 1987, Skibelli, Nissen-Lie and Torjesen 2001). Various rhEPO variants exist (for example, epoetin-α, epoetin-β, darbepoetin-α), which differ from each other and from endogenous EPO in the carbohydrate groups (Skibelli, Nissen-Lie and Torjesen 2001).

During the first 10 years of its therapeutic use, three cases of PRCA have been reported in patients treated with rhEPO (Bergrem et al. 1993, Peces et al. 1996, Prabhakar and Muhlfelder 1997). By 1999, a sudden increase in the number of PRCA was observed. In 2002, Casadevall and co-workers described 21 cases of PRCA, which occurred in patients treated with rhEPO to correct anaemia due to chronic renal failure. They were observed between 1998 and 2001 in different centres throughout Europe (Casadevall et al. 2002). In all these patients, anaemia was secondary to PRCA and neutralizing antibodies were present. All EPO-related PRCA patients showed an initial normal response to rhEPO and then developed severe anaemia, which was resistant to increasing dose as well as to a switch to another EPO. Anaemia appeared at different time points from the beginning of EPO treatment, with a median time of nine months (Bennett et al. 2004). It has been found that the majority of PRCA cases were associated with the subcutaneous administration (Casadevall 2002, Eckardt and Casadevall 2003). The study of the first cases described by Casadevall showed that sera from these patients recognized the endogenous molecule as well as the deglycosylated EPO: in fact, when sera of patients were incubated with the glycosylated and the deglycosylated epoetin, antibodies bound to both forms with the same efficiency. The depletion of IgG in the sera was associated with a reversion of Ab-mediated inhibition of erythroid cell proliferation in vitro. In the majority of PRCA cases, an immunosuppressive treatment after the discontinuation of EPO therapy was required to stop antibody development (Verhelst et al. 2004).

2.3. Immunogenicity of Biopharmaceuticals in Gene-Defective Hosts

2.3.1. The Case of Haemophilia A and B

From the immunological point of view, X-linked disorders represent a special situation because the mutated or deleted gene segments cause an altered immune repertoire and replacement with the wild-type protein is expected to be immunogenic (Figure 2.2). The clinical effects of immunogenicity will vary, depending on the extent of gene mutation: the absence of the gene, as

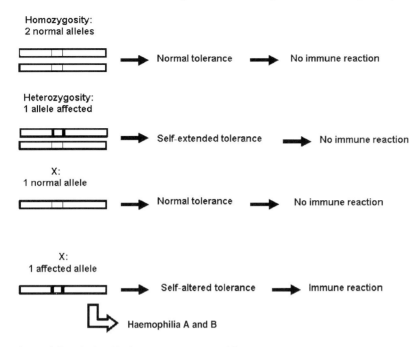

Figure 2.2 Relationship between genome and immune responses.

well as large gene deletions or a premature stop-codon, will have more severe consequences than point mutations.

Haemophilia A is an X-linked genetic disease, and thus males are mainly affected, whereas their mothers are carriers of the defective gene; it is a bleeding disorder caused by a deficiency of blood coagulation factor VIII. The disease results from mutations or deletions that alter the expression and secretion of factor VIII. The malfunction of factor VIII causes a reduced coagulation power, with prolonged post-traumatic bleeding times and spontaneous haemorrhages. Replacement therapy with factor VIII has been successfully used, and initial preparations of factor VIII were natural preparations derived from donated blood. Today, a large number of recombinant DNA-derived factor VIII preparations are available (Kromminga and Schellekens 2005). As expected, substitution therapy results in antibody formation, as the patient's immune system recognizes parts of the factor VIII as a foreign antigen. The immune response is a classical one, with a switch from IgM to IgG and affinity maturation (Opdenakker et al. 2003), discussed in more detail in Chapter 9.

The reported incidence of antibodies to plasma-derived factor VIII is about 20–25% (Ehrenforth et al. 1992, Lusher et al. 1993, Bray et al. 1994). For haemophilia A, it has been described that in about one-third of patients who develop antibodies to factor VIII these antibodies have low titre and are transient (Lusher 2000) and that their blocking effect can be overcome by increasing the dosage of factor VIII. In contrast, in those patients who develop antibodies at high titre, bleeding is a significant problem which requires alternative treatments, such as the use of recombinant factor VIIa or activated prothrombin complex concentrate (APCC).

Recent studies on antibodies to factor VIII show that neutralization may be due to a proteolytic activity (Lacroix-Desmazes et al. 2002), and a correlation between the neutralizing activity of IgG in plasma and the hydrolysis rate of factor VIII by IgG in vitro was observed. Factor VIII can be completely absent in patients with severe haemophilia A. These patients do not benefit from the administration of factor VIII because factor VIII represents a foreign antigen and patients develop an immune response against it. The same occurs in those patients who have factor VIII gene with large deletions or nonsense mutations that cause premature termination, whereas antibody development rarely occurs in patients with only frameshift or missense mutations (Kromminga and Schellekens 2005).

Haemophilia B is another X-linked bleeding disorder caused by a deficiency of blood coagulation factor IX. The prevalence of this disease is much lower than that of haemophilia A, and the incidence of antibodies against factor IX is about 1–3% (Lusher 2000). In contrast with factor VIII, the immune response to factor IX leads to severe allergic reactions and anaphylaxis in about 50% of patients (Lusher 2000). For patients with anti-factor IX antibodies, other treatments are required, such as factor VIIa and APCC (Schellekens and Casadevall 2004).

The experience on haemophiliac patients teaches that with the extent of the gene defect and the severity of the phenotype, the probability of developing neutralizing antibodies increases. Thus, for patients with the most severe disease, substitution therapy or gene therapy will have the highest risk of failure because of the production of neutralizing antibodies, and therapy has to be accompanied by strategies of immunological tolerance induction or immunosuppression (Opdenakker et al. 2003).

2.3.2. The Case of Pompe Disease

Pompe disease is a rare autosomal recessive disorder caused by deficiency of the lysosomal enzyme acid alpha-glucosidase (GAA). The incidence is about 1/40,000. The genetic defect leads to lysosomal glycogen accumulation in different tissues, the most severely affected being the skeletal and cardiac muscles. Different forms of the disease are known, depending on the residual GAA activity. The classical form is the infantile type, characterized by a progressive cardiomyopathy, muscular weakness, respiratory insufficiency and death in the first year of life. The adult form is less severe, as cardiac muscle is usually not affected. Recombinant precursor human acid alpha-glucosidase has been produced in CHO cell cultures and from milk of transgenic rabbits (Van Hove, Yang and Wu 1996, Bijvoet et al. 1999). There are still few data about replacement therapy: in a phase II trial on two affected infants (Klinge et al. 2005) treated with rhGAA for 48 months, results are encouraging, as the therapy was well tolerated and there was an overall improvement in left-ventricular mass and in cardiac and skeletal muscle functions. The two patients developed antibodies against rhGAA, but, according to the authors, no reduction in muscle function was observed. Data from a multicentre, multinational open-label study (Kishnani et al. 2007) on 18 infants affected by Pompe disease, who began treatment with intravenous infusion of rhGAA prior to six months of age, have been published. This study represents the largest cohort of patients with Pompe disease treated with replacement therapy. The study showed that the treatment was safe and effective. One of the 18 patients developed antibodies, which inhibited rhGAA activity in vitro. As the total number of treated patients is limited, no conclusive observations on the effect of antibodies are available. Further long-term studies are required to evaluate the potential of this therapy and the consequences of immunogenicity.

2.4. Adverse Drug Reactions

Drug reactions include all adverse events related to drug administration, regardless of aetiology. They can be classified into two groups: immunologic aetiology and non-immunologic aetiology (Table 2.2). About 20–25% of adverse drug reactions are caused by unpredictable effects, both immune and non-immune mediated, whereas 75–80% of adverse reactions are caused by predictable non-immunological events (Riedl and Casillas 2003). The predominant immune mechanisms leading to drug hypersensitivity are described in the classification by Gell and Coombs (Table 2.3). The risk of drug hypersensitivity can be increased by some patient-related factors, which include female gender (Barranco and Lopez-Serrano 1998), asthma, use of beta-blockers (Lang et al. 1991), specific genetic polymorphism, as well as by some drug-related factors, which include the chemical properties, the molecular weight of the drug and the route of administration. It is known that drugs with great structural complexity are more likely to be immunogenic. However, drugs with a small molecular weight (less than 1,000 daltons) may become immunogenic by coupling with carrier proteins, such as albumin, forming complexes (Riedl and Casillas 2003). Moreover, the route of administration affects the immunogenicity, the subcutaneus route being more immunogenic than the intramuscular and the intravenous routes.

An example of adverse drug reactions presumably secondary to immunogenicity is represented by antibodies to natalizumab, an alfa4-integrin antagonist, used in the treatment of aggressive forms of relapsing multiple sclerosis. In the AFFIRM study (Polman et al. 2006) on 627 patients receiving natalizumab, 37 (6%) had persistent antibodies (detectable on at least two occasions) to the drug, which were associated to an increase in infusion-related adverse events and a loss of clinical efficacy. Comparable findings were obtained in the SENTINEL study (Rudick et al. 2006) conducted on

Table 2.2 Immunological and non-immunological drug reactions.

Immunological	Non-immunological
Type I reaction (IgE mediated)	*Predictable*
Type II reaction (cytotoxic)	Pharmacological side effect
Type III reaction (immune complex)	Secondary pharmacological side effect
Type IV reaction (delayed, cell mediated)	Drug toxicity
Specific T-cell activation	Drug–drug interactions
Fas/Fas ligand-induced apoptosis	Drug overdose
Other	*Unpredictable*
	Pseudoallergic
	Idiosyncratic
	Intolerance

Table 2.3 Drug hypersensitivity reactions: Gell and Coombs classification.

	Type I	Type II	Type III	Type IV
Immune reaction	IgE mediated	Cytotoxic	Immune-complex	Delayed, cell mediated
Mechanism	Drug-IgE complex, with release of histamine from mast cells	Specific IgM or IgG antibodies directed at drug-hapten coated cells	Drug–antibody complexes with complement activation and tissue deposition	MHC presentation of drug molecule to T cells
Timing	Minutes to hours	Variable	1–3 weeks	2–7 days

1171 subjects, in which persistent antibodies to natalizumab were detected in 6% of patients and their presence was associated to a loss of clinical efficacy, as well as an increase in infusion-related adverse events.

2.5. Unknown Effects: Glatiramer Acetate

Glatiramer acetate (GA, also known as copolymer-1, copaxone) is a synthetic random polypeptide of the amino acids alanine, glutamate, tyrosine and lysine in a defined molar ratio and with a molecular weight ranging between 5000 and 9000 dalton.

It was first synthesized more than 30 years ago, in an attempt to mimic the encephalitogenic properties of myelin basic protein (MBP). Surprisingly, it was observed that GA was able to block the induction of experimental autoimmune encephalomyelitis, EAE (Arnon and Aharoni 2004). Subsequently, it was tested in therapeutic trials in patients with MS (Johnson et al. 1995, 1998, 2000), and it has gained marketing approval for the treatment of relapsing-remitting multiple sclerosis, showing a significant reduction in the number of new and enhancing lesions on MRI (Wolinsky et al. 2001, Comi et al. 2001), in relapse rate and a lower rate of disease progression (Johnson et al. 1995, 1998, 2000, 2005).

Development of anti-GA antibodies in treated patients is a known phenomenon, but the clinical meaning of anti-GA is not clear yet. Data from different studies give inconclusive results. The study by Brenner and co-workers (Brenner et al. 2001) showed that anti-GA antibodies developed only in treated patients and not in the placebo group and that antibodies titres peaked after three months, then slowly decreased but remained higher than baseline values. Farina and colleagues (2005) not only observed the presence of anti-GA antibodies in treated patients but also found naturally occurring anti-GA antibodies in some untreated individuals. The authors suggested that these naturally occurring anti-GA antibodies might belong to the low-affinity, poly-reactive pool and observed that the difference between treated and untreated patients was not the mere presence or absence of antibodies, but rather their isotype profile, as treated individuals frequently produced IgG4 antibodies, while unexposed subjects had anti-GA IgM, IgG1 and IgG2.

In a study by the group of Teitelbaum et al. (1996), the authors did not observe any neutralizing activity in serum of GA-treated patients. In contrast, Salama and co-workers (2003) observed neutralization of GA-specific T-cell reactivity in a study which included 42 patients treated with GA for a mean time of three years; 48% of the patients developed anti-GA antibodies, which were expressed at high titre in 33%. The study did not have clinical endpoints, but the authors nonetheless tried to correlate clinical response to GA with the presence of antibodies and observed that patients with high-titre antibodies tend to have a higher relapse rate and a more rapid progression than patients with low antibodies titres. In the study by Brenner and co-workers (2001), all the patients ($n = 130$) developed anti-GA antibodies, which declined after six months, persisting at low titre, but they did not seem to interfere with copolymer activity.

In Theiler's virus model of demyelinating disease (Ure and Rodriguez 2002), anti-GA antibodies seemed to promote remyelination. However, no clinical studies to date have shown either a neutralizing or a beneficial effect of anti-GA antibodies in patients with multiple sclerosis. Depending on route and frequency of administration, anaphylactic reactions may occur. Rauschka and colleagues (2005) described a systemic anaphylactic reaction to GA in a patient who had a history of atopic allergy and high serum IgE concentrations. The patient had a positive skin test to GA and an unusually high concentration of IgG4 antibodies to the drug. These observations suggest that caution is needed in administrating GA to atopic patients with multiple sclerosis.

2.6. Treatment of Multiple Sclerosis Patients Who Have Developed Antibodies Against Interferon-β

Antibody formation against interferon-β (IFNβ) in patients with multiple sclerosis is used here as a good illustration of the clinical aspects of antibody formation against biopharmaceuticals, and includes a discussion on how to prevent or reduce antibody formation. Some of the aspects in this section are discussed in more detail in Chapter 7.

2.6.1. Description of Interferon-β

The gene of IFNβ shows 45% homology with IFNα genes. The protein is composed of 166 amino acids and has a molecular weight of 22,500 dalton. It has several functions, which include antiviral, antiproliferative and immunomodulant activities, such as the regulation of antigen presentation to T lymphocytes (Goodbourn, Didcock and Randall 2000), the stimulation of T helper 2 and the activation of natural killer cells (Nguyen et al. 2002).

It is one of the first-line drugs for the treatment of relapsing-remitting multiple sclerosis (RR-MS). Two types of recombinant IFNβ exist: IFNβ-1a, which is available in two different commercial preparations (Avonex by Biogen-Idec, Cambridge, and Rebif by Serono, Geneva) (Table 2.4) and is obtained from Chinese hamster ovary, and IFNβ-1b (Betaferon, Schering, Berlin), which is generated in *E. coli*. IFNβ-1b and IFNβ-1a have the same receptor binding region, but IFNβ-1b is a non-glycosylated molecule that has a Met-1 deletion and a Cys-17 to Ser mutation (Mark et al. 1984), while IFNβ-1a is a glycosylated polypeptide with the predicted natural amino acid sequence

Table 2.4 Different commercial preparations of IFNβ.

	Avonex	Betaferon	Rebif
Number of amino acids	166	165	166
Production	CHO	*E. coli*	CHO
Dosage/injection	6 MIU (30 μg)	8 MIU (250 μg)	6–12 MIU (22–44 μg)
Route of administrations	i.m.	s.c.	s.c.
Frequency	Once/week	Every other day	Thrice/week

Note: CHO= Chinese hamster ovary; i.m.= intramuscular; s.c.= subcutaneous

(Holliday and Benfield 1997). These differences affect the pharmacokinetic, pharmacodynamic and immunological properties. In particular, the absence of glycosylation causes the formation of aggregates and a reduction of in vitro activity (Runkel 1998).

2.6.2. Prevalence of Neutralizing Antibodies

Randomized, double-blind, placebo-controlled studies have demonstrated the efficacy of IFNβ in the treatment of RR-MS on both clinical and MRI measures (The IFNB MS Study Group 1993, Jacobs et al. 1996, PRISMS 1998, PRISMS-4 2001, Kappos et al. 2005). A percentage of IFN-treated patients can develop neutralizing antibodies (NAbs) against IFNβ during the course of treatment. The percentage of Nabs-positive (NAbs+) patients varies depending on the IFNβ product, the frequency and route of administration and the type of assay used, with Betaferon the most immunogenic and Avonex the least immunogenic (Table 2.5). Factors influencing the development of anti-IFNβ antibodies are not clearly defined as yet. A cross-reactivity of NAbs has been demonstrated (Khan and Dhib-Jalbut 1998, Antonelli et al. 1999, Bertolotto et al. 2000); thus, once NAbs develop, the switch to a different commercial preparation is not clinically useful.

2.6.3. Dynamics of NAbs

The majority of patients become NAbs+ within 6–18 months of treatment, while clinical impact of NAbs is delayed and is not seen until 24 months of therapy (Figure 2.3). It has been suggested that patients on IFNβ-1b tend to become antibody-positive earlier than those on IFNβ-1a and that in NAbs+ patients, the probability of reverting to NAb-negative status is significantly higher in patients treated with IFNβ-1b than in patients treated with IFNβ-1a (Rebif) (Gneiss et al. 2004, Sorensen et al. 2005). Several studies have

Table 2.5 IFNβ immunogenicity.

Type of drug (phase III trials)	Percentage of NAbs+ (2–3 years)
Avonex (Jacobs 1996)	22
Avonex (Rudick 1998)	6
Rebif 22 (PRISMS)	24
Rebif 44 (PRISMS)	12
Rebif 44 (SPECTRIMS)	15
Betaferon (1996)	38
Betaferon (Polman 2003)	28

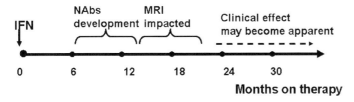

Figure 2.3 Dynamics of NAbs and clinical consequences.

demonstrated that NAbs persist for a long time, despite IFNβ discontinuation. In the study by Polman et al. (2003), 37% of NAbs+ patients reverted to seronegative over three years. In the PRISMS study, 22% reverted to seronegative by four years and 37% by six years, and in a recent Danish study (Petersen et al. 2006), it was shown that patients with NAbs titres above 200 tended to maintain NAb+ status for a median time of 22 months. In a study by our group (Malucchi et al. 2005), spontaneous disappearance of NAbs was only observed in those NAbs+ patients which had low titre of antibodies (<100 TRU), whereas NAbs persisted in patients showing higher titre, despite immunosuppressive treatment.

2.6.4. Effects of NAbs on IFNβ Efficacy

Several studies have demonstrated that the presence of NAbs causes a reduction in IFNβ bioavailability as measured by reduced levels of biologic markers such as neopterin, β2-microglobulin (Rudick et al. 1998), myxovirus resistance protein A (MxA) (Deisenhammer et al. 1999, Kracke et al. 2000, Vallittu et al. 2002) and MxA messenger RNA (Bertolotto et al. 2001, 2003). Besides that, a number of studies have demonstrated that the presence of NAbs is associated with a loss of IFNβ clinical and radiological efficacy (Table 2.6). Betaferon was the first IFNβ approved in the United States for the treatment of RR-MS, as it demonstrated to reduce clinical activity as well as radiological activity in a large study, which involved 372 patients (The IFNβ MS study Group 1993), randomly assigned to receive placebo or the active drug at two different dosages (1.6 MIU and 8 MIU, respectively). Thirty-five percent of patients receiving 8 MIU became NAbs+, and in these patients, the relapse rate in the second and third year of treatment was comparable

Table 2.6 Studies demonstrating a loss of IFNβ clinical and radiological efficacy in NAbs+ patients.

Type of drug	Clinical effect of NAbs relapse rate	MRI effect of NAbs
Avonex (Jacobs 1996)	–/–	–
Avonex (Rudick 1998)	NS/NS	Reduced*
Rebif 22 (PRISMS-4)	Reduced[p]	Reduced[p]
Rebif 44 (PRISMS-4)	Reduced[p]	Reduced[p]
Rebif 44 (SPECTRIMS)	Reduced*	Reduced[p]
Betaferon (1996)	Reduced[p]	Reduced[p]
Betaferon (Polman 2003)	Reduced[p]	Reduced[p]

Note: NS= not significant; *= suggestion; [p]= statistically significant to one of the placebo group (The IFNβ MS Study Group and the University of British Columbia MS/MRI Analysis Group 1996). The loss of efficacy was also radiologically evident, as NAbs+ patients had a significantly higher number of MRI lesions by the second and third years. A negative effect of NAbs was also present in the evaluation of disability progression, even if there was no significant difference between NAbs+ and NAbs negative (Nabs–) patients.

Comparable results are also evident in the Betaferon study on 718 secondary-progressive MS patients (Polman et al. 2003), in which NAbs+ patients had a significantly higher relapse rate and a significantly higher increase in MRI lesion burden than NAbs– patients. Similar evidence arises from other studies in which the other commercial preparations of IFNβ have been used: in the PRISMS-4 study (PRISMS-4 2001) conducted on more than 500 patients treated with Rebif 22 µg or 44 µg for 4 years (or with placebo for two years and then randomly assigned to Rebif 22 or 44), the negative effect of NAbs on clinical and, even more, radiological activities is clearly evident. By the third year of treatment, NAbs+ patients had a significant higher relapse rate than Nabs– (0.81 and 0.5, respectively), as well as about five-fold increase in the mean number of MRI active lesions (Figure 2.4) and three-fold increase in the burden of disease compared to Nabs–. A post hoc analysis by Francis et al. (2005) focused on a subgroup of patients (368 subjects treated with Rebif 22 or 44 from the beginning) of the PRISMS-4. The authors studied two markers of IFN biological activity, represented by β2-microglobulin and neopterin, and the clinical and radiological effects of IFNβ. Interestingly, at one year, the mean increase in the level of these markers from baseline was significant only in Nabs– patients. In addition, upon analysis of the relapse rate during the four years, the authors observed a comparable relapse rate between Nabs– and NAbs+ groups in the first and second years, whereas in the third and fourth years NAbs+ had a significant higher relapse rate. The impact of NAbs was even more evident on MRI results. Also the SPECTRIMS study (2001) on SP-MS patients showed the negative effect of NAbs on clinical and radiological parameters (Li et al. 2001). In the more recent study by Kappos and co-workers (2005) on 802 patients randomly assigned to Avonex 30 or 60 µg for four years, 1.8% and 4.8%, respectively, were NAbs+. Despite the low percentage of NAbs+

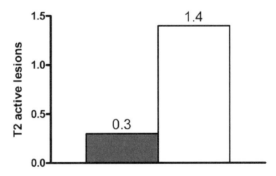

Figure 2.4 Impact of NAbs on MRI: median number of T2-active lesions reported in the PRISMS-4 study (2001). Grey square: Nabs– patients; white square: NAbs+ patients; the difference is statistically significant (*p*<0.001).

patients, the impact of NAbs was dramatically evident, as the annualized relapse rate was 39% higher in NAbs+ than in Nabs– over 12–48 months, time to three-month sustained disability progression was shorter in NAbs+ than in Nabs–, and mean number of MRI active lesions was significantly higher in NAbs+ than in Nabs– patients.

More generally, NAbs have been demonstrated to have a prognostic value, as NAbs+ patients have a higher risk to relapse than Nabs– patients (Sorensen et al. 2003, Malucchi et al. 2004, Tomassini et al. 2006).

As MS is characterized by an unpredictable course, in which, up to date, no clinical or laboratory markers are available, the prognostic character of the detection of NAbs is a useful instrument for the neurologist. Recently, after evaluating NAbs literature, European guidelines regarding antibodies against IFN in MS have been written, giving as an "A level" recommendation that therapy with IFNβ should be discontinued in patients with titres of NAbs >100 (Sorensen et al. 2005).

2.6.5. Possible Strategies to Eliminate NAbs

Up to date no predictive factors of the development of NAbs are known and no guidelines exist about the management of NAbs+ patients. However, as it is evident that NAbs abolish IFNβ efficacy and have a prognostic meaning, some strategies have to be undertaken in NAbs+ patients. As already written above, it is possible that a spontaneous seroreversion occurs, especially in those patients with low titres of antibodies, but several studies (Bellomi et al. 2003, Petersen et al. 2006) showed that NAbs can be a long-lasting phenomenon. Thus, the continuation of IFN therapy after NAbs development, hoping in a spontaneous seroreversion, makes the patient be at risk of taking a useless therapy for many years. Similarly, the switch to a less immunogenic preparation of IFN has no positive effect, as NAbs cross-react with any type of IFNβ.

Hypothetic strategies to eliminate NAbs include the use of plasmapheresis and intravenous immunoglobulins (Sorensen et al. 2005). At present, IgG and plasma exchange are used in the treatment of autoimmune diseases (Yamamoto, Takamatsu and Saito 2007, Zinman, Ng and Bril 2007), but they have no effect on memory or plasma cells, so these treatments could help the elimination of circulating NAbs, but not avoid their development.

Another hypothetic strategy is to increase the dosage of IFN, with the aim of overcoming antibody neutralization, but probably this strategy fails if the NAbs titre is high. Finally, a monoclonal antibody used for the treatment of lymphoma, rituximab, is available. This drug is directed against B cells; thus from a theoretical point of view, it could be used to reduce NAbs titres, but no data exist on this.

2.6.6. Possible Strategies to Prevent Formation of NAbs

An Italian study by Pozzilli and co-workers (2002) evaluated about 160 MS-affected patients, who were treated with IFNβ1a alone or in combination with short pulses of steroids for one year. The authors observed that in the group treated with the combination therapy there was a 50% reduction in the incidence of NAbs development. However, steroids were not able to reduce the titre in NAbs+ patients. In other clinical trials performed on RR- as well as SP-MS-affected patients, a combination therapy (IFN plus immunosuppressive agents) has been used (Fernandez et al. 2002), but no definitive conclusions about the ability in reducing NAbs formation are available. Surely, the modifications in the technical preparation of the drug are of extreme importance in determining drug immunogenicity. This has been demonstrated for Avonex, which in the first study by Jacob and co-workers (1996) induced 22% of NAbs+ patients, whereas in the study by Clanet et al. (2002) induced only 2–3% of NAbs+ patients.

2.6.7. The Costs of Ineffective IFNβ Treatment

As previously stated, IFNβ modifies the natural course of multiple sclerosis, significantly reducing the relapse rate and slowing disease progression. In addition, several studies showed the beneficial effect of IFNβ in delaying the onset of defined multiple sclerosis in patients affected by clinical isolated syndrome (CIS). Thus, there is a large consensus to start IFNβ treatment early.

In Italy, about 52,000 subjects are affected by multiple sclerosis, and about one-third of them receive IFNβ therapy. Consequently, the cost of treatment is about 170 millions euro/year. If we consider that about 15% of treated patients develop NAbs, we can estimate that 2,500 patients are receiving a useless drug and, thus, about 25 millions euro/year are ill spent. This refers only to the Italian situation, whereas, considering the situation in Europe as a whole, the cost obviously increases.

While on one side IFNβ treatment tends to be initiated very early in the disease course, on the other side a percentage of patients are at risk of receiving, for a long period, a useless drug because the identification of IFN non-responder patients by clinical observation often requires several years. Thus, it is clear that the availability of a biological assay which can rapidly identify this group of patients leads to a considerable reduction in therapeutic costs. It also has to be considered that NAbs+ patients would benefit from alternative therapies that have comparable (glatiramer acetate) or lower cost (mithoxantrone, azathioprine) compared to IFNβ.

2.7. Conclusions

At present, proteins are widely used as therapeutic agents; with the development of recombinant DNA techniques, highly purified proteins have been produced. However, even if they are nearly identical to the endogenous proteins, they still may show immunogenicity.

Antibodies against these drugs can have a neutralizing activity which inhibits the efficacy or they can induce changes in pharmacokinetic properties or lead to hypersensitivity reactions. Antibody production seems to be related to many different mechanisms, such as the post-translational modifications, the development of drug aggregates and the use of adjuvants. Antibodies which cause the loss of clinical efficacy or which are directed against the endogenous molecule should be prevented, but at present no failsafe strategy to prevent neutralizing antibodies formation is known. An interesting approach to reduce immunogenicity has been described in a recent work by Tangri et al. (2005), in which the authors tried to reduce EPO immunogenicity by engineering modified forms of the protein with substitutions in the regions containing the epitopes binding to HLA class II molecules; the authors found that the modified forms of EPO were non-immunogenic in vitro; so this strategy could represent one way to limit the immunogenicity of protein drugs. Other strategies include the use of combination therapy, adding steroids to temporarily suppress the immune system.

When antibodies are already present, they may sometimes disappear spontaneously when the treatment is continued, but this process may take years. Intravenous immunoglobulin and plasmapheresis can be used to reduce the antibody burden, but they do not affect memory cells. Considering the potential high costs of such therapies, as well as those adverse events and reduction of drug efficacy, early detection of antibody formation is an important issue in treatment with biopharmaceuticals. Assays for determining antibody formation and type of antibodies are discussed in detail in the Chapter 3.

References

Albertsson-Wikland, K. 1987. Clinical trial with authentic recombinant somatotropin in Sweden and Finland. Acta Paediatr. Scand. (Suppl.) 331:28–34.

Altman, J.J., Pehuet, M., Slama, G., and Tchoapoutsky, C. 1983. Three cases of allergic reaction to human insulin (Letter). Lancet 2:524.

Andersen, O.O. 1973. Insulin antibody formation II: the influence of species difference and method of administration. Acta Endocrinol. 72:33–45.

Antignani, A. and Youle, R.J. 2007. The cytokine, GM-CSF, can deliver BCL-XL as an extracellular fusion protein to protect cells from apoptosis and retain differential induction. J. Biol. Chem. 282(15):11246–11254.

Antonelli, G., Simeoni, E., Bagnato, F., Pozzilli, C., Turriziani, O., Tesoro, R., Di Marco, P., Gasperini, C., Fieschi, C., and Dianzani, F. 1999. Further study on the specificity and incidence of neutralizing antibodies to interferon (IFN) in relapsing remitting multiple sclerosis patients treated with IFN beta-1a or IFN beta-1b. J. Neurol. Sci. 168:131–136.

Arnon, R. and Aharoni, R. 2004. Mechanism of action of glatiramer acetate in multiple sclerosis and its potential for the development of new applications. Proc. Natl. Acad. Sci. USA 101:14593–14598.

Barranco, P. and Lopez-Serrano, M.C. 1998. General and epidemiological aspects of allergic drug reactions. Clin. Exp. Allergy 28(Suppl. 4):61–62.

Bekisz, J., Schmeisser, H., Hernandez, J., Goldman, N.D., and Zoon, K.C. 2004. Human Interferons alpha, beta and omega. Growth Factors 22:243–251.

Bellomi, F., Scagnolari, C., Tomassini, V., Gasperini, C., Paolillo, A., Pozzilli, C., and Antonelli, G. 2003. Fate of neutralizing and binding antibodies to IFN beta in MS patients treated with IFN beta for 6 years. J. Neurol. Sci. 215:3–8.

Bennett, C.L., Luminari, S., Nissenson, A.R., Tallman, M.S., Klinge, S.A., McWilliams, N., McKoy, J.M., Kim, B., Lyons, E.A., Trifilio, S.M., Raisch, D.W., Evens, A.M., Kuzel, D.M., Schumock, G.T., Belknap, S.M., Locatelli, F., Rossert, J., and Casadevall, N. 2004. Pure red cell aplasia and epoetin therapy. N. Engl. J. Med. 351:1403–1408.

Bergrem, H., Danielson, B.G., Eckardt, K.U., Kurtz, A., and Stridsberg, M. 1993. A case of antierythropoietin antibodies following recombinant human erythropoietin treatment. In: Bauer, C., Koch, K.M., and Sciqalla, P., (eds). Erythropoietin: Molecular Physiology and Clinical Application. Marcel Dekker, New York, pp. 265–275.

Berman, E., Heller, G., Kempin, S., Gee, T., Tran, L.-L., and Clarkson, B. 1990. Incidence of response and long-term follow up in a patient with hairy cell leukemia treated with recombinant human interferon alfa-2a. Blood 75:839–845.

Berson, S.A., Yalow, R.S., Bauman, A., Rothschild, M.A., and Newerly, K. 1956. Insulin-I-131 metabolism in human subjects: demonstration of insulin binding globulin in the circulation of insulin treated subjects. J. Clin. Invest. 35:170.

Bertolotto, A., Gilli, F., Sala, A., Audano, L., Castello, A., Magliola, U., Melis, F., and Giordana, M.T. 2001. Evaluation of bioavailability of three types of IFNbeta in multiple sclerosis patients by a new quantitative competitive- PCR method for MxA quantification. J. Immunol. Methods 256:141–152.

Bertolotto, A., Gilli, F., Sala, A., Capobianco, M., Malucchi, S., Milano, E., Melis, F., Marnetto, F., Lindberg, R.L., Bottero, R., Di Sapio, A., and Giordana, M.T. 2003. Persistent neutralizing antibodies abolish the interferon beta bioavailability in MS patients. Neurology 60:634–639.

Bertolotto, A., Malucchi, S., Milano, E., Castello, A., Capobianco, M., and Mutani, R. 2000. Interferon β neutralizing antibodies in multiple sclerosis: neutralizing activity and cross-reactivity with three different preparations. Immunopharmacology 49: 95–100.

Bijvoet, A.G.A., Van Hirtum, H., Kroos, M.A., Van de Kamp, E.H., Schoneveld, O., Visser, P., Brakenhoff, J.P., Weggeman, M., van Corven, E.J., Van der Ploeg, A.T., and Reuser, A.J. 1999. Human α-glucosidase from rabbit milk has therapeutic effect in mice with glycogen storage disease type II. Hum. Mol. Genet. 8:2145–2153.

Blandford, R.L., Sewell, H., Sharp, P., and Hearnshaw, J.R. 1982. Generalized allergic reaction with synthetic human insulin (Comment–Letter). Lancet 2:1468.

Bonetti, P., Diodati, G., Drago, C., Casarin, C., Scaccabarozzi, S., Realdi, G., Ruol, A., and Alberti, A. 1994. Interferon antibodies in patients with chronic hepatitic C virus infection treated with recombinant interferon alpha-2 alpha. J. Hepatol. 20:416–420.

Bray, G.L., Gomperts, E.D., Courter, S., Gruppo, R., Gordon, E.M., Manco-Jonshon, M., Shapiro, A., Scheibel, E., White, G., and Lee, M. 1994. A multicentre study of recombinant factor VIII (recombinate): safety, efficacy, and inhibitor risk in previously untreated patients with hemofilia A. Blood 83: 2428–2435.

Brenner, T., Arnon, R., Sela, M., Abramsky, O., Meiner, Z., Riven-Kreitman, R., Tarcik, N., and Teitelbaum, D. 2001. Humoral and cellular immune responses to Copolymer 1 in multiple sclerosis patients treated with Copaxone®. J. Neuroimmunol. 115:152–160.

Bristol, A. 1993. Recombinant DNA derived insulin analogues as potentially useful therapeutic agents. Trends Biotechnol. 11:301–305.

Carveth-Johnson, A.O., Mylvaganam, K., and Child, D.F. 1982. Generalised allergic reaction with synthetic human insulin (Letter). Lancet 2:1287.

Casadevall, N. 2002. Antibodies against rHuEPO: native and recombinant. Nephrol. Dial. Transplant. 17(Suppl. 5):42–47.

Casadevall, N., Nataf, J., Viron, B., Kolta, A., Kiladjian, J.J., Martin-Dupont, P., Michaud, P., Papo, T., Ugo, V., Teyssandier, I., Varet, B., and Mayeux, P. 2002. Pure red-cell aplasia and antierythropoietin antibodies in patients treated with recombinant erythropoietin. N. Engl. J. Med. 346:469–475.

Chance, R.E., Root, M.A., and Galloway, J.A. 1976. The immunogenicity of insulin preparations. Acta Endocrinol. Suppl. (Copenh) 205:185–198.

Charak, B., Agah, R., and Mazumder, A. 1993. Granulocyte-macrophage colony-stimulating factor-induced antibody-dependent cellular cytotoxicity in bone marrow macrophages: application in bone marrow transplantation. Blood 81: 3474–3479.

Chen, J.W., Frystyk, J., Lauritzen, T., and Christiansen, J.S. 2005. Impact of insulin antibodies on insulin aspart pharmacokinetics and pharmacodynamics after 12-week treatment with multiple daily injections of biphasic insulin aspart 30 in patients with type 1 diabetes. Eur. J. Endocrinol. 153(6):907–913.

Clanet, M., Radue, E.W., Kappos, L., Hartung, H.P., Hohlfeld, R., Sandberg-Wollheim, M., Kooijmans-Coutinho, M.F., Tsao, E.C., Sandrock, A.W., and European IFNbeta-1a (Avonex) Dose-Comparison Study Investigators. 2002. A randomized, double-blind, dose-comparison study of weekly interferon beta-1a in relapsing MS. Neurology 59:1507–1517.

Comi, G., Filippi, M., and Wolinsky, J.S. 2001. European/Canadian multicenter, double-blind, randomized, placebo-controlled study of the effects of glatiramer acetate on magnetic resonance imaging–measured disease activity and burden in patients with relapsing multiple sclerosis. European/Canadian Glatiramer Acetate Study Group. Ann. Neurol. 49:290–297.

Davidson, J.K. and DeBra, D.W. 1978. Immunologic insulin resistance. Diabetes 27:307–318.

Deckert, T. 1985. The immunogenicity of new insulins. Diabetes 34(Suppl. 2):94–96.

Deisenhammer, F., Reindl, M., Harvey, J., Gasse, T., Dilitz, E., and Berger, T. 1999. Bioavailability of interferon beta 1b in MS patients with and without neutralizing antibodies. Neurology 62:1239–1243.

Deleeuw, I., Delvigne, C., and Beckaert, J. 1982. Insulin allergy treated with human insulin (recombinant DNA). Diabetes Care 5(Suppl. 2):168–170.

deShazo, R.D., Levinson, A.I., Boehm, T., Evans, R. III, and Waed, G. Jr. 1977. Severe persistent biphasic local (immediate and late) skin reactions to insulin. J. Allergy Clin. Immunol. 59:161–164.

DeWitt, D.E. and Hirsch, I.B. 2003. Outpatient insulin therapy in type 1 and type 2 diabetes mellitus: a scientific review. JAMA 289:2254–2264.

Dianzani, F., Antonelli, G., Amicucci, P., Cefaro, A., and Pintus, C. 1989. Low incidence of neutralizing antibody formation to interferon-alpha 2b in human recipients. J. Interferon Res. 9(Suppl. 1):S33–S36.

Douglas, D.D., Rakela, J., Lin, H.J., Hollinger, F.B., Taswell, H.F., Czaja, A.J., Gross, J.B., Anderson, M.L., Parent, K., and Fleming, C.R. 1993. Randomized controlled trial of recombinant alpha-2a-interferon for chronic hepatitis C. Comparison of alanine aminotransferase normalization versus loss of HCV RNA and anti-HCV IgM. Dig. Dis. Sci. 38:601–607.

Eckardt, K.U. and Casadevall, N. 2003. Pure red cell aplasia due to anti-erythropoietin antibodies. Nephrol. Dial. Transplant. 18:865–869.

Ehrenforth, S., Kreuz, W., Scharrer, I., Linde, R., Funk, M., Gungor, T., Krackhardt, B., and Kornhuber, B. 1992. Incidence of development of factor VIII and factor IX inhibitors in haemophiliacs. Lancet 339:594–598.

Farina, C., Weber, M.S., Meinl, E., Wekerle, H., and Hohlfeld, R. 2005. Glatiramer acetate in multiple sclerosis: update on potential mechanisms of action. Lancet Neurol. 4:567–575.

Fernandez, O., Guerrero, M., Mayorga, C., Munoz, L., Lean, A., Lugue, G., Hervas, M., Fernandez, V., Capdevila, A., and de Ramon, E. 2002. Combination therapy with interferon beta-1b and azathioprine in secondary progressive multiple sclerosis. A two-year pilot study. J. Neurol. 249:1058–1062.

Figlin, R.A.and Itri, L. 1988. Anti-interfeon antibodies: a perspective. Semin. Hematol. 25:9–15.

Fineberg, S.E. 1994. Insulin allergy and insulin resistance. In: Lebovitz, H.E., (ed). Therapy for Diabetes Mellitus and Related Disorders. American Diabetes Association, Alexandria, Virginia,. pp. 178–184.

Fineberg, S.E., Galloway, J.A., Fineberg, N.S., and Goldman J. 1983. Effects of species of origin, purification levels, and formulation on insulin immunogenicity. Diabetes 32:592–599.

Fineberg, S.E., Huang, J., Brunelle, R., Gulliya, K.S., and Anderson J.H. 2003. Effect of long-term exposure to insulin Lispro on the induction of antibody response in patients with type 1 or type 2 Diabetes. Diabetes Care 26:89–96.

Fireman, P., Fineberg, S.E., and Galloway, J.A. 1982. Development of IgE antibodies to human (recombinant DNA) porcine, and bovine insulins in diabetic subjects. Diabetes Care 5(Suppl. 2):119–125.

Francis, G.S., Rice, G.P., Alsop, J.C., and PRISMS Study Group. 2005. Interferon beta-1a in MS. Results following development of neutralizing antibodies in PRISMS. Neurol. 65:48–55.

Freund, M., von Wussow, P., Diedrich, H., Eisert, R., link, H., Wilke, H., Buchholz, F., LeBlanc, S., Fonatsch, C., Deicher, H., and Poliwoda, H. 1989. Recombinant human interferon (IFN) alpha-2b in chronic myelogenous leukemia: dose dependency of response and frequency of neutralizing anti-interferon antibodies. Br. J. Haematol. 72:350–356.

Frigerio, C., Aubry, M., and Gomez, F. 1997. Desensitization-resistant insulin allergy. Allergy 52:238–239.

Frost, H. 2005. Antibody-mediated side effects of recombinant proteins. Toxicology 209:155–160.

Garcia-Ortega, P., Knobel, H., and Miranda, A. 1984. Sensitization to human insulin (Letter). BMJ 288:1271.

Gneiss, C., Reindl, M., Lutterotti, A., Ehling, R., Egg, R., Khalil, M., Berger, T., and Deisenhammer, F. 2004. Interferon beta: the neutralizing antibody (NAb) titre predicts reversion to NAb negativity. Mult. Scler. 10:507–510.

Goodbourn, S., Didcock, L., and Randall, R.E. 2000. Interferons: cells signalling, immune modulation, antiviral response and virus countermeasures. J. Gen. Virol. 81:2341–2364.

Gossain, V.V., Rouner, D.R., and Homak, K. 1985. Systemic allergy to human (recombinant DNA) insulin. Ann. Allergy 55:116–118.

Grammer, L.C., Roberts, M., Buchanan, T.A., Fitzsimons, R., Metzger, B.E., and Patterson, R. 1987. Specificity of immunoglobulin E and immunoglobulin G against human (recombinant DNA) insulin in human insulin allergy and resistance. J. Lab. Clin. Med. 109:141–146.

Gribben, J.G., Devereux, S., Thomas, N.S., Keim, M., Jones, H.M., Goldstone, A.H., and Linch, D.C. 1990. Development of antibodies to unprotected glycosylation sites on recombinant human GM-CSF. Lancet 335:434–437.

Hanauer, L. and Batson, J.M. 1961. Anaphylactic shock following insulin injection. Diabetes 10:105–109.

Hill, A.D., Redmond, H.P., Austin, O.M., Grace, P.A., and Bouchier-Hayes, D. 1993. Granulocyte-macrophage colony-stimulating factor inhibits tumor growth. Br. J. Surg. 80:1543–1546.

Holliday, S.M. and Benfield, P. 1997. Interferon-b-1a. A Review of its pharmacological proprieties and therapeutic potential in multiple sclerosis. BioDrugs 8: 317–330.

Hooijberg, E., Sein, J.J., van den Berk P.C., Hart, A.A., van der Valk, M.A., Kast, W.M., Melief, C.J., and Hekman, A. 1995. Eradication of large human B-cell tumors in nude mice with unconjugated CD20 monoclonal antibodies and interleukin-2. Cancer Res. 55:2627–2634.

Ishibashi, O., Kobayashi, M., Maegawa, H., Watanabe, N., Takata, Y., Okuno, Y., and Shigeta, Y. 1986. Can insulin antibodies of diabetic patients distinguish human insulin from porcine insulin? Horm. Metab. Res. 18:470–472.

Jacobs, L.D., Cookfair, D.L., Rudick, R.A., Herndon, R.M., Richert, R.T., Salazar, A.M., Fisher, J.S., Goodkin, D.E., Granger, C.V., Simon, J.H., Alam, J.J., Bartoszak, D.M., Bourdette, D.N., Braiman, J., Brownscheidle, C.M., Coats, M.E., Cohan, S.L., Dougherty, D.S., Kinkel, R.P., Mass, M.K., Munschauer, F.E.,

Priore, R.L., Pullicino, P.M., Scherokman, B.J., and Whitham, R.H. 1996. Intramuscular interferon beta-1a for disease progression in relapsing multiple sclerosis. Ann. Neurol. 39:285–294.

Johnson, K.B., Brooks, B.R., Ford, C.C., Goodman, A., Guarnaccia, J., Lisak, R.P., Myers, L.W., Panitch, H.S., Pruitt, A., Rose, J.W., Kachuck, N., and Wolinsky, J.S. 2000. Sustained clinical benefits of glatiramer acetate in relapsing multiple sclerosis patients observed for 6 years. Mult. Scler. 6:255–266.

Johnson, K.B., Brooks, B.R., Cohen, J.A., Ford, C.C., Goldstein, J., Lisak, R.P., Myers, L.W., Panitch, H.S., Rose, J.W., and Schiffer, R.B. 1995. Copolymer 1 reduces relapse rate and improves disability in relapsing-remitting multiple sclerosis: results of a phase III multicenter, double-blind, placebo-controlled trial. Neurol. 45: 1268–1276.

Johnson, K.B., Brooks, B.R., Cohen, J.A., Ford, C.C., Goldstein, J., Lisak, R.P., Myers, L.W., Panitch, H.S., Rose, J.W., Schiffer, R.B., Vollmer, T., Weiner, L.P., and Wolinsky, J.S. 1998. Extended use of glatiramer acetate (Copaxone) is well tolerated and maintains its clinical effect on multiple sclerosis relapse rate and degree of disability. Neurology 50:701–708.

Johnson, K.P., Ford, C.C., Lisak, R.P., and Wolinsky, J.S. 2005. Neurologic consequence of delaying glatiramer acetate therapy for multiple sclerosis: 8-year data. Acta Neurol. Scand. 111(1):42–47.

Jones, G.J. and Itri, L.M. 1986. Safety and tolerance of recombinant interferon alfa-2a (Roferon-A) in cancer patients. Cancer 57:1709–1715.

Kaplan, S.L., Underwood, L.E., August, G.P., Bell, J.J., Blethen, S.L., Blizzard, R.M., Brown, D.R., Foley, T.P., Hintz, R.L., and Hopwood, N.J. 1986. Clinical studies with recombinant-DNA-derived methionyl human growth hormone deficient children. Lancet 1:697–700.

Kappos, L., Clanet, M., Sandberg-Wollheim, M., Radue, E.W., Hartung, H.P., Hohlfeld, R., Xu, J., Bennett, D., Sandrock, A., Goelz, S., and European Interferon beta-1a IM dose-Comparison Study Investigators. 2005. European interferon beta-1a IM dose-comparison study investigators. Neutralizing antibodies and efficacy of interferon beta-1a: a 4-year controlled study. Neurology 65: 40–47.

Khan, O.A. and Dhib-Jalbut, S.S. 1998. Neutralizing antibodies to interferon β-1a and interferon β-1b in MS patients are crossreactive. Neurology 51:1696–1702.

Kishnani, P.S., Corzo, D., Nicolino, M., Byrne, B., Mandel, H., Hwu, W.L., Lesile, N., Levine, J., Spencer, C., McDonald, M., Li, J., Dumontier, J., Halberthal, M., Chien, Y.H., Hopkin, R., Vijayaraghavan, S., Gruskin, D., Bartholomew, D., van der Ploeg, A., Clancy, J.P., Parini, R., Morin, G., Beck, M., De la Gastine, G.S., Jokic, M., Thurberg, B., Richards, S., Bali, D., Davison, M., Worden, M.A., Chen, Y.T., and Wraith, J.E. 2007. Recombinant human acid (alpha)-glucosidase: major clinical benefits in infantile-onset Pompe disease. Neurology 68:99–109.

Klinge, L., Straub, V., Neudorf, U., Schaper, J., Bosbach, T., Gorlinger, K., Wallot, M., Richards, S., and Voit, T. 2005. Safety and efficacy of recombinant acid alpha-glucosidase (rhGAA) in patients with classical infantile Pompe disease: results of a phase II clinical trial. Neuromuscul. Disord. 15:24–31.

Kracke, A., von Wussow, P., Al-Masri, A.N., Dalley, G., Windhagen, A., and Heidenreich, F. 2000. Mx proteins in blood leukocytes for monitoring interferon beta-1b therapy in patients with MS. Neurology 54:193–199.

Kromminga, A. and Schellekens, H. 2005. Antibodies against erythropoietin and other protein-based therapeutics. An overview. Ann. NY Acad. Sci. 1050:257–265.

Kumar, D. 1997. Lispro analog for treatment of generalized allergy to human insulin. Diabetes Care 20:1357–1359.

Kuter, D.J. 2000. Future directions with platelet growth factors. Semin. Hematol. 37:41–49.

Kuter, D.J. 2007. New thrombopoietic growth factors. Blood 109:4607–4616.

Lacroix-Desmazes, S., Bayry, J., Misra, N., Horn, M.P., Villard, S., Pashov, A., Stieltjes, N., d'Oiron, R., Saint-Remy, J.M., Hoebeke, J., Kazatchkine, M.D., Reinbolt, J., Mohanty, D., and Kaveri, S.V. 2002. The prevalence of proteolytic antibodies against factor VIII in Haemophilia A. N. Engl. J. Med. 346:662–667.

Lahtela, J.T., Knip, M., Paul, R., Antone, J., and Salmi, J. 1997. Severe antibody-mediated human insulin resistance: successful treatment with the insulin analog lispro: a case report. Diabetes Care 20:71–73.

Lang, D.M., Alpern, M.B., Visintainer, P.F., and Smith, S.T. 1991. Increased risk for anaphylactoid reaction from contrast media in patients on beta-adrenergic blockers or with asthma. Ann. Intern. Med. 115:270–276.

Li, D.K., Zhao, J.G., Paty, D.W., and University of British Columbia MS/MRI Analysis Research Group, and the SPECTRIMS Study Group. 2001. Randomized controlled trial of interferon beta-1a in secondary progressive MS. MRI results. Neurology 56:1505–1513.

Li, J., Yang, C., Xia, Y., Bertino, A., Glaspy, J., Roberts, M., and Kuter, D. 2001. Thrombocytopenia caused by the development of antibodies to thrombopoietin. Blood 98:3241–3248.

Locatelli, F., Aljama, P., Barany, P., Canaud, B., Carrera, F., Eckardt, K.U., Macdougall, I.C., Macleod, A., Horl, W.H., Wiecek, A., and Cameron, S. 2004. Erythropoiesis-stimulating agents and antibody-mediated pure red cell aplasia: where are we now and where do we go from here? Nephrol. Dial. Transplant. 19:288–293.

Lok, A.S., Lai, C.L., and Leung, E.K. 1990. Morbidity and mortality from chronic hepatitis B virus infection in family members of patients with malignant and nonmalignant hepatitis B virus-related chronic liver diseases. Hepatology 12:1266–1270.

Lundin, K., Berger, L., Blomberg, F., and Wilton, P. 1991. Development of anti-hGH antibodies during therapy with authentic human growth hormone. Acta Paediatr. Scand. 372:167–168.

Lusher, J.M. 2000. Inhibitor antibodies to factor VIII and factor IX: management. Semin. Thromb. Hemost. 26:179–188.

Lusher, J.M., Arkin, S., Abildgaard, C.F., and Schwartz, R.S. 1993. Recombinat factor VIII for the treatment of previously untreated patients with haemophilia A. safety, efficacy, and development of inhibitors. N. Engl. J. Med. 328:453–459.

Malucchi, S., Capobianco, M., Gilli, F., Marnetto, F., Caldano, M., Sala, A., and Bertolotto, A. 2005. Fate of multiple sclerosis patients positive for neutralising antibodies towards interferon beta shifted to alternative treatments. Neurol. Sci. 26:S213–S214.

Malucchi, S., Sala, A., Gilli, F., Bottero, R., Di Sapio, A., Capobianco, M., and Bertolotto, A. 2004. Neutralizing antibodies reduce the efficacy of βIFN during treatment of multiple sclerosis. Neurol. 62:2031–2037.

Mark, D.F., Lu, S.D., Creasey, A.A., Yamamoto, R., and Lin, L.S. 1984. Site-specific mutagene of the human fibroblast interferon gene. Proc. Natl. Acad. Sci. USA 81:5662–5666.

Marshall, M.O., Heding, L.G., Villumsen, J., Akerblom, H.K., Baevre, H., Dahlguist, G., Kiaergaard, J.J., Knip, M., Lindgren, F., and Ludvigsson, J. 1988. Development of insulin antibodies, metabolic control and B-cell function in newly diagnosed insulin dependent diabetic children treated with monocomponent human insulin or monocomponent porcine insulin. Diabetes Res. 9:169–175.

Massa, G., Vanderschueren-Lodeweyckx, M., and Bouillon, R. 1993. Five-year follow up of growth hormone antibodies in growth hormone deficient children treated with recombinant human growth hormone. Clin. Endocrinol. 38:137–142.

Masucci, G., Wersall, P., Raghnammar, P., and Mellstedt, H. 1989. Granulocyte monocyte colony stimulating factor augments the cytotoxic capacity of lymphocytes and monocytes in antibody-dependent cellular cytotoxicity. Cancer Immunol. Immunother. 29:288–292.

Mellstedt, H. 1994. Induction of anti-granulocyte-macrophage colony-stimulating factor antibodies against exogenous nonglycosylated GM-CSF: biological implications. J. Inteferon. Res. 14:179–180.

Nguyen, K.B., Salazar-Mather, T.P., Dalod, M.Y., Van Deusen, J.B., Wei, X.O., Liew, F.Y., Caligiuri, M.A., Durbin, J.E., and Biron, C.A. 2002. Coordinated and distinct roles for IFN-alpha beta, IL-12, and IL-15 regulation of NK cell responses to viral infection. J. Immunol. 69:4279–4287.

Okada, Y., Taira, K., Takano, K., and Hizuka, N. 1987. A case report of growth attenuation during methionyl human growth hormone treatment. Endocrinol. Jpn. 34:621–626.

Opdenakker, G., Van den Steen, P.E., Laureys, G., Hunninck, K., and Arnold, B. 2003. Neutralizing antibodies in gene-defective hosts. Trends Immunol. 24:94–100.

Peces, R., de la Torre, M., Alcazar, R., and Urra, J.M. 1996. Antibodies against recombinant human erythropoietin in a patient with erythropoietin-resistant anaemia. N. Engl. J. Med. 335:523–524.

Pestka, S., Krause, C.D., and Walter, M.R. 2004. Interferons, interferon-like cytokines and their receptors. Immunol. Rev. 202:8–32.

Peters, A., Klose, O., Hefty, R., Keck, F., and Kerner, W. 1995. The influence of insulin antibodies on the pharmacokinetics of NPH insulin in patients with type 1 diabetes treated with human insulin. Diabet Med. 12:925–930.

Petersen, B., Bendtzen, C., Koch-Henriksen, N., Ravnborg, M., Ross, C., Sorensen, P.S., and Danish Multiple Sclerosis Group. 2006. Persistence of neutralizing antibodies after discontinuation of IFNb therapy in patients with remitting-relapsing multiple sclerosis. Mult. Scler. 12:247–252.

Petersen, B., Bendtzen, K., Koch-Henriksen, N., Ravnborg, M., Ross, C., Sorensen, P.S., and Danish Multiple Sclerosis Study Group. 2006. Persistence of neutralizing antibodies after discontinuation of IFNb therapy in patients with relapsing-remitting multiple sclerosis. Mult. Scler. 12:247–252.

Petros, W.P., Rabinowitz, J., Stuart, A.R., Gilbert, C.J., Kanakura, Y., Griffin, J.D., and Peters, W.P. 1992. Disposition of recombinant human granulocyte-macrophage colony-stimulating factor in patients receiving high-dose chemotherapy and autologous bone marrow support. Blood 80:1135–1140.

Polman, C., Kappos, L., White, R., Dahlke, F., Beckmann, K., Pozzilli, C., Thompson, A., Petkau, J., Miller, D., and European Study Group in Interferon Beta-1b in Secondary Progressive MS. 2003. Neutralizing antibodies during treatment of secondary progressive MS with interferon beta-1b. Neurol. 60:37–43.

Polman, C.H., O'Connor, P.W., Havrdova, E., Huthchinson, M., Kappos, L., Miller, D.H., Philips, J.T., Lublin, F.D., Giovannoni, G., Waigt, A., Toal, M., Lynn, F., Panzara, M.A., Sandrock, A.W., and the AFFIRM Investigators. 2006. A randomized, placebo-controlled trial of natalizumab for relapsing multiple sclerosis. N. Engl. J. Med. 354:899–910.

Pozzilli, C., Antonimi, G., Bagnato, F., Mainero, C., Tomassini, V., Onesti, E., Fantozzi, R., Galgani, S., Pasqualetti, P., Millefiorini, E., Spadaro, M., Dahlke, F., and Gasperini, C. 2002. Monthly corticosteroids decrease neutralizing antibodies to IFNbeta1b: a randomized trial in multiple sclerosis. J. Neurol. 249:50–56.

Prabhakar, S.S. and Muhlfelder, T. 1997. Antibodies to recombinant human erythropoietin causing pure red cell aplasia. Clin. Nephrol. 47:331–335.

PRISMS (Prevention of Relapses and Disability by Interferon-β-1a Subcutaneously in Multiple Sclerosis) Study Group. 1998. Randomised double-blind placebo-controlled study of interferon β-1a in relapsing-remitting multiple sclerosis. Lancet 352:1498–1504.

PRISMS-Study Group and the University of British Columbia MS/MRI Analysis Group. 2001. PRISMS-4. Long term efficacy of interferon-beta-1a in relapsing MS. Neurology 56:1628–1636.

Quesada, J.R., Rios, A., Swanson, D., Trown, P., and Gutterman, J.U. 1985. Antitumor activity of recombinant derived interferon alpha in metastatic renal cell carcinoma. J. Clin. Oncol. 3:1522–1528.

Ragnhammar, P., Frodin, J.E., Trotta, P.P., and Mellstedt, H. 1994a. Cytotoxicity of white blood cells activated by granulocyte-colony-stimulating factor, granulocyte/macrophage-colony-stimulating factor and macrophage-colony-stimulating factor against tumor cells in the presence of various monoclonal antibodies. Cancer Immunol. Immunother. 39:254–262.

Ragnhammar, P., Friesen, H.J., Frodin, J.E., Lefvert, A.K., Hassan, M., Osterborg, A., and Mellstedt, H. 1994b. Induction of anti-recombinant human granulocyte-macrophage colony-stimulating factor (Escherichia coli-derived) antibodies and clinical effects in non-immunocompromised patients. Blood 84:4078–4087.

Rauschka, H., Farina, C., Sator, P., Gudek, S., Breier, F., and Schmidbauer, M. 2005. Severe anaphylactic reaction to glatiramer acetate with specific IgE. Neurology 64:1481–1482.

Reeves, W.G. and Kelly, U. 1982. Insulin antibodies induced by bovine insulin therapy. Clin. Exp. Immunol. 50:163–170.

Riedl, M.A. and Casillas, A.M. 2003. Adverse drug reactions: types and treatment options. Am. Fam. Physician 68:1781–1790.

Rini, B., Wadhwa, M., Bird, C., Small, E., Gaines-Das, R., and Thorpe, R. 2005. Kinetics of development and characteristics of antibodies induced in cancer patients against yeast expressed rDNA derived granulocyte macrophage colony stimulating factor (GM-CSF). Cytokine 29:56–66.

Rudick, R.A., Simonian, N.A., Alam, J.A., Campion, M., Scaramucci, J.O., Jones, W., Coats, M.E., Goodkin, D.E., Weinstock-Guttman, B., Herndon, R.M., Mass, M.K., Richert, J.R., Salazar, A.M., Munschauer, F.E., Cookfair, D.L., Simon, J.H., and Jacobs, L.B. 1998. Incidence and significance of neutralizing antibodies to interferon beta-1a in multiple sclerosis. Multiple Sclerosis Collaborative Research Group (MSCRG). Neurology 50:1266–1272.

Rudick, R.A., Stuart, W.H., Calabresi, P.A., Confraveux, C., Galetta, S.L., Radue, E.W., Lublin, F.D., Weinstock-Guttman, B., Wynn, D.R., Lynn, F., Panzara, M.A., Sandrock, A.W., and the SENTINEL Investigators, et al. 2006. Natalizumab plus interferon beta-1a for relapsing multiple sclerosis. N. Engl. J. Med. 354:911–923.

Runkel, L. 1998. Structural and functional differences between glycosylated and non-glycosylated forms of human interferon-β (IFN-β). Pharm. Res. 15:641–649.

Salama, H.H., Hong, J., Zang, Y.C., El-Monqui, A., and Zhang, J. 2003. Blocking effects of serum reactive antibodies induced by galtiramer acetate treatment in multiple sclerosis. Brain 126:2638–2647.

Sasaki, H., Bothner, B., Dell, A., and Fukuda, M. 1987. Carbohydrate structure of erythropoietin expressed in Chinese hamster ovary cells by a human erythropoietin cDNA. J. Biol. Chem. 262:12059–12076.

Schellekens, H. and Casadevall, N. 2004. Immunogenicity of recombinant human proteins: causes and consequences. J. Neurol. 251(Suppl. 2):II4–II9.

Schernthaner, G. 1993. Immunogenicity and allergenic potential of animal and human insulins. Diabetes Care 16:155–165.

Skibelli, V., Nissen-Lie, G., and Torjesen, P. 2001. Sugar profiling proves that human serum erythropoietin differs from recombinant human erythropoietin. Blood 98:3626–3634.

Smith, L.F. 1966. Species variation in the amino acid sequence of insulin. Am. J. Med. 40:662–666.

Sorensen, P.S., Deisenhammer, F., Dudac, P., Hohlfeld, R., Myhre, K.M., Palace, J., Polman, C., Pozzilli, C., and Ross, C. for the EFNS Task Force on Anti-IFN-b Antibodies in Multiple Sclerosis. 2005. Guidelines on use of anti-IFN antibody measurements in multiple sclerosis: report of an EFNS Task Force on IFN-b antibodies in multiple sclerosis. Eur. J. Neurol. 12:817–827.

Sorensen, P.S., Koch-Henriksen, N., Ross, C., Clemmesen, K.M., Bendtzen, K., and Danish Multiple Sclerosis Study Group. 2005. Appearance and disappearance of neutralizing antibodies during interferon-beta therapy. Neurology 65:33–39.

Sorensen, P.S., Ross, C., Clemmesen, K.M., Bendtzen, K., Frederiksen, J.L., Jensen, K., Kristensen, O., Petersen, T., Rasmussen, S., Ravnborg, M., Stenager, E., Koch-Henriksen, N., and the Danish Multiple Sclerosis Study Group. 2003. Clinical importance of neutralizing antibodies against interferon beta in patients with relapsing-remitting multiple sclerosis. Lancet 362:1184–1191.

SPECTRIMS, Secondary Progressive Efficacy Clinical Trial of Recombinant Interferon beta-1a in MS Study Group. 2001. Randomized controlled trial of interferon beta-1a in secondary progressive MS: clinical results. Neurology 56:1496–1504.

Spiegel, R.J., Jacobs, S.L., and Treuhaft, M.W. 1989. Anti-interferon antibodies to interferon-alpha 2b: results of comparative assays and clinical perspective. J. Interferon. Res. 9(Suppl. 1):17–24.

Steis, R.G., Smith, J.W., Urba, W.J., Clark, J.W., Itri, L.M., Evans, L.M., Schoenberger, C., and Longo, D.L. 1988. Resistance to recombinant interferon alfa-2a in hairy cell leukemia associated with neutralizing anti-interferon antibodies. N. Engl. J. Med. 318:1409–1413.

Takano, K., Shizume, K., and Hibi, I. 1989. Turner's syndrome: treatment of 203 patients with recombinant human growth hormone for one year. A multicentre study. Acta Endocrinol. 120:559–568.

Tangri, S., Mothè, B.R., Eisenbraun, J., Sidney, J., Southwood, S., Briggs, K., Zinckgraf, J., Bilsel, P., Newman, M., Chesnut, R., LiCalsi, C., and Sette, A. 2005. Rationally engineered therapeutic proteins with reduced immunogenicity. J. Immunol 174:3187–3196.

Teitelbaum, D., Fridkis-Hareli, M., Arnon, S., and Sela, M. 1996. Copolymer 1 inhibits chronic relapsing experimental allergic encephalomyelitis induced by proteolipid protein (PLP) peptides in mice and interferes with PLP-specific T cell responses. J. Neuroimmunol. 64:209–217.

The IFNB Multiple Sclerosis Study Group. 1993. Interferon beta-1b is effective in relapsing-remitting multiple sclerosis. I. Clinical results of a multicenter, randomized, double-blind, placebo-controlled trial. Neurology 43:655–661.

The IFNβ MS Study Group and the University of British Columbia MS/MRI Analysis Group. 1996. Neutralizing antibodies during treatment of multiple sclerosis with interferon beta-1b:experiences during the first three years. Neurology 47:889–894.

The IFNβ Multiple Sclerosis Study Group. 1993. Interferon beta-1b is effective in relapsing-remitting multiple sclerosis. Clinical results of a multicenter randomized, double-blind, placebo-controlled trial. Neurology 43:655–661.

Tomassini, V., Paolillo, A., Russo, P., Giugni, E., Prosperini, L., Gasperini, C., Antonelli, G., Bastianello, S., and Pozzilli, C. 2006. Predictors of long-term clinical response to interferon beta therapy in relapsing multiple sclerosis. J. Neurol. 253:287–293.

Ure, D.R. and Rodriguez, M. 2002. Polyreactive antibodies to glatiramer acetate promote myelin repair in murine model of demyelinating disease. FASEB J. 16:1260–1262.

Vallittu, A.M., Halminen, M., Peltonieni, J., Ilonen, J., Julkunen, I., Salmi, A., Eralinna, J.P., and Finnish Beta-Interferon Study Group. 2002. Neutralizing antibodies reduce M×A protein induction in interferon-beta-1a-treated MS patients. Neurology 58:1786–1790.

Van Haeften, T.W. 1989. Clinical significance of insulin antibodies in insulin-treated patients. Diabetes Care 9:641–648.

Van Hove, J.L.K., Yang, H.W., and Wu, J.Y. 1996. High level production of recombinant human lysosomal acid α-glucosidase in Chinese hamster ovary cells which targets to heart muscle and corrects glycogen accumulation in fibroblast from patients with Pompe disease. Proc. Natl. Acad. Sci. USA 93:65–70.

Velcovsky, H.G., Beringhoff, B., and Federlin, K. 1978. [Immediate type allergy to insulin (author's translation)]. Immunitat und Infektion 6:146–152.

Velcovsky, H.G. and Federlin, K.F. 1982. Insulin-specific IgG and IgE antibody response in type 1 diabetic subjects exclusively treated with human insulin (recombinant DNA). Diabetes Care 5:126–128.

Verhelst, D., Rossert, J., Casadevall, N., Kruger, A., Eckardt, K.U., and Macdougall, I.C. 2004. Treatment of erythropoietin-induced pure red cell aplasia: a retrospective study. Lancet 363:1768–1771.

von Wussow, P., Freund, M., Block, B., Diedrich, H., Poliwoda, H., and Deicher. H. 1987. Clinical significance of anti-IFN-a antibody titres during interferon therapy. Lancet 2:635–636.

Wadhwa, M., Bird, C., Fagerberg, J., Gaines-Das, R., Ragnhammar, P., Mellstedt, H., and Thorpe, R. 1996. Production of neutralizing granulocyte-macrophage colony-stimulating factor (GM-CSF) antibodies in carcinoma patients following GM-CSF combination therapy. Clin. Exp. Immunol. 104:351–358.

Walford, S., Allison, S.P., and Reeves, W.G. 1982. The effect of insulin antibodies on insulin dose and diabetic control. Diabetologia 22:106–110.

Walsh, G. 2004. Second-generation biopharmaceuticals. Eur. J. Pharm. Biopharm. 58:185–196.

Walsh, G. 2005. Biopharmaceuticals: recent approvals and likely directions. Trends Biotechnol. 553–558.

Witters, L.A., Ohman, J.L., Weir, G.C., Raymond, L.W., and Lowell, F.C. 1977. Insulin antibodies in the pathogenesis of insulin allergy and resistance. Am. J. Med. 63:703–709.

Wolinsky, J.S., Narayana, P.A., Johnson, K.B., and Multiple Sclerosis Study Group and the MRI Analysis Center. 2001. United States open-label glatiramer acetate extension trial for relapsing multiple sclerosis: MRI and clinical correlates. Mult. Scler. 7:33–41.

Yamamoto, K., Takamatsu, J., and Saito, H. 2007. Intavenous immunoglobulin therapy for acquired coagulation inhibitors: a critical review. Int. J. Haematol. 85:287–293.

Zinman, L., Ng, E., and Bril, V. 2007. IV immunoglobulin in patients with myasthenia gravis: a randomized controlled trial. Neurology 68:837–841.

3

Assessment of Unwanted Immunogenicity

Meenu Wadhwa and Robin Thorpe

3.1. Introduction

The success of therapeutic biological medicines, in recent years, has been marred with concerns over unwanted immune responses in recipients of these products (Baert et al. 2003, Koren, Zuckerman and Mire-Sluis 2002). Discontinuation of the megakaryocyte growth and differentiation factor (MGDF) development program by the manufacturer after serious problems with immunogenicity occurred was followed by cases of pure red cell aplasia in some renal failure patients treated with erythropoietin. Both of these incidents were associated with antibodies that neutralized endogenously produced protein (Casadevall et al. 2002, Li et al. 2001) and prompted the biotech industry and regulators to seriously consider the issues of unwanted immunogenicity. Needless to say, a rigorous assessment of immunogenicity is an important consideration in development of biotherapeutic products and necessary for ensuring their safety and efficacy.

The field of unwanted immunogenicity has evolved considerably, bringing significant improvements in our understanding and assessment of immunogenicity. However, the prediction of incidence and clinical significance of immunogenicity remains problematical (see Chapters 2, 4, and 5). The current, most practical and commonly used approach for testing unwanted immunogenicity still remains the detection, measurement and characterization of antibodies generated specifically against the product. New platforms for immunogenicity assessment are continually being exploited to enhance the capability of detecting antibodies, if formed, in patients so that the risks associated with immunogenicity can be managed appropriately during product use. To date, no single assay can provide all the necessary information on the immunogenicity profile of a biotherapeutic. Therefore, a well-devised strategy involving a panel of carefully selected and validated assays for detection and measurement of antibodies is required for evaluation of the unwanted immunogenicity of a therapeutic product (Wadhwa et al. 2003, Mire-Sluis et al. 2004). These antibody responses need to be further correlated with parameters such as pharmacokinetics and/or pharmacodynamics and clinical effects for a detailed assessment of the clinical significance of the induced antibodies (Wadhwa et al. 2003).

3.2. Assays for Detection of Antibodies

Different techniques are available for investigating the presence of antibodies generated against therapeutic proteins in biological fluids. Such methods include binding assays based on immunochemical procedures such as solid or liquid phase immunoassays, radioimmunoprecipitation assays (RIPA) and biophysical methods such as surface plasmon resonance (SPR) (Wadhwa et al. 2003, Thorpe and Swanson 2005). These assays determine the presence (or absence) of antibodies based on the ability of the antibodies to recognize the relevant antigenic determinants in the therapeutic protein. They are capable of generating useful quantitative data provided an appropriate format is used (Wadhwa et al. 2003, Thorpe and Swanson 2005). Despite their use for 'screening' purposes, these assays have certain pros and cons, which are briefly described in Table 3.1. These assays cannot assess the ability of the antibodies to neutralize the biological activity of the therapeutic which is an important element in the assessment of immunogenicity. For evaluation of the neutralizing ability, use of an appropriate non-cell-based competitive ligand binding assay or a cell-based neutralization assay is required.

In this chapter, we have briefly considered the different types of binding assays and cell-based neutralization assays (to distinguish whether the induced antibodies are neutralizing or non-neutralizing) with particular focus on the issues associated with neutralizing antibody assays. Although binding assays also present unique challenges (e.g. the nature of the antigen, type of sample, disease of the patient, any concomitant medication, etc.), these have been discussed in considerable detail elsewhere (Wadhwa et al. 2003, Mire-Sluis et al. 2004).

3.3. Binding Assays

3.3.1. Immunoassays

These assays use the specific interaction of antibody with antigen to provide quantitative information about antibody (or antigen) concentration in unknown samples. Binding assays can be conducted using a variety of formats and/or detection systems. These include direct, indirect, bridging and competitive platforms using radioligand, enzymatic, fluorescent, chemi-luminescent or electrochemical luminescence (ECL) detection systems (Mire-Sluis et al. 2004).

In direct assays, serum or plasma samples are incubated with the antigen which has been previously immobilized directly onto well surfaces of microtitre plates and the bound antibody is detected using either a radio-labelled or an enzyme-labelled anti-immunoglobulin reagent of appropriate specificity. The latter assays, termed enzyme-linked immunosorbent assays (ELISAs), are the most prevalent method for identifying antibodies.

ELISAs rely on the ability of the antigen to be immobilized on a plastic surface. In some cases, this immobilization may alter the antigen conformation and mask epitopes such that antibodies specific to that epitope may not be recognized (Brickelmaier et al. 1999). In such instances, it may be necessary to perform an 'indirect assay' by immobilizing a capturing agent (e.g. a monoclonal antibody specific to the antigen or streptavidin to capture antigen

Table 3.1 Methods used for detection of binding antibodies.

Type of assay	Advantages	Disadvantages
Binding assay – direct format (coating with antigen and detecting with labelled anti-Ig)	Rapid	Prone to spurious binding, 'matrix effects'
	Relatively easy to use	May fail to detect rapidly dissociating antibodies
		Antigen immobilization may mask/alter epitopes
	High throughput 'screening assay' for antibody detection	Species specificity and isotype detection determined by secondary reagent
	Good sensitivity	Detection reagent may differ between control and sample
Binding assay – indirect format (coating with a specific mAb or biotin, etc. followed by antigen)	High through-put	Extensive studies required to demonstrate that the coating mAb does not mask or alter epitopes
	Coating with a specific mAb keeps antigen in oriented position	May fail to detect 'low-affinity' antibodies
	Consistent coating and maintains antigen conformation	Species specificity and isotype detection determined by secondary reagent
Electrochemiluminescence – bridging format	High through-put	Requires two antigen conjugates (biotin and TAG)
	Allows use of high concentrations of matrix	Antigen labelling may alter/denature antigen, mask/alter epitopes

(*Continued*)

Table 3.1 (*Continued*).

Type of assay	Advantages	Disadvantages
	Tolerant to interference from antigen	Requires dedicated equipment, reagents are costly and vendor-specific
	Detection signal consistent during life of TAG conjugate	
Radioimmunoprecipitation assay	Moderate to high through-put	Can be isotype specific, may fail to detect rapidly dissociating antibodies
	Good sensitivity	Requires radiolabelled antigen. Radiolabel may alter/denature antigen, decay of radiolabel may affect antigen stability
	Can be specific	
Surface plasmon resonance	Automated	Expensive. Requires dedicated equipment, reagents are vendor specific
	Provides information on the specificity, isotype, relative binding affinity and relative concentration	May require immobilization of the antigen which may alter the conformation of the native protein
	Enables detection of both 'low-affinity' and high-affinity antibodies	Regeneration step may degrade antigen
	Detection reagent not required	Sensitivity often less than binding assay
	Not species specific	

conjugated to biotin), which can then be used to anchor the therapeutic protein (Brickelmaier et al. 1999). Such assays are fairly sensitive but alternative formats may sometimes be necessary.

Adoption of a 'bridging antibody' format in which antibody is captured by immobilized antigen and detected using a labelled antigen can provide ELISAs with high specificity (antigen must be recognized twice by antibody for detection) and acceptable sensitivity. Use of streptavidin-coated plates for capturing biotinylated antigen and a differently labelled antigen may enhance the sensitivity of the assay (Gross et al. 2006). A bridging assay can overcome some of the problems associated with direct assays, namely, (i) non-specific binding and (ii) the requirement of species-specific reagents when using an animal serum as a positive control for the assay. As a result, this assay is often chosen as the basis for a screening method by product manufacturers.

In general, ELISAs are very amenable to automation, are very robust and reliable; it can be highly sensitive and cheap for routine use. Major limitations are that rapidly dissociating or 'low-affinity' antibodies are not readily detected (as they are washed off), and these assays are prone to significant inhibition by the presence of soluble/circulating antigen. Therefore, use of alternative strategies and/or detection systems may need to be considered.

The availability of ECL detection instruments (Bioveris, Meso Scale Discovery. MSD) has enabled the use of ECL reporters which offer distinct benefits over conventional ELISA formats. A greater dynamic assay range, higher tolerance to sample matrix and circulating antigen are some of the features of this technology. Due to the inclusion of wash steps, the platform is often challenged to detect low affinity antibodies. The Bioveris procedure uses a bead-based approach and provides a solution phase assay while the MSD uses carbon electrode plates which are claimed to have a greater binding capacity than polystyrene. Both instruments are suited for automation and yield high throughput and sensitive assays but this is accompanied by an increased cost in reagents.

3.3.2. Radioimmunoprecipitation Assays (RIPA)

RIPAs can be used to assess serum or plasma samples for the presence of antibodies against relevant antigens. In this assay, serum is incubated with a radiolabelled antigen and antigen–antibody complexes precipitated by addition of an appropriate reagent e.g. immobilized protein A or G or antiglobulin. The precipitate is then assessed for antibodies bound to the antigen by counting the radioactivity present in it. The technique is often coupled with antigen analysis in the precipitate to allow assessment of the antigen components bound by antibody e.g. by SDS PAGE/autoradiography. The procedure is very difficult to automate, and sample throughput is normally slow. RIPAs can be prone to artefacts and the radiolabelling process can mask/denature epitopes recognized by antibodies. Additionally, while protein A and protein G are good for precipitating IgG antibodies and hence commonly used in RIPAs, the early immune response that is identified by the presence of IgM antibodies may not be detected due to less efficient binding to IgM class antibodies. However, these assays can, in some cases, be very sensitive and useful for antibody detection as has been shown for antibodies against erythropoietin (Casadevall et al. 2002, Tacey et al. 2003).

3.3.3. Biosensor-based Immunoassays

This method, unlike most other platforms, does not require the use of a labelled secondary reagent. Although several types of biosensors are available, the vast majority of published biosensor data cites the use of BIAcore instruments (e.g. Biacore 2000 and Biacore 3000) for monitoring the immune response in pre-clinical phases and clinical trials. A possible advantage of Biacore 3000 instrument is the compliance with 21 CFR Part 11 requirement which facilitates the use of this instrument under the conditions of regulatory scrutiny e.g. by US FDA.

The Biacore utilizes surface plasmon resonance to detect the increase in mass at the surface of the sensor chip following binding of an antibody to the antigen immobilized on the sensor chip. This increase in mass is directly proportional to the amount of antigen-binding antibody present in the serum sample being tested (Figure 3.1). The ability of the instrument to monitor the interaction in 'real-time' and provide a continuous signal of the events occurring on the sensor surface enables detection of rapidly dissociating or 'low affinity' antibodies if these are present in the sample (Swanson 2005). Detection of low affinity antibodies is important as these antibodies have the potential to neutralize the therapeutic product and may predict the generation of a later mature immune response. Furthermore, characterization of the antibodies in terms of affinities, antibody class and subclass can also be performed easily (Figure 3.2). These attributes have contributed to the increased use and popularity of this platform in studies on immunogenicity (Swanson 2005).

While the assays described are useful for identifying antibody positive samples, it is important to include an additional confirmatory step in the assessment strategy to ensure that the antibodies generated are specifically targeted to the therapeutic. Some of the procedures that can be used are briefly described in the next section.

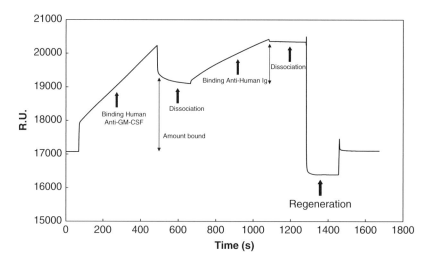

Figure 3.1 A sensorgram showing binding in response units of a human serum to human GM-CSF which has been immobilized (using amine coupling) on the sensor chip. The specificity of this binding has been confirmed using anti-human immunoglobulin as a secondary reagent.

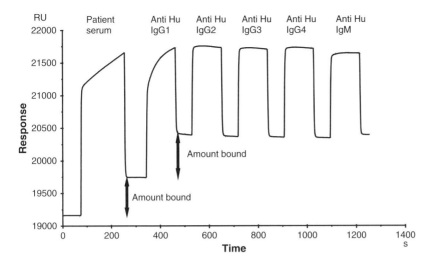

Figure 3.2 Identification of the IgG1 subclass in a sample from a GM-CSF treated patient by evaluation of the binding profile using SPR. For this, serum sample was injected over a GM-CSF immobilized sensor chip followed by sequential injections of specific isotype antibodies.

3.3.4. Confirmation of Antibody Positive Samples

A confirmatory approach can include use of different methods (ELISAs, competitive immunoassays, SPR, etc.), although an assay based on a different scientific principle from that used for the screening assay should usually be considered. It is also necessary to select a confirmatory assay taking into account the limitations and characteristics of the screening assay. In most cases, assay specificity can be demonstrated by addition of free antigen to a serum sample spiked with known amounts of antibody and looking for inhibition of the expected signal. This approach itself can form the basis of a confirmatory assay.

Use of the immunoblotting procedure, which provides information concerning the specificity of the antibodies detected, is valuable as the antibodies may have specificity for other components (e.g. contaminants) in the product and can cause data to be misinterpreted (Wadhwa et al. 1999). For example, very low levels of expression system derived bacterial proteins in rDNA products can cause significant antibody development, whereas the human sequence major protein present (the active principle) may be much less immunogenic (Wadhwa et al. 1999). However, other procedures e.g. analytical radioimmunoprecipitation assays can also be used for specificity studies.

The use of assays described earlier does not obviate the requirement for a functional cell-based neutralization assay. The latter should be incorporated into the strategy for immunogenicity assessment as it has been shown that results from bioassays can often be correlated with the effect of antibodies on clinical response (Wadhwa et al. 1996, 2003, Bertolotto 2004). Some manufacturers conduct neutralization assays at both pre-clinical and clinical level as part of their product development program while others implement these assays at the clinical stage after considering whether the therapeutic is low or high risk.

3.4. Cell-Based Neutralization Assays

The biological activity of a therapeutic is often evaluated using an in vitro cell-based assay based on a functional aspect of the protein or mechanism of action. These assays can be categorized into those that detect signalling responses soon after protein–receptor interaction has occurred (early stage) or those that provide a measurable readout after culmination of a cellular response (late stage). Since these assays assess the cellular response in vitro to a protein, they constitute an ideal and appropriate biological approach for development of a cell-based neutralization assay. It should be realized that different types of bioassay procedures can be used as the basis of a neutralization assay for a biological (Mckay et al. 2005).

A cell-based neutralization assay can be defined as an in vitro assay utilizing cells that interact with or respond to the therapeutic either directly or indirectly in a measurable manner in the presence of test sample for the detection of anti-product neutralizing antibodies (Gupta et al. 2007). The detection of neutralizing antibodies is based on the principle that any sample containing an antibody (of a neutralizing nature) would reduce or abolish the biological activity induced by a known concentration of the therapeutic in a cell-based assay.

Most biological therapeutics can be broadly categorized into agonists or antagonists based on their desired effect in vivo. While agonists (e.g. cytokines, growth factors, hormones, agonistic monoclonal antibodies) induce a response by directly binding to receptors on the target cell surface, therapeutics with antagonistic properties (e.g. soluble receptors, antagonistic Mabs) act by blocking the binding of a ligand to the target receptor expressed on the cell surface. As a result, assay formats and designs of neutralizing antibody assays can vary depending on the biological and the type of assay being used.

3.4.1. Appropriateness of Assay Format and Design

The function-based activity of therapeutic proteins contributes to the unique assay design and critical assay components required for the neutralization assay of these proteins. The simplest assay format is that commonly used for therapeutic proteins with agonistic properties. In these assays, also termed direct neutralizing antibody assays, serial dilutions of the samples (containing antibodies) are prepared in the plates and a constant amount of biological (antigen) is then added to the wells. The mixture is incubated (allowing antigen–antibody interaction), the cells added and the assay continued. Neutralization is assessed by measuring the degree of inhibition of the response induced by the test sample. Therefore, critical assay components include (a) a cell-line responsive to the therapeutic protein, (b) the therapeutic protein, (c) a positive control neutralizing Ab (Nab) and (d) test sample that represents the matrix of the biological samples that require testing. In this assay, there is potential for interactions between the antibody sample and the therapeutic protein, the sample and the cell-line (matrix effects) and also the biological and the cell-line.

For an antibody therapeutic (e.g. anti-cytokine monoclonal antibody), however, the situation is more complex and the interaction of the cytokine with the monoclonal therapeutic also needs to be considered. As assay designs increase in complexity, it is difficult to incorporate all necessary controls and so it is best to adopt a simple assay design if possible. In these assays known as indirect neutralizing antibody assays, serial dilutions of the serum samples are incubated with a mixture containing constant amounts of ligand and therapeutic, the cells added and the assay continued. As for direct assays, neutralization is assessed by measuring the degree of inhibition of the response induced by the test sample. The critical components of this type of neutralization assay for an antagonist include (a) a cell-line that responds to the ligand that is blocked by the therapeutic protein, (b) ligand, (c) therapeutic protein, (d) positive control Nab and (e) test sample.

Irrespective of the format to be used, it is necessary to define the aim of the assay at the outset, for example, a screening assay for providing a positive or negative signal or a quantitative assay. Approaches for assay validation will differ depending on the purpose and the assay design used. A two-tiered approach which involves an initial screening for identification of positive samples in a neutralization assay followed by a quantitative assay for assessment of neutralization potency is preferable as opposed to the screening approach alone. Quantitative procedures are generally more tedious and labour intensive. However, these assays provide data which relates to neutralization of a specific amount of antigen and yield very useful and informative data for comparative purposes. It should be realized that use of properly designed assays to assure confidence that the neutralizing activity can be attributed to specific antibodies is necessary to allow proper interpretation of results obtained from these assays.

While selecting an assay format, consideration should be given to the nature of the product (e.g. a therapeutic protein or a monoclonal antibody), potential interference in the assay from co-medications, dosing regimen and/or disease-specific issues (e.g. presence of rheumatoid factors). Other considerations include the ability to detect antibodies with desired specificities (IgM, IgG subclasses, etc.) and susceptibility to assay interference from circulating product. The potential for assay interference from the biological itself, particularly with monoclonal antibody therapeutics which have longer half-lives than other recombinant proteins, is significant and strategies to minimize this problem are needed (Patton et al. 2005, Lofgren et al. 2006).

3.4.2. Development and Design of a Neutralizing Antibody Assay

Several issues need to be considered during development and design of a neutralizing antibody assay. These include the selection of an appropriate cell-line and end-point, assay controls and the complex interactions between the critical assay components of the assay.

3.4.2.1. Selection of a Cell-line

Often a potency assay for a biological can be used as the basis of a neutralization assay. For example, a neutralization assay for IFN-β can be a modification of the antiviral assays used for potency assessment for interferon. An advantage of choosing a cell-line that is being used for potency assays is that optimization of cell-line maintenance and culture conditions has already been performed. However, these assays need refining for their use as the basis of a neutralization assay as they may not be appropriate or have adequate sensitivity. Therefore, the adaptability of the potency assay to the presence of test sample (appropriate species serum) and response to the therapeutic to yield a sufficiently sensitive assay requires validation. Ideally, the cell-line should yield a functional end-point upon treatment with the therapeutic protein, the assay be simple to perform and the biological end-point tolerant to test sample matrix and perform adequately over a range of concentrations of the protein. With this purpose in mind, an evaluation of cell-lines for use in neutralization assays may be required (Figure 3.3). If multiple cell-lines are available, the responsiveness of the cell-lines to the therapeutic biological and to a dilution series of the positive control antibody can be determined (Figure 3.3). Specificity should also be considered during the selection of the cell-line. Alternative bioassays using different cell-lines e.g. transfected with target receptors may also be used. Cell-lines (natural, engineered) should be well characterized to ensure responsiveness and result in selection of a stable, highly sensitive, suitable assay with good discrimination between signal to noise in the assay matrix. If possible, the selected line (if several are available to choose from) should be able to tolerate serum from different species for use in product development program.

3.4.2.2. Selection of Assay End-point

As stated earlier, assay end-points can utilize early or late biological responses following exposure of the cells to the therapeutic. Examples of assay end-points using early responses include assessment of phosphorylation of intra-cellular substrates or internalization of the therapeutic protein while those

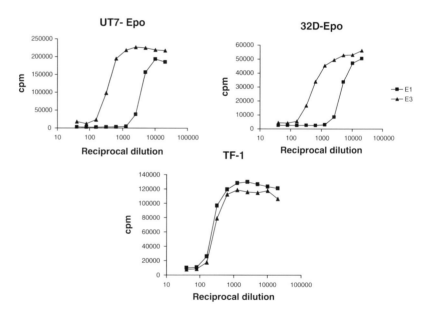

Figure 3.3 The differential sensitivity of three erythropoietin (Epo) responsive cell-lines to inhibition of the biological activity of Epo by Epo antibodies in two different sera (E1, E3) from animals hyperimmunized with Epo is demonstrated. In these assays, Epo was incubated at a concentration of 0.1 IU (for UT-7 and 32-D cells) or 5 IU (for TF-1 cells) with dilutions of the sera at room temperature for 45 min prior to addition of cells. The plates were then incubated for a further 44 h to conduct a direct NAb assay that utilized cell proliferation as the assay end-point. To assess specificity of the antibodies, the serum samples were also titrated in the presence of GM-CSF (1.0 IU); use of this approach did not cause any inhibition (data not shown).

focused on late responses assess parameters such as induction or secretion of cellular proteins, cell proliferation, cell death, etc. Several types of end-points that can be used as the basis of neutralization assays are given in Table 3.2.

3.4.2.3. Selection of Concentration of the Biological

After the cell-line and end-point is selected, the next step is to optimize the assay and select a concentration of the biological that can be routinely used in the assay. In a bioassay, a typical standard curve for the biological consists of a dose range (5–10 points) with a minimum of 4 concentrations in the linear portion of the curve. It is important to evaluate this dose-response curve and select a dose capable of yielding 70–80% of the maximal response with good discrimination between signal to noise in the assay matrix for use in a neutralization assay. The selected concentration should provide a reliable and robust response and should be adequately sensitive to detect clinically relevant neutralizing antibodies. It should be noted that use of a very high dose of the biological will jeopardize the detection of neutralizing antibodies. In contrast, a low dose will not allow valid discrimination between signal and background.

3.4.2.4. Selection of Sample Matrix

It is well established that the sample matrix can influence the responsiveness of cells in a bioassay. It is therefore important to determine the dilution of sample matrix that will have a minimal effect on the cellular response. Since sera are heterogeneous in their content of interfering substances, multiple individual sera are needed for defining the assay matrix. A neutralization assay should be capable of distinguishing antibody from other interfering factors e.g. soluble receptors, binding proteins, complement components, etc. which may confound results. Inclusion of an approach for establishing specificity is useful in determining the presence of interfering substances.

3.4.2.5. Inclusion of Specificity Evaluation

A specificity evaluation is useful for assurance that the inhibitory response is due to presence of specific neutralizing antibodies rather than matrix effects. As this strategy may be useful for discrimination of specific response from interfering factors, it should be developed and implemented simultaneously with the neutralization antibody assay. A specificity assay can be developed using different approaches. For example, evaluation of neutralization activity in the samples can be determined both in the absence (allows determination of interference/background inhibition) and presence of the therapeutic protein or in the presence of the therapeutic protein and another antigen or stimulus (at a concentration capable of inducing a similar cellular response to that of the therapeutic protein in the cell-line used for assay) in the assays. An example of this approach has been described previously in the neutralization assay for detection of Epo antibodies (Wei et al. 2004). Alternatively, the samples can be pre-treated with an absorbing resin e.g. protein G which binds immunoglobulin molecules resulting in immunodepletion (or removal of the antibody molecules) and both the pre- and post-treatment samples assessed for neutralization activity (Menetrier-Caux et al. 1996).

Table 3.2 Types of assays in current use for detection of neutralizing antibodies.

Biological	Therapeutic class	End-point measured	Cells/cell-line used	Format /readout
GM-CSF	Cytokine	Proliferation	TF-1	MTS, Alamar Blue, 3H-thy
IFN-β	Cytokine	Anti-viral Anti-proliferative Reporter gene expression	A549, 2D9 Daudi A549 93D7	CPE/vital dye MTS, Alamar Blue, 3H-thy Luciferase
Epo	Hormone	Colony formation Proliferation	Bone marrow UT-7 Epo, 32DEpoR+	Counting colonies 3H-thy
Anti-TNF TNF antagonist	MoAb, Receptor Ig-fusion	Cytotoxicity	KD4, A375	Cytotoxic effect / MTS
Anti-TGF-β	MoAb	Anti-proliferative	MvLu, TF-1	MTS, Alamar Blue, 3H-thy
CD40 receptor Agonist	MoAb	Receptor upregulation	Daudi	Fluorescence activated cell sorting

3.5. Inclusion of Assay Controls for All Antibody Detection Assays

Inclusion of assay controls, and in particular, positive and negative control antibodies, is vital for monitoring assay performance and for valid interpretation of results. However, initially during product and assay development, an antibody positive human sample is seldom available and so positive controls are generally antisera from hyperimmunized animals. These antisera can be affinity purified and spiked into a suitable matrix for use as a control in the assay. If polyclonal antibodies are not available, monoclonal antibodies can be used as a positive control, either individually or as a cocktail (preferable to individual antibody). As with any assay reagent, such antibodies need to be well characterized i.e. positive control antibody should demonstrate effective binding in binding assays. The positive control antibody for neutralization assays must neutralize the biological activity and show a dose-dependent inhibitory profile which is specific for the therapeutic in the selected assay matrix. For a negative control, an irrelevant antibody from the same animal species which has been affinity purified in the same way as the positive control antibody can be used. Sera from normal healthy individuals or from same disease state can also be used as negative controls in assays but these may contain pre-existing antibodies and other interfering substances which need to be considered (Wadhwa et al. 2003, Mire-Sluis et al. 2004). However, in immunogenicity studies where sera from patients enrolled in clinical trials is being tested for the presence of antibodies, serum samples collected from patients prior to initiation of therapy serve as ideal negative controls (Wadhwa et al. 2003).

3.6. Practicality of the Assay

Easy, fast and robust assays with good reproducibility are generally preferable in comparison with tedious, cumbersome and time-consuming procedures.

3.7. Interpretation and Expression of Results

The nature of results obtained from assays will depend on the assay design used for the assay e.g. a yes/no screening assay or a quantitative assay. Prior to evaluation of samples in antibody assays, it is necessary to clearly define the criteria for interpretation of results i.e. antibody-positive or antibody-negative by determining the 'cut-off' values for each assay and devising appropriate methods (titre value, etc.) for expression of results. In most studies, the antibody content is often expressed as a 'titre' value. However, the 'titre' value which is dependent on a variety of factors is not consistently defined and can often vary between assays and particularly between laboratories.

For neutralization assays, a recommended approach for expressing data is to report results as the 'amount of serum required to neutralize the biological activity induced by a constant amount of the antigen' (Wadhwa et al. 1996). For example, for GM-CSF, the volume of serum required to neutralize the activity of 10 IU of cytokine can be calculated using serum ED50 responses obtained by fitting common asymptotes and slope for all sera analyzed. This approach can also be used to analyze responses to different GM-CSF preparations/products and can be applied to other biologicals.

In some instances, however, it may be necessary to use an antibody standard or reference preparation for expressing the levels of neutralizing antibodies in the test samples relative to the amounts of the neutralizing antibodies in the reference antibody preparation. It may also be possible to express antibody levels using arbitrary units providing that the unitage has been well defined for the reference material. Although this approach is not ideal (the heterogeneous nature of polyclonal antibodies is particularly problematical for this), the use of this strategy may provide relatively precise estimates of antibody levels in the test samples and can reduce variability. This situation is most likely to occur when a number of sequential samples from the same animal or patient are available and it is difficult to include all samples from all patients in the same assays for establishing a valid comparison of antibody levels between different samples/patients.

3.8. Guidance on Optimization, Validation and Standardization of Assays

As a consequence of the challenges involved in antibody assays, there has been considerable progress made by members of the American Association of Pharmaceutical Sciences (AAPS) in formulating recommendations for optimization and development of antibody assays (Mire-Sluis et al. 2004, Gupta et al. 2007). However, it is also necessary to develop validation and standardization criteria that would be appropriate for the antibody assays being developed in various laboratories. It should be realized that the parameters (requiring validation) are unique to each method and its intended use and therefore must be carefully determined on a case-by-case basis.

The EMEA CHMP has recently released draft guidance on immunogenicity assessment of biotechnology-derived therapeutic proteins and recommends using validated antibody assays, characterization of the observed immune response, as well as evaluation of the correlation between antibodies, pharmacokinetics/pharmacodynamics and efficacy and safety. (CHMP, 2007) It also states that the role of immunogenicity in events related to adverse events such as infusion reactions and loss of efficacy should be considered, a view that is also reflected in The International Conference on Harmonization Guideline S6 (1997). Both guidelines recommend the determination of incidence and titre of antibody responses to the biotherapeutic prior to and post-treatment but the EMEA guideline emphasizes post-marketing programs for monitoring of antibodies in recipients and provides general guidance on antibody assays, validation and standardization issues and strategies to be adopted when conducting immunogenicity studies.

3.9. Study Strategy

Careful prospective planning of studies is critical if valid conclusions concerning unwanted immunogenicity are to be derived. When designing immunogenicity studies, it is important to devise a strategy which includes a panel of antibody detection and characterization assays, assays for evaluation of clinical consequences of induced antibodies (if any) and relevant clinical data such that correlations of antibody induction with clinical effects can be made. A simple strategy that can be used for detection of antibodies has previously been described (Wadhwa and Thorpe 2006). It is important to consider identification of appropriate sampling points (in some cases sequential) and include baseline samples (for collection before treatment initiation). The length of such studies will depend on the product, disease and patient group, duration of therapy and desired clinical response.

Studies to date have shown that antibodies may be induced after treatment with several doses of product and that non-neutralizing antibodies usually precede the production of neutralizing responses (Wadhwa et al. 1996, 1999, Ullenhag et al. 2001). In some cases, only a small percentage of patients produce antibodies and only a subpopulation of them develop neutralizing antibodies (Wadhwa et al. 1996, 1999, Ullenhag et al. 2001) which in some instances may be transient. This implies that long-term studies involving analysis of samples from a large number of treated patients may be necessary for a complete assessment of the immunogenicity profile (and its consequences) of a therapeutic protein (Hemmer et al. 2005). For a different disease indication, separate studies in the target population will need to be conducted.

Assessment of relative immunogenicity poses additional problems. Conclusions on the immunogenicity of different products cannot be made by comparing results from published studies because of differences in treatment regimens, sampling protocols and antibody assays used. Data can only be truly comparative if the products have been evaluated in the same trials using the same clinical protocols (i.e. routes of administration and treatment schedules), same sampling procedures and time points (including pre-treatment controls), storage conditions and the antibodies assessed using the same procedures. It is also important to compare and include patients with same clinical abnormalities and same disease stage for both arms of the study. Therefore, clinical studies have to be designed specifically for evaluation of relative immunogenicity if valid conclusions are to be derived, for example, for a biosimilar product relative to the reference (innovator) product. Such data can then be correlated with clinical data on safety and response to the protein therapeutics used.

3.10. Conclusions

Assessment of unwanted immunogenicity of a biological therapeutic is a significant task and achieving valid, useful results involves more than simply ensuring that appropriate tests are performed. Thus, the assays used for assessment of immunogenicity of a biological product (and the criteria used for distinguishing positive from negative or levels of magnitude) have to be carefully selected and validated with due consideration given to assay design, specificity, inclusion of appropriate controls and assay performance. There is no single available method that can provide full information on detection and characterization of antibodies, and therefore implementation of a strategy which incorporates use of a panel of various methods for the assessment of samples is essential. The use of this approach along with data from evaluation of clinical responses will provide a detailed understanding of the profile and significance of antibody responses generated against a therapeutic product.

Acknowledgements. We would like to thank Chris Bird, Isabelle Cludts and Paula Dilger for providing the data for the figures used in this manuscript.

References

Baert, F., Noman, M., Vermiere, S., Assche, G. V., D'Haens, G., Carbonez, A., and Rutgeerts, P. 2003. Influence of immunogenicity on the long-term efficacy of infliximab in Crohn's disease. N. Engl. J. Med. 348:601–608.

Bertolotto, A. 2004. Neutralizing antibodies to interferon beta: implications for the management of multiple sclerosis. Curr. Opin. Neurol. 17:241–246.

Brickelmaier, M., Hochman, P. S., Baciu, R., Chao, B., Cuervo, J. H., and Whitty, A. 1999. ELISA methods for the analysis of antibody responses induced in multiple sclerosis patients treated with recombinant interferon-beta. J. Immunol. Meth. 227:121–135.

Casadevall, N., Nataf, J., Viron, B., Kolta, A., Kiladjian, J. J., Martin-Dupont, P., Michaud, P., Papo, T., Ugo, V., Teyssandier, I., Varet, B., and Mayeux, P. 2002. Pure red cell aplasia and anti-erythropoietin antibodies against human erythropoietin in patients treated with recombinant erythropoietin. N. Engl. J. Med. 346:469–475.

CHMP (Committee for medicinal products for human use). 2007. Guideline on Immunogenicity assessment of biotechnology-derived therapeutic proteins. EMEA/CHMP/BMWP/14327/2006 – draft version released for consultation.

Gross, J., Moller, R., Henke, W., and Hoesel, W. 2006. Detection of anti-EPO antibodies in human sera by a bridging ELISA is much more sensitive when coating biotinylated rhEPO to streptavidin rather than using direct coating of rhEPO. J. Immunol. Meth. 313:176–182.

Gupta, S., Indelicato, S. R., Jethwa, V., Kawabata, T., Marian Kelley, M., Mire-Sluis, A. R., Richards, S. M., Rup, B., Shores, E., Swanson, S. J., and Wakshull E. 2007. Recommendations for the design, optimization, and qualification of cell-based assays used for the detection of neutralizing antibody responses elicited to biological therapeutics. J. Immunol. Meth. 321:1–18.

Hemmer, B., Stuve, O., Kieseier, B., Schellekens, H., and Hartung, H. P. 2005. Immune response to immunotherapy: the role of neutralising antibodies to interferon beta in the treatment of multiple sclerosis. Lancet Neurol. 4:403–412.

International Conference on Harmonization. 1997. Guidance for Industry. S6 Preclinical Safety Evaluation of Biotechnology-Derived Pharmaceuticals. Available at (http://www.fda.gov/cder/guidance/1859fnl.pdf).

Koren, E., Zuckerman, L. A., and Mire-Sluis, A. R. 2002. Immune responses to therapeutic proteins in humans – clinical significance, assessment and prediction. Curr. Pharm. Biotechnol. 3:349–360.

Li, J., Yang, C., Xia, Y., Bertino, A., Glaspy, J., Roberts, M., and Kuter, D. J. 2001. Thrombocytopenia caused by the development of antibodies to thrombopoietin. Blood 98:3241–3248.

Lofgren, J. A., Wala, I., Koren, E., Swanson, S. J., and Jing, S. 2006. Detection of neutralizing anti-therapeutic protein antibodies in serum or plasma samples containing high levels of the therapeutic protein. J. Immunol. Meth. 308:101–108.

Menetrier-Caux, C., Briere, F., Jouvenne, P., Peyron, E., Peyron, F., Banchereau, J. 1996. Identification of human IgG autoantibodies specific for IL-10. Clin. Exp. Immunol. 104:173–179.

McKay, F., Schibeci, S., Heard, R., Stewart, G., and Booth, D. 2005. Analysis of neutralizing antibodies to therapeutic interferon-beta in multiple sclerosis patients: A comparison of three methods in a large Australasian cohort. J. Immunol. Meth. 310:20–29.

Mire-Sluis, A. R., Barrett, Y. C., Devanarayan, V., Koren E., Liu, H., Maia, M., Parish, T., Scott, G., Shankar, G., Shores, E., Swanson, S. J., Taniguchi, G., Wierda, D., and Zuckerman, L. A. 2004. Recommendations for the design and optimization of immunoassays used in the detection of host antibodies against biotechnology products. J. Immunol. Meth. 289:1–16.

Patton, A., Mullenix, M. C., Swanson, S. J., Koren, E. 2005. An acid dissociation bridging ELISA for detection of antibodies directed against therapeutic proteins in the presence of antigen. J. Immunol. Meth. 304:189–195.

Swanson, S. J. 2005. Characterization of an immune response. Dev. Biol. 122:95–101.

Tacey, R., Greway, A., Smiell, J., Power, D., Kromminga, A., Daha, M., Casadevall, N., and Kelley, M. 2003. The detection of anti-erythropoietin antibodies in human serum and plasma: Part I. Validation of the protocol for a radioimmuno-precipitation assay. J. Immunol. Meth. 283:317–329.

Thorpe, R., and Swanson, S. J. 2005. Current methods for detecting antibodies against Erythropoietin and other recombinant proteins. Clin. Diag. Lab. Immunol. 12:28–39.

Ullenhag, G., Bird, C., Ragnhammar, P., Frodin, J. E., Strigard, K., Osterborg, A., Thorpe, R. Mellstedt, H., and Wadhwa, M. 2001. Incidence of GM-CSF antibodies in cancer patients receiving low dose GM-CSF as an adjuvant. Clin. Immunol. 99:65–74.

Wadhwa, M., Bird, C., Fagerberg, J., Gaines-Das, R., Ragnhammar, P., Mellstedt, H., and Thorpe, R. 1996. Production of neutralizing GM-CSF antibodies in carcinoma patients following GM-CSF combination therapy. Clin. Exp. Immunol. 104:351–358.

Wadhwa, M., Skog, A.-L. H., Bird, C., Ragnhammar, P., Lilljefors, M., Gaines-Das, R., Mellstedt, H., and Thorpe, R. 1999. Immunogenicity of Granulocyte-Macrophage Colony Stimulating Factor (GM-CSF) products in patients undergoing combination therapy with GM-CSF. Clin. Can. Res. 5:1353–1361.

Wadhwa, M., Bird, C., Dilger, P., Gaines-Das, R., and Thorpe, R. 2003. Strategies for detection, measurement and characterization of unwanted antibodies induced by therapeutic biologicals. J. Immunol. Meth. 278:1–17.

Wadhwa, M., and Thorpe, R. 2006 Strategies and assays for the assessment of unwanted immunogenic. J. Immunotoxicology 3:115–121.

Wei, X., Swanson, S. J., and Gupta, S. 2004. Development and validation of a cell-based bioassay for the detection of neutralizing antibodies against recombinant human erythropoietin in clinical studies. J. Immunol. Meth. 293:115–126.

Models for Prediction of Immunogenicity

Erwin L. Roggen

4.1. Introduction

4.1.1. Mechanisms of Immunogenicity

Any foreign substance will trigger the highly organised and regulated innate and adaptive networks of cells, and soluble (e.g. antibodies, cytokines) and membrane-associated molecules (e.g. receptors, co-stimulatory factors) that have developed throughout evolution to protect man against phylogenetic distant organisms, and their products. These mechanisms have been extensively reviewed elsewhere (Chapter 1). Therefore, the following paragraphs will only highlight those components of the immune system with relevance to this chapter.

4.1.1.1. The Innate Response

The innate immune system constitutes the primary line of defense. Although non-specific and not conferring long-lasting immunity, a good understanding of these defences is imperative for a proper description of protein immunogenicity as several components of the innate response link innate and adaptive immune networks.

There is growing evidence suggesting that epithelial cells (EC) in the skin and mucosal linings play a critical role in homeostasis and host defence reactions (McKenzie and Sauder 1990, Lambrecht and Hammad 2003a). Trauma of these linings will induce inflammation, a process characterised by release, among others, of eicosanoids (e.g. prostaglandins and leukotrienes) and a variety of cytokines (e.g. interleukin (IL)-1, IL-6, IL-8) by the affected cells, recruitment of innate leukocytes, removal of the offending compound and healing of any damaged tissue (Hietbrink et al. 2006).

Complement is the major humoral component of the innate immune response. In humans, this response is activated by the binding of complement proteins to carbohydrate structures on micro-organisms or by complement binding to antibodies that have attached to such micro-organisms. The result of these interactions is a rapid killing response, resulting in the production of peptides that, among others, attract immune cells (Rus, Cudrici and Niculescu 2005). The relevance of complement-mediated processes for protein immunogenicity is demonstrated by the occurrence of adverse complement-mediated cell lysis induced by specific or cross-reacting IgM and IgG antibody recognising membrane-associated self-antigen or foreign protein adsorbed to the cell surface (Silverstein 1989).

The innate leukocytes include phagocytic cells, among others macrophages, neutrophils and dendritic cells (DC). During the acute phase of inflammation, circulating neutrophils migrate towards the site of inflammation and are usually the first cells to arrive at the affected tissue. Upon arrival, these cells will release a number of factors which further enhance epithelial IL-1 and IL-8 production, resulting in the excretion of the chemokine CCL20 known to attract immature DC (Roggen et al. 2006). Macrophages are versatile cells that reside within tissues and express a phenotype that is generated by the tissue micro-environment (e.g. by EC, fibroblasts and endothelial cells) (Striz et al. 2001). They produce a wide array of enzymes, complement proteins and regulatory factors (e.g. IL-1), and they have the capability to function as antigen-presenting cells. Thus, macrophages determine the outcome of immune responses by instructing both the innate and the adaptive immune systems. Evidence has been presented showing that macrophages with disregulated phenotype are involved in the induction of auto-immunity and allergic sensitisation (Thepen, Kraal and Holt 1996, Stoy 2001, Chen et al. 2003). DC are phagocytes in tissues that are in contact with the external environment (e.g. skin and mucosal linings). Like macrophages, DC link the innate and adaptive immune systems through their antigen-presenting activity and are recognised to play a role in adverse immune responses (Guermonprez et al. 2002, Lambrecht and Hammad 2003b).

4.1.1.2. The Adaptive Response

The adaptive immune response is characterised by the generation of responses that are tailored to specific antigens. The ability to mount these tailored responses is maintained in the body by memory cells, which are promptly reactivated upon a subsequent challenge.

T-cells and B-cells are the major types of effector cells of the adaptive immune system. Since these cells are to protect the host against *foreign* antigens, efficient discrimation of self- and non-self-antigens and removal of the non-self-antigens only are essential for the survival of the host. To make this possible, the majority of T- and B-cells responding to self-proteins are eliminated very early in life from the thymus and bone marrow, respectively, by clonal deletion, receptor editing and functional silencing (central tolerance). The cells escaping from this elimination process into the periphery are controlled during life by other cells such as DC and regulatory $CD^{25+}CD^{4+}$ T-cells (peripheral tolerance) (Sakaguchi et al. 2001, Miller 2005). T-cell tolerance is believed to be the most important mechanism for maintaining B-cell tolerance. There is evidence though suggesting that B-cells can be subjected to positive selection generated and maintained on the basis of their auto-reactivity (Chan, Madaio and Shlomchik 1999, Hayakawa et al. 1999, Zouali 2001). In addition, antigen dose and antigen patterns seem to play an important role in regulating B-cell responsiveness to self-antigens in a T-cell-independent fashion (Bachmann and Zinkernagel 1997).

Among the known subtypes of T-cells, helper T-cells (T_h-cells) are considered to be the most relevant T-cells for protein immunogenicity. These cells recognise linear peptide segments of the protein (T-cell epitopes), resulting from antigen processing by, e.g., macrophages, DC and B-cells, in a class II major histocompatibility complex (MHC) context. Two subsets of T_h-cells have been discriminated based on cytokine production and effector functions. Overall, T_h1-cells produce IL-2, IL-12, interferon (IFN)-γ and tumour necrosis factor (TNF)-β, induce synthesis of antibody that activates complement and activate host defenses mediated by phagocytosis. In contrast, T_h2-cells produce IL-4, IL-5, IL-6, IL-9, IL-10 and IL-13 and are principally responsible for host responses not involving phagocytosis. They greatly facilitate IgE, IgG4 and IgG1 responses, and mucosal immunity by promoting mast cell and eosinophil differentiation, and by facilitating IgA synthesis (Mosmann and Coffman 1989, Kelso 1995).

It is generally recognised that DC exert their key role in protective immunity, as well as adverse immune responses, by their capacity to effectively activate helper T-cells (Guermonprez et al. 2002, Lambrecht and Hammad 2003b). Properly activated mature DC are very efficient at activating, e.g., T_h1- or T_h2-cells, while immature DC stimulation results in anergic T-cells, which in turn act as regulatory T (T_{reg})-cells suppressing the response of other T-cells (Bancherau et al. 2000, Cumberbatch et al. 2005). The mechanisms by which DC shape the differentiation pathway of a naïve T-cell into T_h1- or T_h2-cells are not completely understood. Apparently, the same T-cell epitopes are capable of inducing either T_h1- or T_h2-type responses. Factors that have been reported to affect DC-mediated T_h-cell differentiation include (1) the tissue micro-environment (e.g. cytokines, chemokines and adhesion molecules) established by, e.g., EC, fibroblasts and endothelial cells, (2) the nature of the signals DC provide at the time of antigen presentation (e.g. cytokines, chemokines, soluble receptors, co-stimulatory factors and adhesion molecules), as well as by (3) the activation status of the T-cells (Constant and Bottomly 1997, Kimber et al. 2000, Lanzavecchia and Salusto 2001, Roggen et al. 2006).

B-cells use specific surface antibodies that bind to specific areas on a foreign antigen (B-cell epitopes). In contrast to T-cell epitopes, B-cell epitopes can be linear or conformational (i.e. involving amino acids and amino acid stretches in the structural context of the protein). The antigen–antibody complex is taken up by the cells, and the antigen is processed into T-cell epitopes which are presented in a class II MHC context. Subsequently, B-cells are activated through specific T_h-cell-derived cytokines to divide and secrete antibody into circulation (Kehry and Hodgkin 1994).

4.1.2. Immunogenicity of Therapeutic Proteins

The clinical implications of protein immunogenicity are severe and include (1) impairment of treatment by reduction of the efficacy of the therapeutic protein, (2) auto-immunity if the exogenous drug triggers antibodies recognised by the patient's own endogenous protein, (3) an allergic or anaphylactic response (type 1 hypersensitivity), (4) adverse complement-mediated cell lysis (type 2 hypersensitivity) and (5) inflammation (type 3 hypersensitivity) (Chapter 2).

To minimise the risk, protein drugs of non-human origin were gradually replaced by native and recombinant human proteins, the general idea behind this strategy being that the immunologic response to these proteins, if any at all, would be down-regulated by the mechanisms involved in development and maintenance of central and peripheral tolerance to self-proteins. Unfortunately, antibody production in humans against human proteins has been extensively documented for growth factors, receptors, antagonists, cytokines and hormones (Oberget al. 1989, Peces et al. 1996, Zang et al. 2000, Schellekens 2002). Some of these products such as IFN-β and IL-2, IL-3-granulocyte macrophage colony stimulating factor (GM-CSF) fusion protein PIXY321, GM-CSF and TNF receptor fusion protein were shown to induce antibodies in 88–95% of patients treated with these products (Schellekens 2002).

In general, the frequency and levels of these antibodies vary considerably. This variation seems to be influenced by patient-related, treatment-related and drug-related factors (Table 4.1). With respect to human proteins, the structural and functional integrity of the therapeutic protein seems to be the key issue. There is ample evidence showing that modifications of the protein structure and function, e.g., by glutaraldehyde, DMSO, urea or salt treatment, formulation, glycosylation (among others) or protein engineering may induce structural changes, which have a significant but indirect (i.e. unrelated to changes in the amino acid sequence of T- and B-cell epitopes) impact on antibody-binding and immunogenicity (Janssen, Wauben and Tomassen 1996, Andersson et al. 2001, Hermeling et al. 2004, Wu, Wang and Lu 2004). The availability of well-established assays addressing structural impairment and aggregate formation of the target protein is therefore a prerequisite for controlling the immunogenicity of human therapeutic proteins in humans.

4.2. Testing the Immunogenicity of Therapeutic Proteins Using Animals

It is common practice to assess the immunogenicity of therapeutic proteins in a variety of animal species. For the sake of convenience, the read-out most frequently used is the antibody response launched in these animals upon exposure to the protein, a lack of antibody response being an indication for low probability and a strong antibody response for a high probability of immunogenicity (Wierda, Smith and Zwickl 2001). Analysis of the T-cell repertoire stimulated by the protein is performed, but primarily to acquire an understanding of the host responses related to auto-immunity and sensitisation, and for analysis of the mechanisms governing specificity, induction and expansion of T-cells during the immune response.

Involvement of several experimental animal models in the assessment of the immunogenicity of therapeutic proteins for human usage is dictated by the concern that animal species, as well as different strains of the same species, may differ in antigen presentation, and T- and B-cell epitope recognition. Thus, B- and T-cell epitopes that are recognised in mice, for example, may not be recognised in humans and vice versa (Milich and Leroux-Roels 2003). Consequently, antibodies of non-human origin may or may not be predictive for adverse effects in humans.

Animal testing of therapeutic human proteins should be considered irrelevant, as animals will react with a vigorous immune response to this neo-protein in contrast to humans. In an effort to come around this issue, protocols have been developed for testing the immunogenicity of human therapeutic proteins in transgenic mice with immune tolerance to the native human protein

Table 4.1 Factors influencing the immunogenicity of proteins.

Patient-related factors

Genetic background	– Genetic polymorphism	– Uncommon T- and B-cell epitope recognition – Altered antigen processing – Hyper-reactivity of the immune system – Functional impairment of innate or adaptive immune networks
	– Inherited disorders	
Health status	– Infectious disease – Chronic disease	– Impaired immune homeostasis due to, e.g., ongoing inflammation – Modification of the micro-environment of the immune cells, the nature of the signals provided by DC and the activation state of T-cells
	– Treatment leading to an impaired immune system	– Occurrence of pre-existing antibodies (cross-) reacting with the drug

Treatment-related factors

Route	– sc, id > iv, ip, oral, in, it	– Route of immunisation defines the innate and adaptive immune cells involved in the encounter of the protein drug
Dose	– High dose > low dose	– Tissue-specific antigen processing and T- and B-cell epitope repertoires
Frequency	– High frequency > low frequency	– Tissue-specific micro-environment affects immune cell responsiveness
Duration	– Long term > short term	

Protein-related factors

Phylogenetic distance	– Non-human > human (in humans)	– Phylogenetic distant proteins elicit stronger T- and B-cell responses, while human proteins need to break peripheral tolerance first
Size	– Over 10 kDa >10–5 kDa > under 5 kDa	– Large proteins are generally immunogenic, while smaller proteins are to a lesser extent (if at all) and with lower avidity
Manufacturing and handling	– Impurities	– Antigen uptake, processing and recognition become less effective with decreasing size of the protein
	– Protein modification	– Inappropriate folding of the (human) proteins due to, e.g., incorrect protein modifications, unstability or aggregation enhances the risk for uptake, processing and recognition by DC, T- and B-cells
	– Conformational changes	

Abbreviations and symbols: sc: subcutaneous; id: intradermal; iv: intravenous; ip: intraperitoneal; in: .ntranasal; it: intratracheal; >: more immunogenic than that they express (Stewart et al. 1989, Ottesen et al. 1994, Palleroni et al. 1997, Hermeling et al. 2006). Although the concerns about antibody of non-human origin should be considered also in the case of transgenic animals, these models may predict whether or not a given drug or drug composition is capable of breaking immune tolerance.

While animal testing may be of limiting value for assessing the absolute immunogenic potential of a therapeutic protein, animal models have been proven useful in predicting the relative immunogenicity of similar proteins, such as native and recombinant proteins, or variants of a specific protein (Keil and Wagner 1989, Stewart et al. 1989, Zwickl et al. 1991, Meyer et al. 2000, Wierda, Smith and Zwickl 2001).

4.3. Prediction of Immunogenicity Using In Vitro Techniques

Proper in vitro assessment of the immunogenicity of a therapeutic protein requires that the route of administration and treatment regime are known and that a good understanding of the mode of action is acquired. Indeed, therapeutic proteins may interact directly or indirectly with EC, DC, macrophages, polymorphonuclear cells and T-cells, but intravenous administration of a protein makes it unlikely that it will interact effectively with EC. In contrast, the mucosal route will make EC, DC and macrophages the first cells to see the protein (Stoy 2001, Roggen, Kristensen and Verheyen 2006).

In vitro test formats addressing the interaction between a compound and cells of the innate immune system have been developed and implemented. Some of these test systems are discussed below. It needs to be stressed though that no validated test systems for assessing the immunogenicity of, e.g., proteins are available yet. Various tools for in vitro assessment address the immunogenicity of a protein at epitope level (Walden 1996, Roggen 2006). These tools require the availability of blood samples containing reacting or cross-reacting peripheral blood mononuclear cells and antibody. In the vast majority of the cases, these reactive immune cells and antibodies are obtained from animals or humans treated with the target protein. Thus, its overall immunogenicity is demonstrated. Further analysis of T- and B-cell epitopes will give a better understanding of mechanistic issues, such as specificity, induction and expansion of the respective cells, and their impact on, e.g., auto-immunity and sensitisation to the study protein. Similar to the comparative animal studies, these tools have been proven useful to compare the antigenicity of similar proteins or protein variants with the study protein used to produce the blood samples (Scandella et al. 1988, Alexander et al. 1992, Laroche et al. 2000). When performing such experiments, two important considerations have to be made. First, the use of animal-derived material suffers from the same restrictions discussed for animal experimentation. Second, the occurrence of new epitopes cannot be addressed readily.

In a completely different approach, the immunogenicity of a protein is assessed by identifying promiscuous T-cell epitopes in humans not exposed to the protein of interest (Stickler, Estell and Harding 2000, Warmerdam et al. 2002). Given the central role of T-cells in the development of an immune response, the expectation is that methods based on these promiscuous T-cells may become tools for assessing the immunogenicity of new proteins.

Furthermore, this approach may help us to understand the mechanisms driving the immune responses against self-proteins resulting in a break of tolerance.

4.3.1. Assessing the Impact of Proteins on Innate Cells

The evidence that EC are triggered by compounds to express in vitro surface proteins and soluble mediators, known in vivo to be involved in activation, adhesion, chemotaxis, differentiation and proliferation of innate and adaptive immune cells, has stimulated their use for developing tests addressing the early events in the immune response, especially in skin and respiratory sensitisation (Kimber et al. 2000, Roggen et al. 2006). Biomarkers with the potential of being predictive of the allergenic potency of any protein have not yet been identified. However, macrophage-colony stimulating factor (M-CSF) expression by EC was found to correlate with in vivo allergenicity of proteases in mice. Similarly, granulocyte-colony stimulating factor (G-CSF) seems to be a promising marker for lipase allergenicity (Roggen, Kristensen and Verheyen 2006). These results seem to indicate that in vitro EC-based test systems can provide information on the immunogenic potency of a protein.

It is recognised that DC link innate to adaptive immunity via a process referred to as maturation, which requires CD40 ligation in addition to antigen presentation and CD80/CD86 co-stimulation (Fujii et al. 2004). While much of the early work on DC maturation was performed in vitro, it still is not clear how these biomarkers can be used to assess immunogenicity of proteins in vitro. Promising results have been obtained in the area of skin sensitisation by combining one of these maturation markers with at least one cytokine (e.g. IL-1, IL-8). But despite intensive research, the currently used protocols are not capable of distinguishing strong, moderate and weak contact sensitisers (Kimber et al. 2000). Lindstedt et al. (2005) have demonstrated that proteins in many cases do not induce DC maturation, probably because DC maturation requires antigen challenge in a favourable micro-environment (Constant and Bottomly 1997, Kimber et al. 2000, Lanzavecchia and Salusto 2001, Roggen et al. 2006). Thus, the tool of choice may be an in vitro tests system combining EC and DC in one test. Such immuno-competent tools are currently being developed in a larger European Commission sponsored integrated project (http://www.sens-it-iv.eu).

The central role for macrophages in immune responses was elegantly reviewed by Stoy (2001). Chen et al. (2003) demonstrated in vivo that proteins can enhance the production of inflammatory mediators by macrophages as well as the accessory function of these cells. Furthermore, Radyuk et al. (2003) reported on a test system for studying the role of airway EC and alveolar macrophages in clearance of antrax spores and the prevention of the infection. In spite of these promising results, macrophages have been neglected in the development of cell-based assays for assessing the immuno-genicity of compounds.

4.3.2. Assessing Protein Immunogenicity by T-Cell Epitope Identification

Prediction of the immunogenicity of a therapeutic protein by identification of T-cell epitopes requires a tool allowing for the identification of protein-derived peptides that normally are presented in a class II MHC context.

In general, T-cell reactive peptides can be identified by screening overlapping peptides synthesised according to the known sequence of the target protein, or by screening combinatorial peptide libraries made up of millions of different peptides (Kramer and Scneider-Mergener 1998, Pinilla et al. 1999). The identification of relevant T-cell epitopes is generally based on the specificity analysis of T-cell lines propagated in vitro from peripheral blood mononuclear cells (Walker et al. 1993, Walden 1996, Novak et al. 2001). Alternatively, T-cell reactive peptides can be identified and characterised ex vivo based on the screening of peptide spot libraries using freshly isolated splenocytes in a sensitive enzyme-linked immunospot (ELISPOT) assay (Geginat et al. 2001).

In order to assess their potential to trigger an immune response in a class II MHC context, the selected peptides are covalently bound to the MHC for the generation of class II MHC–peptide complexes (Kotzin et al. 2000, Novak et al. 2001). Alternatively, selected peptides can be loaded exogenously onto empty soluble class II MHC (Reijonen and Kwok 2003). Both techniques were found to be equally effective in staining T-cell clones, but the latter has a higher versatility in providing a large number of different MHC–peptide complexes.

Stickler, Estell and Harding (2000) developed a method using $CD^{4.sup.+}$ T-cells from individuals who were not exposed previously to the protein under study in conjunction with DC derived in vitro. Synthetic peptides constructed to describe the sequence of the protein of interest are co-cultured with DC and $CD^{4.sup.+}$ T-cells, and T-cell proliferation is measured. Typically, data are compiled over a large replicate of human donors to pinpoint immunodominant, usually promiscuous epitope regions. The usefulness of this tool was demonstrated using known food allergens as model proteins (Harding 2003). Provided these data can be further substantiated also outside the field of allergy, this approach could become the first in vitro tool for assessing the immunogenicity of new proteins.

4.3.3. Assessing Protein Immunogenicity by B-Cell Epitope Identification

A variety of relatively simple assays (e.g. direct ELISA, sandwich ELISA, competitive ELISA) for assessing the antigenicity of a protein are available, but only a competitive test format (e.g. two proteins competing for the same antibody) can give information about potential B-cell epitopes. However, this information is very general and mainly comparative.

Methods using monoclonal and polyclonal antibodies for immunoscreening of oligopeptides have been used frequently for acquiring a detailed insight into the antibody-binding amino acid sequences of that protein. These methods are discussed below. Not discussed is an exciting, but yet to be substantiated, method using large repertoires of human Fab immunoglobulin (Ig) fragments as antibody source (Nishikawa, Rapoport and McLachlan 1996, Jakobsen et al. 2004).

4.3.3.1. Identification of Linear B-Cell Epitopes
A frequently used experimental method for investigating B-cell epitopes assesses specific binding of antibodies to sequential overlapping peptides encompassing the entire sequence of the study protein. Eventually, alanine

substitution of every single native amino acid of the antibody-binding peptides may help to identify amino acids in the reactive peptides that are critical for antibody binding (Williams et al. 1998).

Attempts to mimic protein epitopes by means of short synthetic peptides derived from the primary structure of the study protein are bound to select for linear epitopes. Conformational epitopes will not be predicted unless they have a continuous interaction site that is long enough to allow for antibody binding, and which has the highest overall affinity for the antibody. Since protein surface analysis seems to suggest that most antigenic determinants are discontinuous (Barlow, Edwards and Thornton 1986, van Regenmortel and Pellequer 1994), peptide scanning may not provide the expected information on the overall antigenicity of the study protein.

4.3.3.2. B-Cell Epitope Mapping by Phage Libraries Expressing Random Oligopeptides

In contrast to other methods, epitope mapping by phage display screening involves specific monoclonal or polyclonal antibodies, but not necessarily the antigen. The overall advantage of this technology is believed to be that it allows for identification of linear and conformational epitopes.

It is generally known that a considerable fraction of the peptides derived by using not only polyclonal antisera but also monoclonal antibodies may represent irrelevant amino acid sequences. This problem can be successfully addressed by applying a multiple sequence alignment algorithm (PILEUP) together with a matrix for scoring amino acid substitutions based on physico-chemical properties to generate guide trees depicting relatedness of selected peptides (Davies et al. 1999). Alternatively, competitive immunoscreening of phage-displayed random oligopeptide libraries was shown to reduce the level of irrelevant phages from 90 to 10% of the total number of phages obtained by biopanning (Mittag et al. 2006).

Since immunoscreening of phage-displayed oligopeptides is biased towards those regions of an epitope with the highest overall affinity for the antibody, the identified amino acid sequence may not reflect the entire epitope (van Regenmortel 1998). Identification of antibody-binding sequences by immuno-screening of phage-displayed oligopeptides is also complicated by biases imposed primarily by the viral morphogenesis process (Rodi, Soares and Makowski 2002).

Finally, localisation of the sequences in the three-dimensional structure of the target protein may not always be straightforward and is often subjective. In order to eliminate subjectivity, a number of methods were developed. In the EPIMAP method, mimotopes discovered by phage display are individually aligned against their parent antigen via a dynamic programming algorithm revealing segments that are close in three-dimensional space in the native structure, e.g., of IL-10 (Mumey et al. 2006). Proper mapping can also be accomplished by applying feedback-restrained molecular dynamics (FRMD) to the peptide pool as shown for an erythropoietin analog (Cachau et al. 2003).

In spite of the various pitfalls, both linear and conformational epitopes have been identified by localisation of immuno-selected peptides on the three-dimensional structure of a number of proteins (Parhami-Seren, Keel and Reed 1997, Williams et al. 1998, Davies et al. 1999, Ganglberger et al. 2000, Hantusch et al. 2004). Recently, Mittag et al. (2006) demonstrated how this technique can be used for predicting cross-reactivity and potential allergenicity of novel foods. Furthermore, selection of phage-displayed peptide mimics by competitive immunoscreening with serum IgE from allergic patients in combination with computer-based mapping of the peptide mimics onto the surface of the three-dimensional allergen structure showed useful to investigate IgE epitope specificity in individual patients.

4.4. Prediction Using BioInformatics

Using one or a combination of the approaches described above, potential T- and B-cell epitopes have been identified for a considerable number of proteins. These data were collected in various databases and used to develop a number of computer-based tools aiming at assessing the antigenicity of proteins (Table 4.2). The common overall expectation for each of these methods is that they can predict antigenicity of any relevant protein.

4.4.1. Physicochemical and Structural Scales for Predicting B-Cell Epitopes from the Primary Structure of the Protein

A classical approach to epitope prediction is to utilise the tools that were developed for protein identification and analysis (Gasteiger et al. 2005). Some of these tools have been assessed individually (Pellequer, Westhof and van Regenmortel 1994) or in combination (Jameson and Wolf 1988, Alix 2000, Odorico and Pellequer 2003, Saha and Raghava 2004, Blythe and Flower 2005, Batori et al. 2006, Roggen 2006) to predict B-cell epitopes from the primary amino acid sequence of the study protein (Table 4.2). The combination of scales showed little improvement over single-based methods, as an inadequate predictive value of 50–60% was the result.

Interestingly, algorithms for predicting amino acid stretches defining in a protein structure hairpin turns and non-specific turns, but not helical turns, were shown to have a 70% prediction efficacy for antigenicity (Pellequer, Westhof and van Regenmortel 1994). This observation seems to fit with the evidence that continuous antigenic sites are often located in or nearby turns of proteins (Mendz and Moore 1985).

Machine learning tools (e.g. ABCpred, Bepipred, SPA) attempt to extract characteristics of an epitope from a set of learning examples and generalise them in a classification algorithm (Table 4.2). ABCpred was trained on 700 epitopes from the Bcipep database and 700 randomly selected peptides represented by 10- to 20-amino-acid-long stretches. The method achieved a modest maximum accuracy of 66% (Saha and Raghava 2006). Bepipred, combining scores from the Parker hydrophilicity scale and a hidden Markov model trained on linear epitopes, revealed a small but significant increase in area under the receiver operating characteristic curve A_{ROC}) as compared to earlier scale-based methods (Larsen, Lund and Nielsen 2006). Finally, the SPA algorithm yielded a degree of accuracy that was greatly increased over single-parameter methods when tested on epitope sequences obtained from a high-quality proprietary database as well as publicly accessible databases. This algorithm combines common single amino acid propensity scales with neighbourhood parameters reflecting the probability that a given stretch of amino acids exists within a predefined proximity of a specific amino acid residue (Sollner and Mayer 2006).

Table 4.2 Epitope prediction tools, databases and data sets.

Name	URL/e-mail	Description
ABCpred	http://www.imtech.res.in/raghava/abcpred	Sequence-based machine-learning tool for the prediction of continuous epitopes
AntiJen	http://www.jenner.ac.uk/AntiJen/	Database of binding data for various types of proteins, including B-cell epitopes
Bcipep	http://www.imtech.res.in/raghava/bcipep/	Database of B-cell epitopes of varying immunogenicity
Bepipred	http://www.cbs.dtu.dk/services/BepiPred	Sequence-based tool for the prediction of continuous epitopes
BEPITOPE	jlpellequer@cea.fr	Sequence-based tool for the prediction of continuous epitopes
BIMAS	http://thr.cit.nih.gov/molbio/hla_bind/	Prediction server facilitating the prediction of class I molecules
CEP	http://bioinfo.ernet.in/cep.htm	Structure-based tool for the prediction of continuous and discontinuous epitopes
CTLPred	http://imtech.res.in/raghava/ctlpred/	Prediction server facilitating the prediction of class I molecules
DiscoTope	http://www.cbs.dtu.dk/services/DiscoTope	Sequence-/structure-based tool for the prediction of discontinuous epitopes
EMT	elro@novozymes.com	Computer-based B-cell epitope mapping tool for linear and conformational epitopes
EPIMAP	mumey@cs.montana.edu	Phage-display-based tool for the identification of discontinuous epitopes
Epipredict	http://www.epipredict.de/Prediction/prediction.html	Prediction server facilitating the prediction of class II molecules
Epitome	http://www.rostlab.org/services/epitome	Database of antigenic residues and interacting antibodies
Epitope binding	http://hlaligand.ouhsc.edu/prediction.htm	Prediction server facilitating the prediction of class I molecules
HIV database	http://hiv-web.lanl.gov/content/immunology/	Database of HIV-specific immune epitopes
HLADR4Pred	http://www.imtech.res.in/raghava/hladr4pred	Prediction server facilitating the prediction of class II molecules
IEDB	http://www.immuneepitope.org	Database of T- and B-cell epitopes and non-epitopes
IEDB B-cell epitope	http://www.immuneepitope.org/tools/bcell/iedb_input	Sequence-based tool for the prediction of continuous epitopes
LPPEP	http://zlab.bu.edu/zhiping/lppep.html	Prediction server facilitating the prediction of class I molecules
MAPPP	http://www.mpiib-berlin.mpg.de/MAPPP/binding.html	Prediction server facilitating the prediction of class I molecules
MHCPred	http://www.jenner.ac.uk/MHCPred/	Prediction server facilitating the prediction of class I molecules
MHC2Pred	http://www.imtech.res.in/raghava/mhc2pred/	Prediction server facilitating the prediction of class II molecules
MHC-Thread	http://www.csd.abdn.ac.uk/~gjlk/MHC-Thread/	Prediction server facilitating the prediction of class II molecules
MMPred	http://www.imtech.res.in/raghava/mmbpred/	Prediction server facilitating the prediction of class I molecules
MPID-T	http://surya.bic.nus.edu.sg/mpidt	Database containing structural descriptors for in-depth characterisation of TcR
Net MHC	http://www.cbs.dtu.dk/services/NetMHC	Prediction server facilitating the prediction of class I molecules
nHLAPred	http://www.imtech.res.in/raghava/nhlapred/	Prediction server facilitating the prediction of class I molecules

(Continued)

Table 4.2 (*Continued*).

Name	URL/e-mail	Description
Pellequer data set	jlpellequer@cea.fr	Data set consisting of 82 epitopes in 14 protein sequences
PREDEP	http://margalit.huji.ac.il/Teppred/mhc-bind/index.html	Prediction server facilitating the prediction of class I molecules
PREDICT	http://research.i2r.a-star.edu.sg/predict-demo/	Prediction server facilitating the prediction of class I and class II molecules
PROPRED	http://www.imtech.res.in/raghava/propred	Prediction server facilitating the prediction of class II molecules
ProPred1	http://imtech.res.in/raghava/propred1/	Prediction server facilitating the prediction of class I molecules
RANKPEP	http://mif.dfci.harvard.edu/Tools/rankpep.html	Prediction server facilitating the prediction of class I and class II molecules
SPA	johannes.soellner@emergentec.com	Programme for the parametrisation of peptide sequences use with machine-learning algorithms
SVMHC	http://www-bs.informatik.uni-tuebingen.de/Services/SVMHC	Prediction server facilitating the prediction of class I molecules
SYFPEITI	http://syfpeiti.de/	Prediction server facilitating the prediction of class I and class II molecules

It is generally believed that algorithms based on physicochemical characteristics and structural features will address predominantly linear epitopes.
Conformational epitopes may be identified if the epitope comprises a primary
(contiguous) interaction site such as a loop or protruding region of the protein.
However, none of these methods can predict conformational epitopes lacking
such a primary site, nor can they predict hidden antigenic amino acids brought
into contact with paratope residues by specific antigen–antibody interactions
(Alexander et al. 1992, Nair et al. 2002).

4.4.2. Predicting B-Cell Epitopes from the Three-Dimensional Structure of the Protein

A number of novel tools employing the three-dimensional structure of a
protein have been reported recently (Table 4.2). The conformational epitope
prediction (CEP) server calculates the relative accessible surface area (RSA)
for each residue in the structure and determines which regions of the
protein molecule are sufficiently exposed to act as antigenic determinants.
Additionally, regions distant in the primary sequence, but close in three-
dimensional space, are condensed into one epitope. In a data set consisting
of 63 antigen–antibody complexes, the algorithm correctly identified 76% of
the epitopic residues (Kulkarni-Kale, Bhosle and Kolaskar 2005).

The DiscoTope algorithm combines scores from a probability matrix with
a measure of the surface area to predict with a fair degree of accuracy the
location of conformational epitope residues. Using the A_{ROC} as an indicator,
the algorithm achieved a score of 0.711 (Haste-Andersen, Nielsen and Lund
2006).

4.4.3. Predicting Immunogenicity of the Unknown by Similarity with the Known

Alternative methods have based the prediction of epitopes on similarities
between primary amino acid sequences (for T- and B-cell epitopes) and
three-dimensional structures (for B-cell epitopes) of proteins with known
and unknown antigenicity. In general, the strength of these systems is the
coupling of structural predictions with multiple alignments, performed on
a sequence subset extracted following a similarity search, using BLAST,
PSI-BLAST, SSEARCH, FASTA or PattInProt (e.g. http://pbil.ibcp.fr/NPSA,
http://fermi.utmb.edu/SDAP/index.html).

In contrast to predictions used to identify T-cell epitopes (Brusic, Bajic and
Petrovsky 2004, De Groot 2006), the quality of the B-cell epitope predictions
is widely considered to be too poor to be employed as a reliable tool by
immunologists (Blythe and Flower 2005). This difference in predictivity may
be related to the fact that similarity is not defined accurately enough for B-cell
epitopes. Aalberse (2000) has suggested that at least 70% amino acid identity
is required across the full length of the protein sequence. However, cross-
reactivity between tropomyosins of crustacean, mollusc and insect has been
documented, while the overall sequence identity between these proteins is
only 50–60% (Santos et al. 1999, Leung and Chu 2001). Similarly, a 57–67%
sequence identity was demonstrated to be sufficient for IgE cross-reactivity
between the major birch pollen allergen Bet v 1 and Bet v 1 homologues
of fruits and nuts (Vieths, Scheurer and Ballmer-Walker 2002, Mittag et al.

2006). Yet the lowest reported sequence identity (38–48%) resulting in cross-reactivity has been for Bet v 1 homologues in vegetables (Vieths, Scheurer and Ballmer-Walker 2002).

Hileman and co-workers (2002) proposed to add an additional search for matches of eight amino acids to the FASTA search, to add a margin of safety when assessing the potential allergenicity of a protein. This suggestion was based on a study comparing the protein sequences of 6 insecticidal proteins, 3 common low-allergenic food proteins and 50 corn proteins using the FAST algorithm and by searching for matches of contiguous identical stretches of 6, 7 and 8 amino acids of length. They recognised however that additional work is required to evaluate specific threshold criteria (e.g. percentage of sequence similarity) to improve bioinformatics as a tool for prediction of, e.g., allergenicity.

4.4.4. T- and B-Cell Epitope Mapping Based on Amino Acid Motifs

4.4.4.1. Identification of T-Cell Epitopes

Today there is a wealth of servers available over the World Wide Web, facilitating the prediction of T-cell epitopes from the sequence of the target protein (Table 4.2). Some of these servers allow for the prediction of epitopes for alleles belonging to class I or a class II MHC context, while other facilitate prediction for both classes.

MHC class I-restricted T-cell epitopes are effectively described by relatively strict peptide-binding motifs of individual class I MHC molecules (Rammensee et al. 1999). This knowledge allows the educated guessing of epitopes and thus greatly reduces the number of synthetic peptides required for epitope identification. It has to be stressed that regarding the identification of class II MHC-restricted T-cell epitopes the less strict binding requirements generally result in a lower predictive value of MHC class II motifs (Sinigaglia and Hammer 1994).

A new database (MPID-T) for sequence–structure–function information on T-cell receptor (TcR)–peptide–MHC interactions has been made available. MPID-T contains structural descriptors for in-depth characterisation of TcR, peptide and MHC interactions. The ultimate purpose of this tool is to enhance the understanding of the binding mechanisms underlying TcR–peptide–MHC (Tong et al. 2006).

4.4.4.2. Identification of B-Cell Epitopes

Batori et al. (2006) were the first to provide evidence suggesting the existence of general antibody-binding motifs using chicken lysozyme (Gal d 4) as model protein. This observation was further substantiated by epitope mapping performed on antigenically known industrial enzymes ($N = 8$), environmental allergens ($N = 4$), food allergens ($N = 7$) and therapeutic proteins ($N = 2$) (Greenbaum et al. 2007). The computer-based epitope mapping tool revealed a high sensitivity (>80%) and positive predictive value (75–100%), depending on the minimum RSA of the amino acids included in the mapping. These results seem to be in line with previous observations (Hopp and Woods 1981, O'Lorcain, Talebi and Mulcohy 1996, Alix 2000), indicating that the most exposed amino acids are most likely to be involved in antigenic determinants. The current data seem to suggest that a 40% minimum RSA is an acceptable lower cut-off for mapping, giving balanced sensitivity and positive predictive value. As yet, only Ara h 2 epitope 4 (Stanley et al. 1997) and the Bet v 1 epitope reported by Mirza et al. (2000) were shown to require amino acids with at least 10 and 30% minimum RSA, respectively. Thus, the EMT seems to accommodate the fact that epitopes are three-dimensional entities with various degrees of accessibility. Comparison of the predictive efficacy of the EMT and existing prediction scales, after normalisation of the various scales in terms of sensitivity, revealed a superior performance of the EMT which increased with decreasing sensitivity and increasing positive predictive value (Roggen 2006).

4.5. Conclusion

The objective of this chapter was to give an overview on the models currently available for prediction of protein immunogenicity. It should be clear from the text that the current status of immunogenicity prediction is far from ideal and the ultimate need of the research and regulatory community is access to better prediction tools.

At present, animals still are required to carry out research and regulatory testing. The main issue related to animal experimentation is the relevance of the resulting data for predicting safety in humans. Typically, the predictivity of animal testing is increased by assessing the immunogenicity of the pharmaceutical protein in a number of animal species, ranging from mice to primates, and eventually man.

The growing understanding of the molecular and cellular immune networks that are affected upon challenge with a protein has raised the expectation that in the near future tools will be made available that allow for in vitro immunogenicity testing. Currently, two types of assays are envisaged. The first type addresses the innate (non-specific) responses elicited in EC and DC upon contact with a study protein. While promising results were obtained, none of these test formats was validated to predict protein immunogenicity. The second group of assays wants to identify the T- and B-cell epitopes encoded by the amino acid sequence of the protein. These in vitro alternative methods require the availability of specific serum and are therefore limited to assessment of cross-reactivity. No information is provided with regard to new epitopes.

These classical epitope mapping methods have identified a significant number of T- and B-cell epitopes which were collected in a variety of databases. The B-cell epitope databases have been used to evaluate the predictive power of tools originally developed to analyse physicochemical and structural features from the primary structure of the study protein. Unfortunately, prediction of antigenicity from the sequence of a protein using any of these tools alone or in combination is inaccurate. T- and B-cell epitopes can be addressed by comparing amino acid sequence and structural similarities. It is believed that proteins having a similar structure and at the same time sharing a substantial part of the amino acid sequences share antigenic properties. The problem with this approach is that the minimal sequence similarity required to make this work still has to be defined. Finally, a number of computer-based epitope mapping tools have been demonstrated to identify T- and B-cell epitopes with various degrees of accuracy. For these tools to be accepted as prediction tools for research and regulation, it is imperative that they are evaluated on high-quality training and testing data sets.

References

Aalberse, R. C. 2000. Structural biology of allergens. J. Allergy Clin. Immunol. 106:228–238.

Alexander, H., Alexander, S., Getzoff, E. D., Tainer, J. A., Geysen, H. M., and Lerner, R. A. 1992. Altering the antigenicity of proteins. Proc. Natl. Acad. Sci. USA 89:3352–3356.

Alix, A. J. 2000. Predictive estimation of protein linear epitopes by using the program PEOPLE. Vaccine 18:311–314.

Andersson, K., Choulier, L., Hamalainen, M. D., van Regenmortel, M. H., Altshuh, D., and Malmqvist, M. 2001. Predicting the kinetics of peptide-antibody interactions using multivariate experimental design of sequence and chemical space. J. Mol. Rec. 14:62–71.

Bachmann, M. F., and Zinkernagel, R. M. 1997. Neutralizing antiviral B cell responses. Ann. Rev. Immunol. 15:235–270.

Bancherau, J., Briere, F., Caux, C., Davoust, J., Lebecque, S., Liu, Y. J., Pulendran, B., and Palucka, K. 2000. Flow-cytometry screening for the modulation of receptor-mediated endocytosis in human dendritic cells: implications for the development of an in vitro technique for predictive testing of contact sensitisers. J. Immunol. Methods 203:171–180.

Barlow, D. J., Edwards, M. S., and Thornton, J. M. 1986. Continuous and discontinuous protein antigenic determinants. Nature 322:747–748.

Batori, V., Friis, E. P., Nielsen, H., and Roggen, E. L. 2006. An in silico method using an epitope motif database for predicting the location of antigenic determinants on proteins in a structural context. J. Mol. Rec.19:21–29.

Blythe, M. J., Flower, D. R. 2005. Benchmarking B cell epitope prediction: underperformance of existing methods. Protein Sci. 14:246–248.

Brusic, V., Bajic, V. B., Petrovsky, N. 2004. Computational methods for prediction of T-cell epitopes—a framework for modelling, testing, and applications. Methods 34:436–443.

Cachau, R. E., Gonzalez-Sapienza, G., Burt, S. K., Ventura, O. N. 2003. A new addition to the structural bioinformatics toolbox: 3D models of short bioactive peptides from multiple sequences using feedback restrained molecular dynamics (FRMD). Cell. Mol. Biol. (Noisy-le-grand) 49:973–983.

Chan, O. T., Madaio, M. P., and Shlomchik, M. J. 1999. B-cells are required for lupus nephritis in the polygenic fas-intact MRL model of systemic autoimmunity. J. Immunol. 163:3592–3596.

Chen, C.-L., Lee, C.-T., Liu, Y.-C., Wang, J.-Y., Lei, H.-Y., and Yu, C.-K. 2003. House dust mite Dermatophagoides farinae augments proinflammatory mediator production and accessory function of alveolar macrophages: implications for allergic sensitisation and inflammation. J. Immunol. 170:528–536.

Constant, S. L., and Bottomly, K. 1997. Induction of T_h1 and T_h2 CD[4.sup.+] T-cell responses: the alternative approaches. Ann. Rev. Immunol. 15:297–322.

Cumberbatch, M., Clelland, K., Dearman, R., and Kimber, I. 2005. Impact of cutaneous IL-10 on resident epidermal Langerhans' cells and the development of polarised immune responses. J. Immunol. 175:43–50.

Davies, J. M., Scealy, M., Cai, Y., Whisstock, J., Mackay, I. R., and Rowley, M. J. 1999. Multiple alignment and sorting of peptides derived from phage-displayed random peptide libraries with polyclonal sera allows discrimination of relevant phagotopes. Mol. Immunol. 36:659–667.

De Groot, A. S. 2006. Immunomics: discovering new targets for vaccines and thera-peutics. Drug Discov. Today 11:203–209.

Fujii, S.-i., Liu, K., Smith, C., Bonito, A. J., and Steinman, R. M. 2004. The linkage of innate to adaptive immunity via maturing dendritic cells in vivo requires CD40 ligation in addition to antigen presentation and CD80/86 costimulation. J. Exp. Med. 199:1607–1618.

Ganglberger, E., Grunberger, K., Sponer, B., Radauer, C., Breiteneder, H., Boltz-Nitulescu, G., Scheiner, O., and Jensen-Jarolim, E. 2000. Allergen mimotopes for 3-dimensional epitope search and induction of antibodies inhibiting human IgE. FASEB J. 14:2177–2184.

Gasteiger, E., Hoogland, C., Gattiker, A., Duvaud, S., Wilkins, M. R., Appel, R. D., and Bairoch, A. 2005. Protein identification and analtsis tools on the ExPASy server. In: The Proteomics Protocols Handbook, ed. J. M. Walker, Vol. 715, pp. 571–607, Tonkawa, NJ: Humana Press.

Geginat, G., Schenk, S., Skoberne, M., Goebel, W., and Hof, H. 2001. A novel approach of direct ex vivo epitope mapping identifies dominant and subdominant CD4 and CD8 T cell epitopes from *Listeria monocytogenes*. J. Immunol. 166: 1877–1884.

Greenbaum, J. A., Haste-Andersen, P., Blythe, M., Bui, H.-H., Cachau, R., E., Crowe, J., Davies, M., Kolaskar, A. S., Lund, O., Morrison, S., Mumey, B., Ofran, Y., Pellequer, J.-L., Pinilla, C., Ponomarenko, J. V., Raghava, G. P. S., van Regenmortel, M. H. V., Roggen, E. L., Sette, A., Schlessinger, A., Sollner, J., Zand, M., and Peters, B. 2007. Towards a consensus on datasets and evalu-ation metrics for developing B cell epitope prediction tools. J. Mol. Rec. 20:75–82.

Guermonprez, P., Valladeau, J., Zitvogel, L., Théry, C., and Amigorena, S. 2002. Antigen presentation and T cell stimulation by dendritic cells. Annu. Rev. Immunol. 20:621–67.

Hantusch, B., Krieger, S., Untermayr, E., Scholl, I., Knittelfelder, R., Flicker, S., Spitzauer, S., Valenta, R., Boltz-Nitulesen, G., Scheiner, O., and Jensen-Jarolim, E. 2004. Mapping of conformational IgE epitopes on Phl p 5a by using mimotopes from a phage display library. J. Allergy Clin. Immunol. 114:1294–1300.

Harding, F. A. 2003. A human dendritic cell-based method to identify CD[4.sup.+]T-cell epitopes in potential protein allergens. Environ. Health Perspect. 111:251–254.

Haste-Andersen, P., Nielsen, M., and Lund, O. 2006. Prediction of residues in discon-tinuous B-cell epitopes using protein 3D structures. Protein Sci. 15:2558–2567.

Hayakawa, K., Asano, M., Shinton, S., Gui, M., Allman, D., Stewart, C., Silver, J., and Hardy, R. 1999. Positive selection of natural autoreactive B-cells. Science 285:113–116.

Hermeling, S., Crommelin, D. J., Schellekens, H., and Jiskoot, W. 2004. Structure-immunogenicity relationships of therapeutic proteins. Pharmacol. Res. 21:897–903.

Hermeling, S., Schellekens, H., Maas, C., Gebbink, M. F., Crommelin, D. J., and Jiskoot, W., 2006. Antibody responses to aggregated human interferon-α 2a in wild type and transgenic tolerant mice depends on type and level of aggregation. J. Pharm. Sci. 95:1084–1096.

Hietbrink, F., Koenderman, L., Rijkers, G. T., and Leenen, L. P. H. 2006. Trauma: the role of the innate immune system. World J. Emergency Surg. 1:15–25.

Hileman, R. E., Silvanovitch, A., Goodman, R. E., Rice, E. A., Holleschak, G., Astwood, J. D., and Hefle, S. L. 2002. Bioinformatic methods for allergenicity assessment using a comprehensive allergen database. Int. Arch. Allergy Immunol. 128:280–291.

Hopp, T. P., and Woods, K. R. 1981. Prediction of protein antigenic determinants from amino acid sequences. Proc. Natl. Acad. Sci. USA 78:3824–3828.

Jakobsen, C. G., Bodtger, U., Kristensen, P., Poulsen, L. K., and Roggen, E. L. 2004. Isolation of high-affinity human IgE and IgG antibodies recognising Bet v 1 and Humicola lanuginosa lipase from combinatorial phage libraries. Mol. Immunol. 41:941–953.

Jameson, B. A. and Wolf, H. 1988. The antigenic index: a novel algorithm for predicting antigenic determinants. CABIOS 4:181–186.

Janssen, R., Wauben, M. H., and Tomassen, J. 1996. Quaternary structure of a carrier protein influences antigenicity and immunogenicity of an inserted T-cell determinant. Intl. Immunol. 8:829–845.

Kehry, M. and Hodgkin, P. 1994. B-cell activation by helper T-cell membranes. Crit. Rev. Immunol. 14:221–238.

Keil, W. and Wagner, R. R. 1989. Epitope mapping by deletion mutants and chimeras of two vesicular stomatitis virus glycoprotein genes expressed by a vaccinia virus vector. Virology 170:392–407.

Kelso, A. 1995. T_h1 and T_h2 subsets: paradigm lost? Immunol. Today 16:374–379.

Kimber, I., Cumberbath, M., Dearman, R. J., Bhushan, M., and Griffiths, C. E. M., 2000. Cytokines and chemokines in the initiation and regulation of epidermal langerhans cell mobilisation. Br. J. Dermatol. 142:401–412.

Kotzin, B. L., Falta, M. T., Crawford, F., Rosloniec, E. F., Bill, J., Marrack, P., and Kappler, J. 2000. Use of soluble peptide-DR4 tetramers to detect synovial T cells specific for cartilage antigens in patients with rheumatoid arthritis. Proc. Natl. Acad. Sci. USA 97:291–296.

Kramer, A. and Schneider-Mergener, J. 1998. Synthesis and screening of peptide libraries on continuous cellulose membrane supports. Methods Mol. Biol. 87:25–39.

Kulkarni-Kale, U., Bhosle, S., and Kolaskar, A. S. 2005. CEP: a conformational epitope prediction server. Nucleic Acids Res. 33:W168–W171.

Lambrecht, B. N. and Hammad, H. 2003a. The other cells in asthma: dendritic cells and epithelial cells crosstalk. Curr. Opin. Pulm. Med. 9:34–41.

Lambrecht, B. N. and Hammad, H. 2003b. Taking our breath away: dendritic cells in the pathogenesis of asthma. Nat. Rev. Immunol. 3:997–1003.

Lanzavecchia, A. and Salusto, F. 2001. Regulation of T cell immunity by dendritic cells. Cell 106:263–266.

Laroche, Y., Heymans, S., Capaert, S., De Cock, F., Demarsin, E., and Collen, D. 2000. Recombinant staphylokinase variants with reduced antigenicity due to elimination of B-lymphocyte epitopes. Blood 96:1425–1430.

Larsen, J. E., Lund, O., and Nielsen, M. 2006. Improved method for predicting linear B-cell epitopes. Immunome Res. 2:2.

Leung, P. S. and Chu, K. H. 2001. cDNA cloning and molecular identification of the major oyster allergen from the Pacific oyster Crassostera gigas. Clin. Exp. Allergy 31:1287–1294.

Lindstedt, M., Schiott, A., Johnsen, C. R., Roggen, E. L., Johansson-Lindbom, B., and Borrebaeck, C. A., 2005. Individuals with occupational allergy to detergent enzymes display a differential transcriptional regulation and cellular immune response. Clin. Exp. Allergy 35:199–207.

McKenzie, R. C. and Sauder, D. N. 1990. Keratinocyte cytokines and growth factors. Immunodermatology 8:649–661.

Mendz, G. L. and Moore, W. J. 1985. NMR studies of myelin basic protein. Conformation of a peptide that is an antigenic determinant for B-cell reactivity. Biochem. J. 229:305–313.

Meyer, D. L., Schultz, J., Lin, Y., Henry, A., Scanderson, J., Jackson, J. M., Goshorn, S., Rees, A. R., and Graves, S. S. 2000. Reduced antibody response to streptavidin through site-directed mutagenesis. Protein Sci. 10:491–503.

Milich, D. R. and Leroux-Roels, G. 2003. Immunogenetics of the response to HBsAg vaccination. Autoimmun. Rev. 2:248–257.

Miller, J. F. 2005. Principles of immunological tolerance. Transfus. Med. Hemother. 32:322–331.

Mirza, O., Henriksen, A., Ipsen, H., Larsen, N., Wissenbach, M., Spangfort, M., and Gajhede, M. 2000. Dominant epitopes and allergic cross-reactivity: complex formation between a Fab fragment of amonoclonal murine IgG antibody and the major allergen from birch pollen Bet v 1. J. Immunol. 165:331–338.

Mittag, D., Batori, V., Neudecker, P., Wiche, R., Friis, E. P., Ballmer-Weber, B. K., Vieths, S., and Roggen, E. L. 2006. A novel approach for investigation of specific and cross-reactive IgE epitopes on Bet v 1 and homologous food allergens in individual patients. Mol. Immunol. 43:79–89.

Mosmann, T. R., and Coffman, I. L. 1989. T_h1 and T_h2 cells: different patterns of lymphokine secretion lead to different functional properties. Ann. Rev. Immunol. 7:145–173.

Mumey, B., Ohler, N., Angel, T., Jesaitis, A., and Dratz, E. 2006. In Proceedings of High Performance Computing in Genomics, Proteomics, and Transcriptomics, Springer-Verlag: Sorrento.

Nair, D. T., Singh, K., Siddiqui, Z., Niyak, B. P., Rao, K. V., and Salunke, D. M. 2002. Epitope recognition by diverse antibodies suggests conformational convergence in an antibody response. J. Immunol. 168:2371–2382.

Nishikawa, T., Rapoport, B., and McLachlan, S. 1996. The quest for the auto-antibody immunodominant region on thyroid peroxidase: guided mutagenesis based on a hypothetical three-dimensional model. Endocrinology 137:1000–1006.

Novak, E. J., Liu, A. W., Gebe, J. A., Falk, B. A., Nepom, G. T., Koelle, D. M., and Kwok, W. W. 2001. Tetramer-guided epitope mapping: rapid identification and characterisation of immunodominant CD4+ T-cell epitopes from complex antigens. J. Immunol. 166:6665–6670.

Oberg, K., Alm, G., Magnusson, A., Lundqvist, G., Theodorsson, E., Wide, L., and Wilander, E. 1989. Treatment of malignant carcinoid tumors with recombinant intereron alfa-2b: development of neutralizing interferon antibodies and possible loss of antitumor activity. J. Natl. Cancer Inst. 81:531–535.

Odorico, M., and Pellequer, J.-L., 2003. BEPITOPE: predicting the location of continuous epitopes and patterns in proteins. J. Mol. Rec. 16:20–22.

O'Lorcain, P., Talebi, A., and Mulcohy, G. 1996. B-cell epitope mapping within the MA16 antigenic sequence found in Eimeria acervulina merozoites and sporozoites. Vet. Parasitol. 66:147–157.

Ottesen, J. L., Nilsson, P., Jami., Weilguny, D., Dührkop, M., Bucchini, D., Havelund, S., and Fogh, J. M. 1994. The potential immunogenicity of human insulin and insulin analogues evaluated in a transgenic mouse model. Diabetologia 37:1178–1185.

Palleroni, A. V., Aglione, A., Labow, M., Brunda, M. J., Pestka, S., Sinigaglia, F., Garotta, G., Alsenz, J., and Braun, A. 1997. Interferon immunogenicity: preclinical evaluation of interferon-a 2a. J. Interferon Res. 17:S23–S27.

Parhami-Seren, B., Keel, T., and Reed, G. L. 1997. Sequences of antigenic epitopes of Streptokinase identified via random peptide libraries displayed on phage. J. Mol. Biol. 271:333–341.

Peces, R., de la Torre, M., Alcazar, R., and Urra, J. M. 1996. Antibodies against recombinant human erythropoietin in a patient with erythroietin-resistant anemia. N. Engl. J. Med. 335:523–524.

Pellequer, J. L.,Westhof, E., and van Regenmortel, M. H. 1994. Epitope predictions from the primary structure of proteins. In: Peptide Antigens: A Practical Approach, ed. G. B. Wisdom, pp. 7–25, Oxford: IRL Press.

Pinilla, C., Martin, R., Gran, B., Appel, J. R., Boggiano, C., Wilson, D. B., and Houghten R. A. 1999. Exploring immunological specificity using synthetic peptide combinatorial libraries. Curr. Opin. Immunol. 11:193–202.

Radyuk, S., Mericko, P. A., Popova, T. G., Grene, E., and Alibek, K. 2003. In vitro generated respiratory mucosa: a new tool to study inhalation anthrax. Biochem. Biophys. Res. Comm. 305:624–632.

Rammensee, H. G., Bachmann, J., Emmerich, N. P., Bachor, O. A., and Stevanovic, S. 1999. SYFPEITHI: database for MHC ligands and peptide motifs. Immunogenetics 50:213–219.

Reijonen, H., and Kwok, W. W. 2003. Use of HLA class II tetramers in tracking antigen-specific T-cells and mapping T-cell epitopes. Methods 29:282–288.

Rodi, D. J., Soares, A. S., and Makowski, L. 2002. Quantitative assessment of peptide sequence diversity in M13 combinatorial peptide phage display libraries. J. Mol. Biol. 322:1039–1052.

Roggen, E. L. 2006. Recent developments with B-cell epitope identification for predictive studies. J. Immunotox. 3:1–13.

Roggen, E. L., Kristensen Soni, N., and Verheyen, G. 2006. Respiratory immunotoxicity: an in vitro assessment. Toxicol. In Vitro 20:1249–1264.

Roggen, E. L., Lindstedt, M., Borrebaeck, C., and Verheyen, G. 2006. Interactions between dendritic cells and epithelial cells in allergic disease. Toxicol. Lett. 162: 71–82.

Rus, H., Cudrici, C., and Niculescu, F. 2005. The role of the complement system in innate immunity. Immunol. Res. 33:103–112.

Saha, S., and Raghava, G. P. 2004. BcePred: prediction of continuous B-cell epitopes in antigenic sequences using physicochemical properties. ICARIS:197–204.

Saha, S. and Raghava, G. P. 2006. Prediction of continuous B-cell epitopes in an antigen using recurrent neural network. Proteins 65:40–48.

Sakaguchi, S., Sakaguchi, N., Shimizu, J., Yamazaki, S., Sakihama, T., Itoh, M., Kuniyasu, Y., Nomura, T., Toda, M., and Takahashi, T. 2001. Immunologic tolerance maintained by CD25+CD4+ regulatory T-cells: their common role in controlling autoimmunity, tumor immunity and transplantation tolerance. Immunol. Rev. 182:18–32.

Santos, A. B., Chapman, M. D., Aalberse, R. C., Vailes, L. D., Ferriani, V. P., Oliver, C., Rizzo, M. C., Naspitz, C. K., and Arruda, L. K. 1999. Cockroach allergens and asthma in Brazil: identification of tropomyosin as a major allergen with potential cross-reactivity with mite and shrimp allergens. J. Allergy Clin. Immunol. 104: 329–337.

Scandella, D., DeGraaf, M. S., Mattingly, M., Roeder, D., Timmons, L., and Fulcher, C. A. 1988. Epitope mapping of human factor VIII inhibitor antibodies by deletion analysis of factor VIII fragments expressed in E. coli. Proc. Natl. Acad. Sci. USA 85:6152–6156.

Schellekens, H. 2002. Immunogenicity of therapeutic proteins: clinical implications and future prospects. Clin. Ther. 24:1720–1740.

Silverstein, A. M. 1989. A History of Immunology, Academic Press: San Diego.

Sinigaglia, F. and Hammer, J. 1994. Defining rules for the peptide-MHC class II interaction. Curr. Opin. Immunol. 6:52–56.

Sollner, J. and Mayer, B. 2006. Machine learning approaches for prediction of linear B-cell epitopes on proteins. J. Mol. Rec. 19:200–208.

Stanley, J. S., King, N., Burks, A. W., Huang, S. K., Sampson, H., Cockrell, G., Helm, R. M., West, C. M., and Bannon, G. A. 1997. Identification and mutational analysis of the immunodominant IgE binding epitopes of the major peanut allergen Ara h 2. Arch. Biochem. Biophys. 342:244–253.

Stewart, T. A., Hollingshead, P. G., Pitts, S. L., Chang, R., Martin, L. E., and Oakley, H. 1989. Transgenic mice as a model to test the immunogenicity of proteins altered by site-specific mutagenesis. Mol. Biol. Med. 6:275–281.

Stickler, M. M., Estell, D. A., and Harding, F. A. 2000. CD[4.sup.+]T-cell epitope determination using unexposed human donor peripheral blood mononuclear cells. J. Immunother. 23:654–660.

Stoy, N. 2001. Macrophage biology and pathobiology in the evolution of immune responses: a functional analysis. Pathobiology 69:179–211.

Striz, I., Slavcev, A., Kalanin, J., Jaresova, M., and Rennard, S. I. 2001. Cell-cell contacts with epithelial cells modulate the phenotype of human macrophages. Inflammation 254:241–246.

Thepen, T., Kraal, G., and Holt, P., G. 1996. The role of alveolar macrophages in regulation of lung inflammation. In: Cytokines and Adhesion Molecules in Lung Inflammation, eds. M. Chignard, M. Pretolani, P. Renesto, B. B. Vargaftig, Vol. 796, pp. 200–232, NewYork: Annals of the New York Academy of Sciences.

Tong, J. C., Kong, L., Tan, T. W., and Ranganathan, S. 2006. MPID-T: database for sequence-structure-function information on T-cell receptor/peptide/MHC interactions. Appl. Bioinformatics 5:111–114.

van Regenmortel, M. H. 1998. Mimotopes, continuous paratopes and hydropathic complementarity: novel approximations in the description of immunochemical specificity. Dispers. Sci. Technol. 19:1199–1219.

van Regenmortel, M. H. and Pellequer, J. L. 1994. Predicting antigenic determinants in proteins: looking for unidimensional solutions to the three-dimensional problem? Peptide Res. 7:224–228.

Vieths, S., Scheurer, S., and Ballmer-Weber, B. 2002. Current understanding of cross-reactivity of food allergens and pollen. Ann. N. Y. Acad. Sci. 964:47–68.

Walden, P. 1996. T-cell epitope determination. Curr. Opin. Immunol. 8:68–74.

Walker, P. R., Smerdon, R., Haron, J., and Lehner, T. 1993. Mapping major and minor T-cell epitopes in vitro and their immunogenic or tolerogenic effect in vivo in non-human primates. Immunology 80:209–216.

Warmerdam, P. A., Vanderlick, K., Vandervoort, P., De Smedt, H., Plaisance, S., De Maeyer, M., and Collen, D. 2002. Staphylokinas-specific cell-mediated immunity in humans. J. Immunol. 168:155–161.

Wierda, D., Smith, H. W., and Zwickl, C. M. 2001. Immunogenicity of biopharmaceuticals in laboratory animals. Toxicology 158:71–74.

Williams, S. C., Badley, R. A., Davis, P. J., PujK, W. C., and Meloen, R. H. 1998. Identification of epitopes within beta lactoglobulin recognised by polyclonal antibodies using phage display and PEPSCAN. J. Immunol. Meth. 213:1–17.

Wu, K. J., Wang, C. Y., and Lu, H. K. 2004. Effect of glutaraldehyde on the humoral immunogenicity and structure of porcine dermal collagen membranes. Arch. Oral Biol. 49:305–311.

Zang, Y. C., Yang, D., Hong, J., Tejada-Simon, M. V., Rivera, V. M., and Zhang, J. Z. 2000. Immunoregulation and blocking antibodies induced by interferon beta treatment in MS. Neurology 55:397–404.

Zouali, M. 2001. B-cell tolerance to self in systemic auto-immunity. Arch. Immunol. Ther. Exp. 49:361–365.

Zwickl, C. M., Cocke, K. S., Tamura, R. N., Holzhausen, L. M., Brophy, G. T., Bick, P. H., and Wierda, D. 1991. Comparison of the immunogenicity of recombinant and pituitary human growth hormone in rhesus monkeys. Fundam. Appl. Toxicol. 16:275–287.

Immunogenicity of Biopharmaceuticals: Causes, Methods to Reduce Immunogenicity, and Biosimilars

Marco van de Weert and Eva Horn Møller

5.1. Introduction

The immune response to biopharmaceuticals is still an elusive process, governed by a large number of factors. In this chapter an overview is given of several of the factors implicated in the development of an immune response, and the potential strategies to reduce immunogenicity are discussed. Finally, the implications of the complex immune response to the development of biosimilars are described in Section 5.4.

The factors most commonly associated with immunogenicity of biopharmaceuticals are listed in Table 5.1 (Hermeling et al. 2004, Schellekens 2002a, Schellekens 2002b, Schellekens and Casadevall 2004). Those related to the analytical aspects of immunoassays will not be discussed here, and the reader is referred to Chapter 3 for a more in-depth discussion on these aspects. The other factors can be subdivided into three subheadings: structural characteristics of the biopharmaceutical, product-related factors, and patient-related factors. Although most of the discussion will be focused around protein-based biopharmaceuticals, several of the aspects discussed are also of relevance to other biopharmaceuticals. Wherever possible, we have tried to include some references to those other biopharmaceuticals.

5.2. Causes of Immunogenicity

5.2.1. Structural Characteristics of the Biomacromolecule

Perhaps the most easily understandable factor responsible for an immune response to biopharmaceuticals is the level of non-self of the biopharmaceutical. That is, how similar is the biopharmaceutical to the endogenous compound? As discussed in Chapter 1, non-native sequences of large biomacromolecules are registered as foreign, and thus usually result in a rapid immune response. The history of biopharmaceutical development counts

Table 5.1 Factors of importance and their effect on the measured immune response to biopharmaceuticals.

Factor affecting the immune response	Effect on immune response
Similarity to endogenous compound	Non-human structures are generally more likely to yield a strong immune response
Genotype of the patient	Variable, individuals may react differently to various antigens
Immune status of the patient	An impaired immune system will reduce the immune response to biopharmaceuticals
Route of administration	s.c. administration is generally more immunogenic than i.m. or i.v.
Frequency and duration of administration	Frequent and long-term use are more likely to result in an immune response
Dose	Higher dose increases the potential for an immune response
Types of antigens expressed on surface	Not all non-human antigens result in equally strong immune responses
Structure and stability	Misfolded and/or degraded biopharmaceuticals may be more antigenic
Product-related impurities	May generate a "danger" signal
Assay methods	See Chapter 3
Timing and frequency of sampling	See Chapter 3
Titer expression	See Chapter 3

many examples of this type of immune responses, and several examples are given in the case study chapters. The oldest known example is that of insulin (Chapter 8), which has been in use since the 1920s and until the 1980s was exclusively of animal origin. In the past, essentially all patients that used insulin developed antibodies at one point in time, often requiring increasing doses of insulin to offset the reduced efficacy. A more current example is the use of monoclonal antibodies with non-human sequences (Cheifetz and Mayer 2005, Hwang and Foote 2005), of which a few examples are discussed in Chapters 10 and 11.

It is important to realize that the treatment of genetic diseases in which little or no endogenous protein is expressed also may result in an immune response. In these cases the protein is to some extent non-natural to the human body, and no self-tolerance has developed. Well-known examples are the immune responses to Factor VIII in a certain proportion of hemophilia A patients (Chapter 9), and to growth hormone in some growth hormone-deficient patients. In the case of hemophilia A, this immune response may render treatment with Factor VIII useless for some patients. Further treatment is then only possible using factor VIIa. For growth hormone, no serious side-effects of antibody formation have been reported.

Immunogenicity may also be caused by structural changes of the protein, which results in non-natural presentation of certain amino acids on the surface of the protein. From a theoretical perspective, partially unfolded monomeric proteins may elicit an immune response, if this partial unfolding results in exposure of antigen sites. It is unknown whether such a mechanism plays any role in the immunogenicity development, and this will also be difficult to determine; many partially unfolded molecules tend to aggregate rapidly, forming a non-native aggregate, which is itself potentially immunogenic. Immunogenicity of aggregates is discussed in more detail in Section 5.2.2.

Similarity of the protein to the endogenous species does not only include the amino acid sequence, but also its glycosylation pattern. A number of studies have shown that non-human carbohydrate residues may be immunogenic (Benatuil et al. 2005, Bolgiano et al. 2001, Cobb and Kasper 2005, Siddiqui et al. 2007). For example, 1–8% of all circulating antibodies in humans is reported to be reactive to the carbohydrate epitope αGal (Galα1-3Galβ1-4GlcNAc-R) (Benatuil et al. 2005). An additional potential danger of non-native glycosylation patterns, including absence thereof, includes the exposure of otherwise protected antigen sites on the protein. Experimental evidence is growing that altered glycosylation patterns of self-proteins is implicated in the development of several autoimmune disease. This should serve as a potential warning signal for biopharmaceuticals containing non-native glycosylation pattern.

The known immunogenicity of certain carbohydrate residues also shows the potential danger of administering non-protein compounds containing such residues. Glycosylation has been considered as a potential alternative to PEGylation (see Section 5.3.2), but its potential immunostimulatory effects means that careful design is required.

Increased immunogenicity caused by deviations from the endogenous structure may also be observed for oligonucleotides. A known method to increase the immunogenicity of DNA-based vaccines is the incorporation of so-called CpG motifs (Klinmann, Xie, and Ivins 2006), i.e., unmethylated dinucleotides of cytosine and guanine. These motifs are alien to the human body and usually result in a very efficient and direct immune response. It is obvious that such immunostimulatory activity may be highly undesirable when oligonucleotides are used for treatment purposes. There have been few studies on the immunogenicity of oligonucleotide-based therapeutics, and generally, there is much more focus on the potential immunogenicity of the required vectors to achieve proper delivery. However, it has been shown that even small interference RNA (siRNA) can stimulate the immune system (Schlee, Hornung, and Hartmann 2006). The recognition of RNA is probably an important factor in the innate defense system against viral infection. Thus, one should not expect that immunogenicity is not a problem for oligonucleotide-based drugs.

5.2.2. Aggregates and Array Structures

Many proteins have a tendency to form non-native associates, generally referred to as aggregates. Such aggregation may take place through partially unfolded intermediates, resulting in non-covalently linked aggregates, or through chemical reactions, such as disulfide scrambling or dityrosine formation (Chi et al. 2003, Wang 2005). Aggregates are heavily implicated in the immune response to a variety of protein drugs, and high levels of aggregates will generally cause great concern for regulatory agencies (Rosenberg 2006). Recently, studies on transgenic animals and immunotolerant mice have shown that aggregates of therapeutic proteins invoke an immune response (Hermeling et al. 2006, Maas et al. 2007, Purohit, Middaugh, and Balasubramanian 2006). Hermeling et al. (2006) observed that such an immune response was most reactive to the native protein, interferon-β, if the aggregates were composed of more native-like protein. This may explain why Purohit et al. (2006) did not observe cross-reactivity for recombinant human Factor VIII, as they challenged their animal model with protein aggregates prepared by heat stress. The latter often results in a significant change in protein structure.

Maas et al. (2007) have shown that the presence of fibrils, i.e., large and highly ordered protein aggregates, is linked to the immune response to biopharmaceuticals. The immunogenicity related to the presence of fibrils may be explained by array presentation, as discussed further below. However, fibrils contain protein molecules that usually are structurally different from the native protein. Thus, fibrils, and potentially also certain aggregates, may represent a "danger signal" rather than being directly involved in the immune response to the native protein. Frequent administration of the "danger signal" together with the native protein may then result in the body labeling the native protein as foreign, as discussed further in Section 5.2.3.

The most prevalent hypothesis to explain the immunogenicity of protein aggregates is the "array" hypothesis (Bachmann and Zinkernagel 1997, Bhanot 2004, Dintzis et al. 1989, Rosenberg 2006, Smith et al. 2006, Sulzer and Perelson 1997). The human immune system is specialized in recognizing proteins that are presented in some type of array format, such as is the case on viral capsids and bacterial cell walls. A number of studies in animals have shown that a very efficient immune response can be obtained by artificially creating such array structures, for example by linking proteins to a polymeric backbone. Aggregates may represent such an array structure themselves, and it has been suggested that the immunogenicity of Eprex (see also Chapter 6) may be related to the protein, rhEPO, being expressed as an array on micelles of the added surfactant (Hermeling et al. 2003). Others have criticized this hypothesis, and proposed leachates as the main cause of the immune response (see Section 5.2.3) (Heavner 2006, Sharma et al. 2004).

Arrays have also been used to explain why certain adjuvants are such potent immunostimulators: adsorption of the protein to the surface of these adjuvants results in an array presentation of the protein. Moreover, the array hypothesis may explain the (transient) immune response to long-circulating liposomes (Ishida et al. 2006b, Ishida et al. 2006a, Judge et al. 2006, Semple et al. 2005, Wang et al. 2005). The surface of these liposomes is modified with the polymer polyethylene glycol (PEG), which is meant to reduce protein adsorption to the surface and subsequent uptake by mainly the liver (known as opsonization). PEGylation of liposomes generally increases their circulation time with many factors upon the first injection, but when injected again within a few weeks after the first injection, a rapid clearance is observed. It has been shown that this is caused by IgM-type antibodies against the PEG-liposomes expressed after the first injection (Ishida et al. 2006b). These IgM antibodies have a limited expression period, and clearance is not observed when injecting, e.g., six weeks or more after the first injection.

The observed clearance of PEG-liposomes and the array hypothesis are a potential concern for several advanced drug delivery systems. In a number of approaches, antibodies, or other biopharmaceuticals, are coupled to larger structures containing a drug compound, in order to target the whole system to diseased sites. For example, liposomes can be modified to present compounds like antibodies or carbohydrates on their surface, which allow them to be bound to cells overexpressing certain antigens or receptors. In theory, this will result in an array presentation, and may thus lead to an immune response.

5.2.3. Product-Related Factors

As described in the previous sections, the similarity of the biopharmaceutical to the endogenous compound plays an important role in immunogenicity development. Studies in these areas have been reasonably comprehensive, allowing general conclusions to be drawn from the data. More elusive is the effect of the so-called product-related factors. These factors constitute the additional compounds other than the active ingredient found in the final product, such as degradation products, process- or product-related impurities, and additives.

The best summative description of those product-related factors that facilitate the immune response would be "danger signals" (see also Chapter 1). That is, the compound(s) itself activates the immune system, and due to their co-administration with the biopharmaceutical, the immune system also attacks the biopharmaceutical. The "danger signal" has also been implicated in the activity of various adjuvants, which enhance the otherwise weak immunogenicity of the intended vaccine.

It is unfortunately not always clear which compounds may result in a "danger signal", mainly due to the lack of systematic studies in this area (cf. Sharma 2007a, Sharma 2007b, Sharma 2007c). This makes it difficult to predict the importance of certain impurities. For example, leachates from injection devices have been implicated by the manufacturer as the potential cause of the enhanced immunogenicity of Eprex (Sharma et al. 2004). However, multiple actions were taken to reduce the immunogenicity, making it difficult to ascertain that leachates were indeed the main factors. Others have, for example, criticized the animal studies that were claimed to prove the involvement of the leachates (Schellekens and Jiskoot 2006). The variety of hypotheses put forward to explain the enhanced immunogenicity of Eprex shows the limited knowledge with respect to the factors that cause an immune response. Further research into this area is therefore required in order to clarify which impurities or additives may lead to potent immune responses.

5.2.4. Patient-Related Factors

Apart from the various factors introduced by the product, characteristics of the patients also play an important role. For example, the immune system of patients may differ genetically, resulting in a varying strength of the response to any immune stimulus. Moreover, the disease may reduce the activity of the immune system, and hence reduce the potential for an immune response to the biopharmaceutical. An additional factor is the required dose, and dosing regime, to treat the disease. Intuitively one can understand that high doses of a biopharmaceutical will increase the amount of both potential immunogenic biopharmaceutical as well as the possible "danger signals" in the formulation. Added with more frequent administration of both, there is a higher chance of triggering the immune system to take action. The above-mentioned rapid clearance of PEGylated liposomes upon frequent injections clearly shows the importance of the administration frequency.

Finally, the route of administration is of great importance to the potential of an immune response. In military terms, the human body has its main line of defense at the outer perimeter. That is, immunocompetent cells are mainly found in areas that are the first to be exposed to infiltrating parasites or unwanted substances, such as the skin and mucosa. As a result, the strength of an immune response to an antigen can be ordered by route of administration as subcutaneous (s.c.) > intramuscular (i.m.) > intravenous (i.v.). In many aspects this is rather unfortunate, as subcutaneous administration is the most amenable route for self-administration by patients. Intramuscular and intravenous administration require significantly more expertise, and are thus much less suited for self-administration.

The relationship between route of administration and immunogenicity is well known from the field of vaccines, and there is no reason to assume it is not valid for ordinary biopharmaceuticals. This is an important aspect, since there is an increasing focus on alternative routes of administration for both vaccines and biopharmaceuticals. For example, nasal and oral vaccine delivery are being investigated with increasing vigor, and similar routes are considered for biopharmaceuticals. If an efficient immune response is obtained for vaccines through these alternative routes, this should be considered as a potential warning for the delivery of biopharmaceuticals through the same route.

5.3. Methods for Reducing Immunogenicity

A wide scope of actions can be taken against the unwanted immunogenicity of a biopharmaceutical. Between the production of the drug product and the handling of the biopharmaceutical prior to administration, caution and consideration can to a large extent prevent or minimize adverse events. In an effort to minimize the unwanted immunogenicity of biopharmaceuticals, all factors as summarized in Table 5.1 should be considered as a whole.

5.3.1. Optimizing the Structure

The primary sequence of a protein, or the nucleotide sequence of a DNA or RNA molecule, has great impact on its interaction with the immune system. For proteins that are conformationally unstable, point mutations may be used to increase stability or to introduce sites for protein modification (Section 5.3.2). However, altering single amino acids in the protein sequence may also lead to immunogenicity against the protein. For example, the conversion of tyrosine into 3-nitrotyrosine (Ohmori and Kanayama. 2005) and of arginine into citrulline (Lundberg et al. 2005), respectively, gave powerful responses from the immune system. Point mutations should thus be considered carefully with regard to the prospect of unwanted immunogenicity versus the expected advantages. Conservative amino acid replacements will, however, be unlikely to foster new immunogenic epitopes.

The purity of the protein or oligonucleotide must be validated. This can be controlled during the production by optimizing cell lines and purification procedures. Uncontrolled, even when minor, impurities from the host cells can be strongly immunogenic and their presence can delay or terminate the entire early development of a biopharmaceutical.

The intrinsic immunogenicity of partial sequences in a biological molecule can be predicted with the help of epitope mapping, as has been considered in detail in chapter 4. Thus, in silico and in vitro studies can give indications of particularly immunogenic epitopes. This is a helpful instrument for de-immunization during the design and the early clinical development of the biopharmaceutical.

For many therapeutical antibodies, it is evident that the immunogenicity decreases as sequences are changed from murine to chimeric to fully human sequences (Weiner 2006). A few examples are treated in more detail in Chapters 10 and 11. Thus, if the protein has a murine sequence or epitope, the immunological profile might be improved by progressing toward more humanized sequences. Humanized and human antibodies can, however, still elicit considerable immunogenic responses (Presta 2006, Hwang and Foote 2005). The marketed fully human antibody adalimumab (Humira®) elicited human anti-human antibodies (HAHAs) in 12% of the patients treated (Abbott: Adalimumab Product Approval Information).

In case of therapeutic antibodies, the target for the antibody is also a determinant for unwanted immunogenicity. Targeting the antibody against B-cell markers should generally yield antibodies with less anti-antibody responses (AARs) as compared to non-B-cell markers (Hwang and Foote 2005).

Changing the quaternary structure or shifting the quaternary structure equilibrium of a protein might also have influence on unwanted immunogenicity. If the native protein exists in a monomer–multimer equilibrium, a shift in this equilibrium might affect its immunostimulatory effect. Usually, monomeric proteins unfold more easily than proteins in native conglomerates, and this could theoretically cause a more pronounced immunogenicity. However, insulin Lys-Pro, which is predominantly monomeric, is comparable to human insulin with regard to immunogenicity.

5.3.2. Modification of the Biomacromolecule

A well-established method for masking a protein against the immune system is the covalent attachment of a polyethylene glycol (PEG) molecule to the biological molecule. The modification with PEG has advantages other than the reduction of unwanted immunogenicity, such as better solubility, reduced clearance through the kidneys, improved stability toward, e.g., proteinases, and improved physical stability (Veronese and Pasut 2005). The choice of PEG size and shape, position of the PEGylation site(s), and number of PEGs attached depends on the aim of the PEGylation as well as on the structural and biological characteristics of the biomacromolecule in question. PEGs in the size range from 1 to 100 kDa have been explored for therapeutical use. The PEG architectures can be linear, multi-arm, or branched.

The covalent attachment of PEG to the protein can be accomplished using different activating groups, different linkers, and by targeting different amino acids. It is important for the retention of biological activity to control the number and positions of the PEGs. The sites for PEGylation can be selected using epitope mapping, such that particularly immunogenic epitopes are masked.

The easiest and most often encountered method is to couple a PEG reagent to the side chain amino group of a lysine or to the N-terminal of the protein.

The PEGylation of amino groups can to some extent be controlled by the pH during the coupling. A more precise method is to target a thiol group in the protein. PEG-maleimide is a popular reagent for this purpose, and gives a stable linkage. If a cysteine is not already present in the protein, it can be engineered into the sequence. The targeting of the PEG reagent to the wanted amino acid side chain is also governed by the size and structure of the PEG, as well as by the physical structure of the protein. Monographs on PEGylation chemistry and strategies are widely available.

The success of the PEGylation approach is remarkable, as evidenced by the numerous PEGylated biopharmaceuticals on the market. These include the G-SCF derivative Neulasta® (Amgen), which is PEGylated with a single 20 kDa PEG on the N-terminal; Pegvisomant, a growth hormone antagonist which is PEGylated with 4–6 5kDa PEGs on lysine residues; and the PEGylated oligonucleotide Macugen® (Pfizer), which has been PEGylated with a 40 kDa branched PEG. Despite this success it should be kept in mind that PEGylated proteins can still cause immunogenicity and antigenicity (Li et al. 2001).

Other polymers with comparable characteristics, e.g., dendrimers, can potentially be employed in the same manner in order to mask a protein and decrease its immunogenicity. The carbohydrate polymer polysialic acid has been much investigated and is a potential successor to PEG (Gregoriadis et al. 2005).

Glycosylation may also reduce, or enhance, the immunogenicity of a biomacromolecule. The absence of the natural glycosylation pattern in a protein has been thought to cause a swift development of neutralizing antibodies (Gribben et al. 1990, Schellekens 2004). Another, related reason for a diminished immunogenicity of glycosylated proteins can be that glycosylated proteins are often more stable toward misfolding and aggregation, examples being interferon-β (Runkel et al. 1998) and rhEPO (Tsuda et al. 1990, Narhi et al. 2001). On the other hand, some glycans will enhance immunogenicity, for example the plant glycans xylose and alpha-1,3-fucose (Bardor et al. 2003). Hence, for example plant production of biopharmaceuticals implies a humanization of the glycans (Lerouge et al. 2000). The challenge of engineering and analyzing glycosylation is a cornerstone of biopharmaceutical drug design (reviewed by, e.g., Sinclair and Elliot 2005, Brooks 2004).

5.3.3. Improving the Formulation

Since the development of an immunogenic response is thought to be linked to the chemical and physical construct of the molecule, the stability of the biomacromolecule in the formulation is paramount. Thus, the chemical and physical stability of the formulation should be optimized to yield as little degradation products as possible. For biopharmaceuticals, this entails the proper choice of buffer and pH, cosolvents, additives and excipients, and proper packaging and device design and materials.

A particular aspect of the latent immunogenicity of biopharmaceuticals is the so-called leachables or leachates. Leachables are a common denomination of organic and inorganic compounds that can leak out of packaging materials and contaminate a biopharmaceutical preparation. The presence of leachables in biopharmaceuticals is a source of concern for two reasons: they can be detrimental to the stability of the biological molecule and they can act as a "danger signal" or adjuvant that may provoke an immunogenic response to, e.g., an endogenous protein. The focus on leachables has been especially on the container closures as a source of impurities (Sharma 2007b), particularly after the outbreak of Eprex-related PRCA.

Concentrations in the ppm range of various compounds leaking from the packaging material can be damaging to the stability. Certain metal ions are, e.g., known to have a negative effect on the physical stability of proteins such as alpha-synuclein (Binolfi et al. 2006) and GLP-1 derivatives (Christensen et al. 2007).

Plasticizers, curing agents, and antioxidants are also among the compounds that can leak from container closures or other primary packaging materials. Clearly, good and detailed specifications of the primary packaging and meticulous quality control of the delivered goods are means to optimize the quality of biopharmaceuticals and to limit possible immunogenicity.

The choice of material for and the design of the primary and secondary packaging are important. Protection from light is generally helpful, since photodegradation is a stepping stone for biopharmaceutical denaturation. Also, since proteins are known to adsorb to surfaces and may irreversibly denature at those surfaces, it can be advantageous to minimize surface contacts as much as possible, both to the air–liquid surface and to the liquid–material surface. A proper choice of material for the primary packaging may reduce adsorption and increase the physical stability of the therapeutic molecule.

5.3.4. Clinical Measures

Much can be done to counter the unwanted immunogenicity of biopharmaceuticals in the clinical step. To begin with, the handling of the biopharmaceutical is of crucial importance for the frequency of immunogenicity-related adverse effects in the patients. Improper storage temperatures, repeated freezing–thawing events, shaking, or exposure to sunlight can all affect the quality of the product in one way or another. Qualified cold-chain logistics and quality assurance on the entire storing and shipping procedure is a necessity for any company in the field of biotechnology products intended for human or animal use.

It is important to realize that the generally delicate nature of biopharmaceuticals demands delicate handling. Shaking or heating an ampoule with a biopharmaceutical drug can lead to formation of denatured or aggregated protein. Package inserts with description of correct handling procedures may be helpful, but education of the health professionals in the handling of biotechnology products will remain an important issue in the future.

As mentioned in Section 5.2.4, the dosing schedule is likewise an important factor. Repeated challenge of the immune system with a biopharmaceutical gives a higher incidence of immunogenicity than a bolus injection given just once. Often, however, this is difficult to manipulate, since the pharmacology of the drug will to a large extent govern the dosing schedule.

The route of administration has a large significance. Administration by the intravenous route will rarely, if ever, lead to the induction of neutralizing antibodies, but in adverse cases may result in an anaphylactic shock. A marketing approval for i.v. administration should in most cases be possible even if risk of immunogenicity development is high. Since s.c. administration is more patient-friendly, it is often an important parameter of competition on the market. Subcutaneous administration is known to provoke adverse immunologic events, the reason for this being the large number of immune cells in the skin. Thus if the target disease justifies an s.c. administration, it is the more important to optimize all other factors in order to secure a good immunogenicity profile.

In summary, biopharmaceuticals are much more fragile than small molecule drugs. The causes for unwanted immunogenicity and antigenicity of biopharmaceuticals are still not very well understood. For the pharma company that works in the field of biopharmaceuticals, it is therefore necessary to exert a very high level of quality control in *every* step from production to patient in order to minimize the frequency of antibody formation to a biopharmaceutical. This should be done, not only during the clinical development of the biopharmaceutical, but equally so in the post-marketing phase.

5.4. Biosimilars

5.4.1. Biosimilar Development

In the low molecular weight drugs market, patent expiry often leads to the development of one or more generic products. These generics are significantly cheaper than the original, or innovator, product. There are three main reasons for this reduced price. First, the generics manufacturer has much lower costs in the initial research and development of the drug. Whereas the innovator product has come from a long and tedious elimination process of sometimes thousands of potential candidates, the generics manufacturer knows exactly which compound to produce, and to a large extent also the most appropriate formulation and route of administration. Second, marketing costs are significantly lower. Physicians need to be convinced that the innovator product is a useful product in the treatment of a disease, but the generics manufacturer only needs to make physicians and/or pharmacists aware that there is a generic. Third, the generic usually only needs to be bioequivalent to the innovator product. That is, if the active compound is chemically equivalent to the innovator product and shows the same pharmacokinetic and pharmacodynamic profile, it is assumed that safety and efficacy are also equal. This results in a significant reduction in clinical trials, and hence much lower costs of the final product.

It is highly attractive, from an economic perspective, to approach the market for biopharmaceuticals in a similar way. Biopharmaceuticals are generally very expensive, and even a modest reduction in price of these products can save billions of euros in health care costs. Unfortunately, most biopharmaceuticals are highly complex molecules, making it essentially impossible to assure the presence of a chemically and physically equivalent molecule (Belsey et al. 2006, Schellekens 2002a, Schellekens 2004). Moreover, it is almost impossible to characterize all degradation products and their safety profile. Even manufacturers of innovator products frequently obtain different profiles for their active compound, also in cases where seemingly trivial changes are made (Sharma 2007c). Full structural characterization and equivalence is not possible, implying that similar bioequivalence does not assure the same efficacy and safety profile of the biogeneric. The complex nature of the immune response to biopharmaceuticals, discussed in Section 5.2, shows how small differences may have big and unpredictable effects. The risk assessment required in the development of biopharmaceuticals is discussed in more detail in Chapter 13.

As biopharmaceuticals are so complex, truly generic products are considered impossible, and one rather speaks of biosimilars or follow-on biologicals. The European Union has made a political decision in 2004 to allow these biosimilars on the market, forcing the European regulatory agencies to make guidelines. A concerted effort has resulted in several relevant guidelines that require the biosimilar to be compared to an already marketed product, both structurally as well as clinically (EMEA 2005). That is, efficacy and safety need to be tested and compared to an already marketed product. Schellekens (2004) has noted that this requirement may actually result in more and more complex clinical trials, involving larger numbers of patients, than development of the innovator product required. For example, a rhEPO biosimilar may need to be tested over a period of several years on tens of thousands of patients, to assure that no PRCA cases occur. Thus, economical benefits may be limited for some biosimilars.

The possibility of getting biosimilars approved was put to test in 2006, and saw a victorious outcome for the generics manufacturers: the European Medicines Evaluation Agency approved Sandoz's Omnitrope as a biosimilar (EMEA 2006a), soon followed by Valtropin (EMEA 2006b); both products are recombinant human growth hormone biosimilars. Earlier, the Australian regulatory agencies had approved Omnitrope under its own set of regulations. However, it was not all good news, as BioPartners GmbH had Alpheon, a recombinant interferon alpha-2a biosimilar, rejected by the EU (EMEA 2006c).

The situation in the USA is less clear than in the EU. Officially, the FDA does not have any provisions for biosimilars (or follow-on biologicals) (Beers and Tsang 2007, Chamberlain 2004, Dove 2001). Nevertheless, Omnitrope was approved in the USA in 2006, based on an application that involved comparison with a competitor product, Pfizer's Genotropin (Beers and Tsang 2007). The FDA maintains that it did not consider Omnitrope as a biosimilar, but invoked §505(b)(2), which allows products to be approved that are not considered true generics but sufficiently similar to already marketed products. This paragraph only applies to a small handful of biopharmaceuticals, which were approved under the Federal Food, Drug, and Cosmetic Act (FFDCA). Most other biopharmaceuticals have been, and are, approved under the Public Health Safety Act (PHSA), which puts stricter demands on new drug applications. Thus, further biosimilar approvals in the USA in the near future are probably restricted to those products approved under the FFDCA, while new legislation is required for products approved under the PHSA.

5.4.2. Potential Differences Between Biosimilars and the Innovator Product

The highly complex manufacturing process of biological products makes it inherently impossible to produce exact copies. That is, the level of impurities from the production process as well as the degradation product profile of the biosimilar may all differ from the innovator product. This implies that one can never assure full bioequivalency, including safety profile, between the biosimilar and the innovator product without clinical studies.

It may be argued that biosimilars may well be safer. In the past few decades, significant improvements have been made in understanding many crucial aspects of the production process, as well as the potential danger factors for immunogenicity development. In fact, production processes have been improved to such an extent, that it may be difficult to produce a product which is as "bad" as the innovator product with respect to the amount of degradation products and impurities. However, since the production host, site, and facilities will differ, there may be other degradation products and impurities in the biosimilar product. Their potential to cause an immune response may be larger than those in the innovator product, thus offsetting the possible smaller amount of degradation products and impurities. In addition, the use of other formulation principles, materials, and procedures during storage and administration may affect the level of degradation products upon the actual administration of the biosimilar. The case study on rhEPO (Chapter 6) shows the profound, in this case positive, effect of changes in packaging material, storage procedures, and route of administration. Thus, only clinical studies will be able to show that the biosimilar product is truly as safe and efficacious as the innovator product. If those are as extensive as for a innovator product, filing the product as a biosimilar would not be beneficial.

While the discussion above may appear to paint a rather bleak picture for biosimilar development, the recent approvals of Omnitrope and Valtropin shows that it is not an impossible task. Probably the most important factor for successful development of a biosimilar is a proven trackrecord of the innovator product. Both Omnitrope and Valtropin contain a protein drug to which there are essentially no reported serious adverse immune responses. Other such generally safe protein drugs, such as recombinant human insulin, may thus also be developed as biosimilars, whereas a rhEPO biosimilar may be much less likely. Indeed, Pliva has abandoned its advance program to develop a rhEPO biosimilar due to the expected costs for the clinical trials.

5.5. Conclusions

There is a wide range of factors involved in the immune response to biopharmaceuticals. It is still unknown which of these factors are the most important, but there is a slowly increasing effort to study this in more detail. So far, these studies indicate that structural equality between biopharmaceutical and native compound is insufficient to assure the absence of an immune response. Impurities and degradation products, especially those resulting in an array presentation of the biopharmaceutical, can result in a highly undesirable immune response. The unpredictability in this immune response will remain the main hurdle for the development of biosimilars, until all factors causing an immune response are clarified, or until a robust and predictive cell or animal model is developed.

References

Bachmann, M. F. and Zinkernagel, R. M. 1997. Neutralizing antiviral B cell responses. Ann. Rev. Immunol. 15:235–270.
Bardor, M., Faveeuw, C., Fitchette, A. C., Gilbert, D., Galas, L., Trottein, F., Faye, L., and Lerouge, P. 2003. Immunoreactivity in mammals of two typical plant glyco-epitopes, core alpha(1,3)-fucose and core xylose. Glycobiology 13:427–434.

Beers, D. O. and Tsang, L. 2007. US rules on biosimilars – what has changed? www.practicallaw.com/5-205-4376. Access date August 2007.

Belsey, M. J., Harris, L. M., Das, R. R., and Chertkow, J. 2006. Biosimilars: initial excitement gives way to reality. Nat. Rev. Drug Discov. 5:535–536.

Benatuil, L., Kaye, J., Rich, R. F., Fishman, J. A., Green, W. R., and Iacomini, J. 2005. The influence of natural antibody specificity on antigen immunogenicity. Eur. J. Immunol. 35:2638–2647.

Bhanot, G. 2004. Results from modeling of B-cell receptors binding to antigen. Progress Biophys. Mol. Biol. 85:343–352.

Binolfi, A., Rasia, R. M., Bertoncini, C. W., Ceolin, M., Zweckstetter, M., Griesinger, C., Jovin, T. M., and Fernandez, C. O. 2006. Interaction of alpha-synuclein with divalent metal ions reveals key differences: a link between structure, binding specificity and fibrillation enhancement. J. Am. Chem. Soc. 128:9893–9901.

Bolgiano, B., Mawas, F., Yost, S. E., Crane, D. T., Lemercinier, X., and Corbel, M. J. 2001. Effect of physico-chemical modification on the immunogenicity of *Haemophilus influenza* type b oligosaccharide-CRM$_{197}$ conjugate vaccines. Vaccine 19:3189–3200.

Brooks, S. A. 2004. Appropriate glycosylation of recombinant proteins for human use: implications of choice of expression system. Mol. Biotechnol. 28:241–255.

Chamberlain, P. 2004. Biogenerics: Europe takes another step forward while the FDA dives for cover. Drug Discov. Today 9:817–820.

Cheifetz, A. and Mayer, L. 2005. Monoclonal antibodies, immunogenicity, and associated infusion reactions. Mt. Sinai J. Med. 72:250–256.

Chi, E. Y., Krishnan, S., Randolph, T. W., and Carpenter, J. F. 2003. Physical stability of proteins in aqueous solution: mechanism and driving forces in nonnative protein aggregation. Pharm. Res. 20:1325–1336.

Christensen, S., Moeller, E. H., Bonde, C., and Lilleoere, A. M. 2007. Preliminary studies of the physical stability of a glucagon-like peptide-1 derivate in the presence of metal ions. Eur. J. Pharm. Biopharm. 66:366–371.

Cobb, B. A. and Kasper, D. L. 2005. Coming of age: carbohydrates and immunity. Eur. J. Immunol. 35:352–356.

Dintzis, R. Z., Okajima, M., Middleton, M. H., Greene, G., and Dintzis, H. M. 1989. The immunogenicity of soluble haptenated polymers is determined by molecular mass and hapten valence. J. Immunol. 143:1239–1244.

Dove, A. 2001. Betting on biogenerics. Nat. Biotech. 19:117–120.

EMEA. 2005. Guideline on similar biological medicinal products. CHMP/437/04.

EMEA. 2006a. European public assessment report (EPAR) – Omnitrope. EMEA/H/C/607.

EMEA. 2006b. European public assessment report (EPAR) – Valtropin. EMEA/H/C/602.

EMEA. 2006c. Questions and answers on recommendation for refusal of marketing application for Alpheon. EMEA/190896/2006.

Gregoriadis, G., Jain, S., Papaioannou, I., and Laing, P. 2005. Improving the therapeutic efficacy of peptides and proteins: a role for polysialic acids. Int. J. Pharm. 300:125–130.

Gribben, J. G., Devereux, S., Thomas, N. S., Keim, M., Jones, H. M., Goldstone, A. H., and Linch, D. C. 1990. Development of antibodies to unprotected glycosylation sites on recombinant human GM-CSF. Lancet 335:434–437.

Heavner, G. A. 2006. Rebuttal letter. Pharm. Res. 23:643–644.

Hermeling, S., Crommelin, D. J. A., Schellekens, H., and Jiskoot, W. 2004. Structure-immunogenicity relationships of therapeutic proteins. Pharm. Res. 21:897–903.

Hermeling, S., Schellekens, H., Crommelin, D. J. A., and Jiskoot, W. 2003. Micelle-associated protein in epoietin formulations: a risk factor for immunogenicity? Pharm. Res. 20:1903–1907.

Hermeling, S., Schellekens, H., Maas, C., Gebbink, M. F. B. G., Crommelin, D. J. A., and Jiskoot, W. 2006. Antibody response to aggregated human interferon alpha2b in wild-type and transgenic immune tolerant mice depends on type and level of aggregation. J. Pharm. Sci. 95:1084–1096.

Hwang, W. Y. K., and Foote, J. 2005. Immunogenicity of engineered antibodies. Methods 36:3–10.

Ishida, T., Ichihara, M., Wang, X. Y., and Kiwada, H. 2006a. Spleen plays an important role in the induction of accelerated blood clearance of PEGylated liposomes. J. Control. Release 115:243–250.

Ishida, T., Ichihara, M., Wang, X. Y., Yamamoto, K., Kimura, J., Majima, E., and Kiwada, H. 2006b. Injection of PEGylated liposomes in rats elicits PEG-specific IgM, which is responsible for rapid elimination of a second dose of PEGylated liposomes. J. Control. Release 112:15–25.

Judge, A., McClintock, K., Phelps, J. R., and MacLachlan, I. 2006. Hypersensitivity and loss of disease site targeting caused by antibody responses to PEGylated liposomes. Mol. Ther. 13:328–337.

Klinmann, D. M., Xie, H., and Ivins, B. E. 2006. CpG oligonucleotides improve the protective immune response induced by the licensed anthrax vaccine. Ann. N. Y. Acad. Sci. 1082:137–150.

Lerouge, P., Bardor, M., Pagny, S., Gomord, V., and Faye, L. 2000. N-glycosylation of recombinant pharmaceutical glycoproteins produced in transgenic plants: towards an humanisation of plant N-glycans. Curr. Pharm. Biotechnol. 1:347–354.

Li, J., Yang, C., Xia, Y., Bertino, A., Glaspy, J., Roberts, M., and Kuter, D. J. 2001. Thrombocytopenia caused by the development of antibodies to thrombopoietin. Blood 98:3241–3248.

Lundberg, K., Nijenhuis, S., Vossenaar, E. R., Palmblad, K., van Venrooij, W. J., Klareskog, L., Zendman, A. J., and Harris, H. E. 2005. Citrullinated proteins have increased immunogenicity and arthritogenicity and their presence in arthritic joints correlates with disease severity. Arthritis Res. Ther. 7:R458–R467.

Maas, C., Hermeling, S., Bouma, B., Jiskoot, W., and Gebbink, M. F. B. G. 2007. A role for protein misfolding in immunogenicity of biopharmaceuticals. J. Biol. Chem. 282:2229–2236.

Narhi, L. O., Arakawa, T., Aoki, K., Wen, J., Elliott, S., Boone, T., and Cheetham, J. 2001. Asn to Lys mutations at three sites which are N-glycosylated in the mammalian protein decrease the aggregation of Escherichia coli-derived erythropoietin. Protein Eng 14:135–140.

Ohmori, H., and Kanayama, N. 2005. Immunogenicity of an inflammation-associated product, tyrosine nitrated self-proteins. Autoimmun. Rev. 4:224–229.

Presta, L. G. 2006. Engineering of therapeutic antibodies to minimize immunogenicity and optimize function. Adv. Drug Deliv. Rev. 58:640–656.

Purohit, V. S., Middaugh, C. R., and Balasubramanian, S. V. 2006. Influence of aggregation on immunogenicity of recombinant human factor VIII in hemophilia A mice. J. Pharm. Sci. 95:358–371.

Rosenberg, A. S. 2006. Effects of protein aggregates: an immunologic perspective. AAPS J. 8(3):59.

Runkel, L., Meier, W., Pepinsky, R. B., Karpusas, M., Whitty, A., Kimball, K., Brickelmaier, M., Muldowney, C., Jones, W., and Goelz, S. E. 1998. Structural and functional differences between glycosylated and non-glycosylated forms of human interferon-beta (IFN-beta). Pharm. Res. 15:641–649.

Schellekens, H. 2002a. Bioequivalence and the immunogenicity of biopharmaceuticals. Nat. Rev. 1:457–462.

Schellekens, H. 2002b. Immunogenicity of therapeutic proteins: clinical implications and future prospects. Clin. Therap. 24:1720–1740.

Schellekens, H. 2004. How similar do 'biosimilars' need to be? Nat. Biotech. 22: 1357–1359.

Schellekens, H., and Casadevall, N. 2004. Immunogenicity of recombinant human proteins: causes and consequences. J. Neurol. 251:II/4–II/9.

Schellekens, H., and Jiskoot, W. 2006. Eprex-associated pure red cell aplasia and leachates. Nat. Biotech. 24:613–614.

Schlee, M., Hornung, V., and Hartmann, G. 2006. siRNA and isRNA: two edges of one sword. Mol. Ther. 14:463–470.

Semple, S. C., Harasym, T. O., Clow, K. A., Ansell, S. M., Klimuk, S. K., and Hope, M. J. 2005. Immunogenicity and rapid blood clearance of liposomes containing polyethylene glycol-lipid conjugates and nucleic acid. J. Pharmacol. Exp. Therap. 312:1020–1026.

Sharma, B. 2007a. Immunogenicity of therapeutic proteins. Part 1: impact of product handling. Biotechnol. Adv. 25:310–317.

Sharma, B. 2007b. Immunogenicity of therapeutic proteins. Part 2: impact of container closures. Biotechnol. Adv. 25:318–324.

Sharma, B. 2007c. Immunogenicity of therapeutic proteins. Part 3: impact of manufacturing changes. Biotechnol. Adv. 25:325–331.

Sharma, B., Bader, F., Templeman, T., Lisi, P., Ryan, M., and Heavner, G. A. 2004. Technical investigations into the cause of the increased incidence of antibody-mediated pure red cell aplasia associated with Eprex. Eur. J. Hosp. Pharm. 5:86–91.

Siddiqui, N. I., Idakieva, K., Demarsin, B., Doumanova, L., Compernolle, F., and Gielens, C. 2007. Involvement of glycan chains in the antigenicity of Rapana thomasiana hemocyanin. Biochem. Biophys. Res. Commun. 361:705–711.

Sinclair, A. M., and Elliott, S. 2005. Glycoengineering: the effect of glycosylation on the properties of therapeutic proteins. J. Pharm. Sci. 94:1626–1635.

Smith, M. L., Lindbo, J. A., Dillard-Telm, S., Brosio, P. M., Lasnik, A. B., McCormick, A. A., Nguyen, L. V., and Palmer, K. E. 2006. Modified *Tobacco mosaic virus* particles as scaffolds for display of protein antigens for vaccine applications. Virology 348:475–488.

Sulzer, B. and Perelson, A. S. 1997. Immunons revisited: binding of multivalent antigens to B cells. Mol. Immunol. 34:63–74.

Tsuda, E., Kawanishi, G., Ueda, M., Masuda, S., and Sasaki, R. 1990. The role of carbohydrate in recombinant human erythropoietin. Eur. J. Biochem. 188:405–411.

Veronese, F. M., and Pasut, G. 2005. PEGylation, successful approach to drug delivery. Drug Discov. Today 10:1451–1458.

Wang, W. 2005. Protein aggregation and its inhibition in biopharmaceutics. Int. J. Pharm. 289:1–30.

Wang, X. Y., Ishida, T., Ichihara, M., and Kiwada, H. 2005. Influence of the physicochemical properties of liposomes on the accelerated blood clearance phenomenon in rats. J. Control. Release 104:91–102.

Weiner, L. M. 2006. Fully human therapeutic monoclonal antibodies. J. Immunother. 29:1–9.

Case Study: Immunogenicity of rhEPO

Arno Kromminga and Gilbert Deray

6.1. Abstract

Erythropoietin is an endogenous growth factor that is required for erythropoiesis. The hormone consists of a single acidic polypeptide chain of 165 amino acids and three N-linked and one O-linked carbohydrate side chains. Autoantibodies against endogenous EPO are extremely rare in humans. Since its introduction as a drug for the treatment of renal and non-renal anemia, antibodies against recombinant human erythropoietin were observed in low frequencies in single cases only. Due to a steep increase in the number of patients developing anti-erythropoietin antibodies during the course of therapy from 1999 to 2004 there is an increased interest in the observation of patients treated with erythropoietin. Moreover, new products as well as modified versions of the natural hormone have entered the market. In addition, modified versions with optimized features as well as peptides mimicking the erythropoietin action are under development and will enter clinical trials soon. These aspects make it essential to screen patients for the presence of anti-EPO antibodies. Despite the lack of a common calibrator, screening assays for the detection of anti-erythropoietin antibodies are available.

6.2. Description of Erythropoietin

6.2.1. Structure and Function

Human erythropoietin (EPO) is an acidic polypeptide consisting of 165 amino acids with a molecular mass of 30.4 kD (Jelkmann 2007). The carbohydrate moiety consists of three tetra-antennary N-linked (Asn 24, Asn 38 and Asn 83) and one O-linked chains (Ser 126) and constitutes up to 40% of the molecular mass (Sasaki et al. 1988). The glycosylation pattern is diverse and leads to a certain degree of heterogeneity. The structure and length of the sialic acids directly affect the biological activity and plasma half-life time of the hormone. It is noteworthy that some N-glycosidic chains are targets of sulfation, of which the biological function is still unknown.

EPO is a member of an extensive cytokine family that includes growth hormone, somatropin, prolactin, interleukins 2 through 7 as well as "colony stimulating factors" (G-CSF, M-CSF and GM-CSF). The hormone is mainly synthesized in the endothelial kidney cells (85–90%). Only minor amounts are produced in other cell types including hepatocytes and other tissues like brain, uterus, testis and even hair follicles (10–15%). The serum concentration (2–24 mIU/ml) is maintained by a feedback mechanism based on the tissue O_2 pressure (pO_2), which depends on the hemoglobin concentration, the arterial pO_2, the O_2 affinity of the hemoglobin and the rate of the blood flow. High serum concentrations of EPO are found in various tumors including renal tumors, hepatic tumors, cerebellar hemangioblastoma and adrenal tumors as a consequence of a reduced oxygen availability, i.e., the synthesis of EPO is stimulated by hypoxia. Decreased serum concentration of EPO in the serum is found in different forms of terminal and pre-terminal kidney insufficiencies as well as anemia of unknown origin like chronic infections, autoimmune diseases, AIDS, hypothyroidism, etc.

During erythropoiesis in the bone marrow EPO binds to its erythropoietin receptor (EPOR) on erythroid progenitor cells, which leads to their final differentiation to erythrocytes via the JAK-STAT-signal pathway. In this way each day more than 200 billion erythrocytes are produced. In addition to the mere erythropoiesis, EPO is also involved in apoptotic processes and stimulates the generation of megakaryocytes. It was shown that EPOR is expressed in numerous cell types including neurons, astrocytes, myocytes and hair follicles (D'Andrea and Zon 1990). The EPO/EPOR interaction was observed in various non-erythroid tissues in the context of cell differentiation, chemotaxis, angiogenesis, activation of intracellular calcium and inhibition of apoptosis. Some studies have demonstrated the neuroprotecting and neurotrophic effects of EPO (Marti et al. 2000, Ehrenreich et al. 2002).

6.2.2. Manufacturers of Recombinant Human EPO and EPO Variants

Since the first launch of recombinant human EPO in 1989 by Amgen, many different recombinant EPO preparations have reached the market. Besides the well-established recombinant EPO preparations, there are also numerous novel preparations under development. In 1989 Amgen launched the first recombinant human EPO preparation (Epogen, epoetin a). Johnson & Johnson has developed, under a license from Amgen, a variant named epoetin β which is known under the names Procrit (in USA) and Eprex (outside USA) or Erypo (in Europe). In 1990 Boehringer Mannheim (now Roche) brought an EPO preparation (epoetin β) under the name of NeoRecormon on the market. Although both preparations are produced in CHO cells, epoetin a and epoetin β show a slightly different molecular mass due to some differences in the glycosylation pattern. Additional variants were developed, like epoietin ω (Elanex Pharmaceuticals) which shows differences in glycosylation due to its production in BHK kidney cells.

Genetically modified EPO versions were developed to achieve optimized pharmacokinetic characteristics compared to natural endogenous human EPO or other recombinant versions (Bunn 2007). Realizing that glycosylation is an important factor for the circulation time of EPO in human plasma, Amgen produced in 2001 a modified EPO preparation (Aranesp, darbepoetin a) with a threefold prolonged serum half-life. This was achieved by the substitution of five amino acids generating additional glycosylation sites. Furthermore, in 2004 Amgen has introduced an Aranesp analog under the name of AMG114 which was shown to have a half-life time in human serum of up to 131 hours.

Besides protein engineering, chemical modification is an alternative approach to optimize protein characteristics. Roche has developed a variant of EPO with a half-life time of 135 hours by the method of PEGylation. In addition, this product, called CERA (continuous erythropoiesis receptor activator), seems to show different binding kinetics to its receptor compared with endogenous EPO. Other manufacturers also work on the generation of PEGylated variants of EPO, some using different expression systems. Moreover, by introducing other chemical modifications like carbamylation the function of EPO can be modified.

A third approach to optimize protein characteristics is a variation in the route of administration. Usually EPO is administered subcutaneously or intravenously. An alternative is an administration method by inhalation. Syntonix (a subsidiary of Biogen Idec) developed an EPO–Fc fusion protein which uses the FcRn pathway for pulmonary delivery.

In the last few years several companies have developed synthetic peptides that mimic the biological erythropoietic action of EPO. Besides synthetic homologs of the native EPO form, peptides were developed with no homologies to the EPO peptide sequence. A synthetic cyclic peptide-based erythropoiesis-stimulating agent (Hematite™) has been produced by Affymax (Palo Alto, CA, USA). The PEGylated synthetic product has recently entered the clinical study phase (Fan et al. 2006). Another synthetic EPO mimetic peptide from Aplagen (Baesweiler, Germany), which is coupled to a macromolecule, is currently under development and has entered the pre-clinical phase. Besides pharmacokinetic and (possibly) pharmacodynamic improvements, these synthetic products are not targets of an immune response by anti-EPO antibodies and therefore could be used to treat EPO-induced PRCA patients. Whether or not these peptides are themselves targeted by the immune systems and may induce an adverse immune response is not known yet.

6.3. Immune Reactions

The development and validation of assays to detect human anti-EPO antibodies in serum or plasma has been hampered a long time by the lack of purified antibodies as assay calibrators. Four types of assays have been published and used for the detection of binding antibodies against EPO: a radioimmunoprecipitation assay (RIPA), a direct ELISA, a bridging ELISA and an SPR analysis using the BIAcore technology.

6.3.1. Radioimmunoprecipitation Assay

The analysis of anti-EPO antibodies by radioimmunoprecipitation (RIP) makes use of radioactive 125-iodinated recombinant human erythropoietin (Casadevall et al. 2002a, Tacey et al. 2003). Antibodies in the serum of patients are bound by protein G immobilized on sepharose beads. Antibodies with reactivity against EPO are detected by the measurement of radioactivity in the precipitate. The amount of radioactive counts is correlated with the antibody concentration. The availability and preparation of an affinity-purified human antibody to EPO enabled the establishment of a RIP assay that is calibrated with a human standard. The lower limit of detection of this RIP is 8 ng/ml, the precision ranges from 5.8 to 15.3%. The mean coefficient of variation ranged from 6.1 to 16.6% for antibody concentrations between 7.8 and 500 ng/ml. Both the sensitivity and specificity of this assay are >98%.

6.3.2. Enzyme-Linked Immunosorbent Assays (ELISA)

ELISA methods have long been hampered by the lack of specificity. ELISA methods used for the detection of anti-EPO antibodies are either performed in a direct or bridging format. In direct ELISAs antibodies in serum samples are detected after binding to immobilized antigen on the surface of microtiterplates by adding a enzyme-labeled secondary antibody. Several modifications of this assay have been performed and published (Tzioufas et al. 1997, Sipsas et al. 1999, Castelli et al. 2000, Schett et al. 2001). Improved ELISA formats like the bridging type of ELISA have significantly increased the specificity of the method (Kientsch-Engel et al. 1990, Urra et al. 1997, Swanson et al. 2004, Gross et al. 2006). One of the ELISAs (Kientsch-Engel et al. 1990) includes control material to assess the function of the test and uses a competitive pre-adsorption using rhEPO to determine the specificity of the measured immune reaction. Most recently an optimized bridging ELISA was published, which demonstrated a high sensitivity of 10 ng/ml and high specificity (Gross et al. 2006). This assay detects anti-EPO antibodies by bridging two separately labeled rhEPO-molecules by one anti-EPO Ab. A rabbit polyclonal anti-EPO IgG serves as reference material for this ELISA. It should be mentioned that this rabbit antibody preparation may react different than antibodies of human origin due to different affinities.

6.3.3. Surface Plasmon Resonance (SPR)

The SPR analysis for the detection of anti-EPO antibodies using BIAcore analysis is a label-free real-time binding assay. The sensitivity of this method (approximately 400 ng/ml) is usually lower than the sensitivity of screening assays like RIPA and ELISA, but SPR is superior for the exact characterization of the antibodies (Swanson et al. 2004, Mason et al. 2003). While immunoassays detect the end-state concentration of antibodies, SPR detects the kinetic process of binding and gives avidity data. As in immunoassays the antigen is immobilized on a solid surface, i.e., a sensor chip, and the interaction with the ligand, i.e., antibodies, is detected by an increase in accumulating mass. For the analysis of antibody isotypes or subclasses a secondary (label-free) anti-immunoglobulin is added.

6.3.4. Bioassays for NAbs

The neutralizing capacity of binding anti-EPO antibodies is assessed by cellular assays which use an EPO-dependent cell line (TF-1, UT-7) or bone marrow biopsies. An EPO-dependent subclone of the human acute myeloid leukemia UT-7 cell line (ACC 137) originally derived from bone marrow of a 64-year-old male patient with acute myeloid leukemia can be used for the detection of neutralizing anti-EPO antibodies. Some investigators use a subclone of the TF-1 human erythroleukemic cell line. The most sensitive, but most difficult to obtain, assay is the use of erythroid cells from bone marrow (Casadevall et al. 2002a).

6.4. Clinical Relevance and Therapeutic Consequences

Anemia is an almost universal finding in patients with end-state renal disease (Eschbach and Adamson 1985). The uncomplicated anemia of patients with chronic renal failure (CRF) is normocytic and normochronic (Besarab, Ross, and Nasca 1995). The bone marrow of such patients is usually "normocellular", without the compensatory increase in erythroid activity expected for the degree of anemia.

The primary cause of anemia in patients with chronic kidney disease (CKD) is insufficient production of EPO by the diseased kidneys (Eckardt 2001, Eschbach 1989). Additional factors which may cause or contribute to the anemia include: iron deficiency, needle punctures, blood retention in the dialysis instrument, gastrointestinal bleeding, severe hyperparathyroidism, inflammation and shortened red blood cell survival (NKF-K/DOQI 2001). If left unattended, these factors will influence the outcome of rhEPO treatment in all pre-dialysis patients with CRF.

Dialysis patients have an age-adjusted death rate estimated to be 3.5 times higher than that of the general population (Foley et al. 1996). A considerable proportion of this excess mortality can be explained by the high prevalence of non-renal comorbid conditions, such as diabetes mellitus and cardiovascular disease among patients reaching end-stage renal disease (ESRD) therapy. In recent years, there has been a growing realization that factors which are unrelated to baseline comorbid illnesses may be causes or markers of poor outcome in dialysis patients. For example, it is generally accepted that a low serum albumin concentration, the amount of solute removal during dialysis and anemia are independent predictors of mortality in these patients (Collins, Ma, and Keshavish 1994).

When untreated the anemia of CKD is associated with a number of physiologic abnormalities, including decreased tissue oxygen delivery and utilization, increased cardiac output, cardiac enlargement, ventricular hypertrophy, angina, congestive heart failure, decreased cognition and mental acuity and impaired immune responsiveness (NKF-K/DOQI 2001, Foley et al. 1996, Collins, Ma, and Keshavish 1994).

During the last 15 years evidence-based clinical practice recommendations have been developed to guide appropriate anemia management. Current evidence supports that hemoglobin (Hgb) levels greater than 11 g/dl improve outcome. The target may need to be varied for patients with CRF with specific comorbidities. However, the optimal Hgb level and upper limit of the desired range has not yet been clearly elucidated. Differences in opinion exist when interpreting evidence, and some support Hgb level normalization whereas others do not. Two large randomized clinical trials examining greater Hgb values showed more cardiovascular complications and a trend towards greater mortality in pre-dialyzed or ESRD patients randomized to "normal" Hgb (Besarab et al. 1998, Singh et al. 2006). Another recent trial showed no increase in mortality in pre-dialyzed patients whose hemoglobin was normalized (Drüeke et al. 2006). From these trials it was concluded that Hb concentrations greater than 12 g/dl are not recommended in patients with severe cardiovascular disease.

Two decades have passed since the first patients with ESRD were treated with rhEPO (Winearls et al. 1986). Prior to 1990 the treatment of renal anemia was highly unsatisfactory, relying on iron supplementation, repeated blood transfusions and occasionally androgen therapy. Many patients were transfusion dependent. Therefore, they were exposed to the risks of transmission of infectious agents (particularly viral), sensitization to histocompatibility antigens and iron overload.

Two forms of rhEPO became available around 1990, and in 2001 another erythropoietin agent called darbepoietin alfa was licensed to treat renal anemia (Mac Dougall 2002). These EPO agents may be given intravenously (i.v.) or subcutaneously (s.c.). In peritoneal dialysis, and for transplanted and pre-dialysis patients, epoetin should be administered s.c. In dialyzed patients it may be administered by both routes. For normal as well as CKD patients s.c. administration of EPO (and not darbepoetin) has more favorable pharmacodynamics than i.v. administration, despite the incomplete absorption of EPO following s.c. administration (bioavailability approximately 20%) (Kaufman et al. 1998).

The frequency of administration of EPO is influenced by many factors. In hemodialyzed patients receiving epoetin alfa or epoetin beta i.v., the drug should be given three times a week during both the correction and the maintenance phases. The dosing frequency of epoetin beta may be reduced to once weekly or every two weeks when administered s.c. (Locatelli et al. 2004).

6.4.1. Pure Red Cell Aplasia

Recombinant human EPO has a relatively wide therapeutic window and is usually well tolerated. Possible adverse events related to epoetin use include hypertension, seizures, increased clotting tendency and pure red cell aplasia (PRCA). PRCA is a progressively developing, severe isolated anemia, with sudden onset and almost complete absence of red blood cell precursors from an otherwise normal bone marrow (Casadevall et al. 2002a, Eckardt and Casadevall 2003, Bennett et al. 2004, Krantz 1974, Casadevall 2002b, Verhelst et al. 2004). PRCA is usually an autoimmune disorder in which immunoglobulin (IgG) antibodies are directed against erythroid progenitors or precursors. PRCA usually arrives spontaneously or in association with thymoma, lymphoid proliferation or an immune-related disorder such as lupus erythematosus or rheumatoid arthritis. The disease may also develop secondary to drugs or viral infection, such as those of the B19 parvovirus or hepatitis B virus. EPO-induced PRCA is caused by the development of anti-EPO antibodies. These antibodies cross-react with the patient's endogenous EPO and lead to a more severe form of anemia than before the onset of EPO therapy. Despite the widespread use of EPO in cancer-related anemia and other types of anemia, virtually all cases of antibody-positive PRCA occurred in patients with renal anemia.

The renal anemia-related PRCA cases occurred mainly in patients receiving epoetin alfa (EPREX®/ERYPO®, Ortho Biotech) outside of the USA, although a limited number received an other EPO product or a combination of products (Boven et al. 2005, Mac Dougall 2005) (Figure 6.1). Antibodies generated against rhEPO cross-react with endogenous EPO, and mandate that treatment with EPO of any brand is discontinued, although, recently there have been reports of cases of EPO-associated PRCA in which re-challenge has been successful. PRCA patients require repeated blood transfusions, and immunosuppressant therapy with corticosteroids and cyclophosphamide or

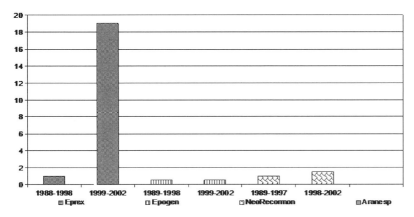

Figure 6.1 Antibody-mediated PRCA per patient-years (rate per 100,000 patient-years) for different EPO products.

cyclosporine has been used to control antibody formation (Mac Dougall 2005, Asari and Gokal 2004). Antibody titers have been observed to slowly decrease in most patients after rhEPO was stopped.

The incidence rate for patients with subcutaneous exposure to Eprex in pre-filled syringes with polysorbate 80 was found to be 4.61/10 000 patients per year, which is much higher than that of other EPO formulations (Krantz 1974, Asari and Gokal 2004). Between January 1998 and April 2004, 175 cases of EPO-associated PRCA were reported for Eprex, 11 cases for NeoRecormon and 5 cases for Epogen (Bennett et al. 2004). Between 2001 and 2003, the estimated exposure-adjusted incidence was down to 18 cases per 100 000 patient-years for the Eprex formulation without human serum albumin, 6 per 100 000 patient-years for the Eprex formulation with human serum albumin, 1 case per 100 000 patient-years for NeoRecormon and 0.2 case per 100 000 patients-years for Epogen (Mac Dougall 2005). The exposure-adjusted incidence thus decreased by 83% worldwide (Bennett et al. 2004), after procedures were adopted to ensure appropriate storage, handling and administration of Eprex to patients with chronic kidney disease (Figure 6.2).

The cause of Eprex-associated PRCA has not been solved in detail, although several hypotheses have been raised including:

• Formation of micelles
• Silicon droplets in the pre-filled syringes
• Leachates from rubber stoppers
• Aggregation
• Mishandling

None of theories per se explain solely the steep increase of immune response. Micelles are very unstable and their potential formation does not explain the epidemiological data. There are some inconsistent anecdotal reports of silicon-induced immune responses, but in general silicon is inert and does not explain the immune reaction against Eprex. Leachates from the rubber stoppers in pre-filled syringes acting as adjuvants have been brought up by the manufacturer as the most probable cause, but also this hypothesis is not covered by experimental data. The epidemiological difference in countries like Germany and France can be explained by differences in s.c. administration.

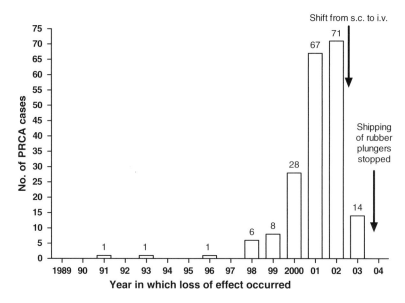

Figure 6.2 Incidence of anti-EPO antibodies/PRCA in the period 1989–2004.

While in Germany patients are treated in hospitals by nephrologists, French patients administer the drug themselves at home. This may lead to an increased risk of mishandling by non-compliance with the strict recommendations of the manufacturer. Subsequently aggregates may have formed, which induced the immune response by breaking the immune tolerance. Formation of aggregates seems to be the most likely explanation for the Eprex-induced PRCA.

6.5. Biosimilars

A generation of biotechnology-derived therapeutic agents is reaching the end of their patent lives, heralding the market entry of biosimilars. For nephrologists who are used to prescribing biopharmaceuticals such as EPO or interferon to their patients, the issue of emerging biosimilars is of particular importance. Most patients are receiving EPO with a clear understanding of the efficacy and safety of the drug. Because nephrologists are satisfied with the current treatment, both in terms of efficacy and safety, there is thus a full responsibility both from drugs agencies scientists and nephrologists to review the safety profile and efficacy of the biosimilar products.

In this context it has to be underlined that recombinant therapeutics are complex products and have little in parallel with traditional biogenerics. Therefore, even perfectly respected, current EMEA guidelines will still leave clinicians with unresolved issues.

6.5.1. EMEA Guideline on Biosimilar Medicinal Products Containing Recombinant Erythropoietins

A guideline for the approval of biosimilars has been published in 2005 by the EMEA, which includes non-clinical and clinical issues (Wiecek and Mikhail 2006). An updated version of the EMEA guideline will be published soon (http://www.emea.europa.eu/pdfs/human/biosimilar/1432706en.pdf).

Non-clinical studies are recommended to be comparative and designed to detect differences in response to the biosimilar and reference product. Any alterations in reactivity between the biosimilar and the reference product should be assessed. In vivo, the erythrogenic effect of the biosimilar and the reference product should be quantitatively compared in an appropriate animal assay. Clinical studies should include PK, PD and should be performed in single dose cross-over studies using s.c. and i.v. administration.

Equivalent therapeutic efficacy between the biosimilar and the reference product should be demonstrated in at least two adequately powered randomized, double-blind, parallel group clinical trials. Clinical safety should come from at least 300 patients treated for at least 12 months. In addition, a pharmacovigilance plan should be presented to address immunogenicity and potential rare serious adverse events. Finally, extension of indication from the sensitive clinical model (renal failure) to other indications can be granted. The EMEA has therefore provided a valuable base for EU legislation to biosimilars. Currently such legal framework does not exist in the USA for the approval of biosimilars.

Not only initial efficacy but maintaining batch to batch consistency (comparability) is an ongoing challenge, since biological manufacturing processes involve many steps from cloning the desired gene, via selection of a suitable cell-type fermentation and purification, to formulation of the end product (Kuhlmann and Covic 2006, Schellekens 2005, Schellekens 2002). Testing of 12 batches of EPO from five manufacturers showed variations in the potencies from 68 to 119% of specifications. Different potencies even between product samples from the same manufacturer were demonstrated (Kelley et al. 2005). Such variability in the efficacy may have major clinical impact. Lack of efficacy will result in a high number of patients below the target Hb ($> 11 \, g/dl$), and therefore lead to adverse outcome. Low hemoglobin is not the only concern; potencies above the specifications may result in high hemoglobin above the target, which may result in an increased risk of cardiovascular morbidity (Besarab et al. 1998, Singh et al. 2006). That is why EMEA guidances clearly specify that "exaggerated pharmacodynamic responses" may result in hypertension and thrombotic complications.

Batch to batch variability may also result in hemoglobin cycling. The phenomenon of cyclic fluctuations in hemoglobin levels (hemoglobin cycling) is a common occurrence in EPO-treated hemodialysis patients, but has not yet been widely studied. It is closely associated with frequent EPO dose changes due to EPO variability, and may have a major adverse impact on patient outcome, since wide movement of hemoglobin values is not a part of normal homeostasis (Swanson et al. 2004, Hoesel et al. 2004, Thorpe and Swanson 2005, Kromminga and Schellekens 2005).

Before conducting clinical studies, pre-clinical (both in vitro and in vivo) comparability is mandatory to assess PK and PD of the biosimilar. Also, manufacturing processes, which are highly elaborate and sophisticated, will have to guarantee consistency in the production of these drugs, not only to provide initial comparability but also the same efficacy over time (Kuhlmann and Covic 2006). For example, the extent of glycosylation is notably sensitive to changes in cell growth conditions, such as culture pH, the availability of precursors and nutrients, and the presence or absence of various cytokines and hormones. Glycosylation can affect the half-life of EPO and therefore its potency; increasing the degree of sialylation and glycosylation decreases renal clearance rate and increases EPO in vivo activity (Kuhlmann and Covic 2006, Stoffel et al. 2007, Weber et al. 2002).

Several clinical trials have demonstrated correction of anemia with biosimilar EPO preparations used in either open-label or controlled studies (Stravitz et al. 2005). As expected from pre-clinical data, correction of anemia differed between EPO alfa and biosimilar epoetins in each of the comparative studies. Differences in the in vitro and in vivo potencies were observed in those trials, and the EPO preparations were either more or less potent in vivo compared with in vitro studies.

Equally important is safety. Safety data obtained from open-label and controlled studies of biosimilar generally have shown good tolerability of treatment. However, unacceptable levels of bacterial endoxins were identified in 3 of 12 biosimilar epoetin samples obtained from five different laboratories (Stravitz et al. 2005) in studies comparing biosimilar EPO with epoetin alfa. Similar adverse event profiles were noted.

Immunogenicity is a critical issue in biotechnologically derived medicine. Most biopharmaceuticals induce immune responses (Kessler, Goldsmith, and Schellekens 2006) but the formation of antibodies often has no or minor clinically relevant consequences. However, in some cases the consequences can be severe and potentially lethal, causing a loss of efficacy or even to autoimmune processes. Occasionally, antibodies result in enhanced efficacy of the product (Hoesel et al. 2004). The risk of immune responses against EPO was made clear by cases of PRCA in patients receiving epoetin alfa. The PRCA cases were associated with a breakdown of immune tolerance to EPO treatment resulting in neutralizing antibodies directed against not only the recombinant protein but also endogenous EPO.

According to the EMEA guidelines on immunogenicity, safety of biosimilars should be addressed through safety data from at least 300 patients and a pharmacovigilance plan. In order to compare immunogenicity of products, animal models, sensitive and specific assay for detecting high-affinity antibodies, and large clinical trials are necessary. Standardized animal models are not available. Moreover, due to the lack of a common calibrator different assays may reveal different results from different laboratories (Mac Dougall 2005). To detect a difference in PRCA incidence between two products, data from around 40 000 patient-years of treatment are necessary. However, EMEA only recommends safety data from at least 300 patients and with at least 12-month immunogenicity data. PRCA is a rare, but serious complication, which will therefore not be detected with pre-marketing evaluations. Guidelines from the EMEA state that a pharmacovigilance plan for post-marketing monitoring should be included in the data package submitted for drug approval. Nevertheless, existing pharmacovigilance strategies were slow in detecting and reacting to the rise in PRCA cases. This questions the appropriateness of the current system for the continuous post-marketing evaluation.

6.6. Conclusion

Treatment with rhEPO may induce an immune response and lead to the formation of anti-EPO antibodies. These antibodies may lead to the clinical manifestation of PRCA, a severe form of anemia. The rise of EPO-induced

PRCA cases in the period of 1998–2004 has made health authorities, manufacturers and clinicians aware of the risk of adverse immune reactions and the importance of the analysis of anti-EPO antibodies. Screening analysis has therefore become more important after the development and production of EPO biosimilars, because those products are already available in some countries and may be marketed in Europe and USA before all issues are resolved.

Reliable and sensitive screening assays for the detection of anti-EPO antibodies are available, although attempts to generate a common calibrator for those assays are still not successful. As recommended by some guidelines, positive results in the screening results have to be confirmed by a more specific confirmatory assay. In addition, a more detailed characterization of the antibodies is desirable. The neutralizing capacity of anti-EPO antibodies has been shown by a cellular assay using cell lines or bone marrow derived cells that are unequivocally dependent on EPO.

References

Asari, A. and Gokal, R. 2004. Pure red cell aplasia secondary to epoetin alpha responding to darbepoeitin alpha in a patient on peritoneal dialysis. J. Am. Soc. Nephrol. 15:2204–2207.

Bennett, C. L., Luminari, S., Nissenson, A. R., Tallman, M. S., Klinge, S. A., McWilliams, N., McKoy, J. M., Kim, B., Lyons, E. A., Trifilio, S. M., Raisch, D. W., Evens, A. M., Kuzel, T. M., Schumock, G. T., Belknap, S. M., Locatelli, F., Rossert, J., and Casadevall, N. 2004. Pure red cell aplasia and epoetin therapy. N. Engl. J. Med. 351:1403–1408.

Besarab, A., Ross, R. P., and Nasca, T. J. 1995. The use of recombinant human erythropoietin in predialysis patient. Current Opin. Nephrol. Hypertens. 4:155–161.

Besarab, A., Bolton, W. K., Browne, J. K., Egrie, J. C., Nissension, A. R., Okamoto, D. M., Schwab, S. J., and Goodkin, D. A. 1998. The effects of normal as compared with low hematocrit values in patients with cardiac disease who are receiving hemodialysis and epoetin. N. Engl. J. Med. 339:584–590.

Boven, K., Stryker, S., Knight, J., Thomas, A., van Regenmortel, M., Kemeny, D. M., Power, D., Rossert, J., and Casadevall, N. 2005. The increased incidence of pure red cell aplasia with an Eprex formulation in uncoated rubber stopper syringes. Kidney Int. 67:2346–2353.

Bunn, H. F. 2007. New agents that stimulate erythropoiesis. Blood 109:868–873.

Casadevall, N., Nataf, J., Viron, B., Kolta, A., Kiladjian, J. J., Martin-Dupont, P., Michaud, P., Papo, T., Ugo, V., Teyssandier, I., Varet, B., and Mayeux, P. 2002a. Pure red-cell aplasia and antierythropoietin antibodies in patients treated with recombinant erythropoietin. N. Engl. J. Med. 346:469–475.

Casadevall, N. 2002b. Antibodies against rhuEPO: Native and recombinant. Nephrol. Dial. Transplant. 17(Suppl. 5):42–47.

Castelli, G., Famularo, A., Semino, C., Machi, A. M., Ceci, A., Cannella, G., and Melioli, G. 2000. Detection of anti-erythropoietin antibodies in haemodialysis patients treated with recombinant human-erythropoietin. Pharmacol. Res. 41: 313–318.

Collins, A. J., Ma, J. Z., and Keshavish, P. 1994. Urea index and other predictors of hemodialysis patient survival. Am. J. Kidney Dis. 23:272–282.

D'Andrea, A. D. and Zon, L. I. 1990. Erythropoietin receptor. Subunit structure and activation. J. Clin. Invest. 86:681–687.

Drüeke, T. B., Locatelli, F., Clyne, N., Eckardt, K. U., Macdougall, I. C., Tsakiris, D., Burger, H. U., and Scherhab, A. 2006. Normalization of hemoglobin level in patients with chronic kidney disease and anaemia. N. Engl. J. Med. 355:2071–2083.

Eckardt, K. U. and Casadevall, N. 2003. Pure red cell aplasia due to anti-erythropoietin antibodies. Nephrol. Dial. Transplant. 18:865–869.

Eckardt, K. U. 2001. Anemia in end stage renal disease: Pathophysiological considerations. Nephrol. Dial. Transplant. 16(Suppl. 7):2–8.

Ehrenreich, H., Hasselblatt, M., Dembowski, C., Cepek, L., Lewczuk, P., Stiefel, M., Rustenbeck, H. H., Breiter, N., Jacob, S., Knerlich, F., Bohn, M., Poser, W., Ruther, E., Kochen, M., Gefeller, O., Gleiter, C., Wessel, T. C., De Ryck, M., Itri, L., Prange, H., Cerami, A., Brines, M., and Siren, A. L. 2002. Erythropoietin therapy for acute stroke is both safe and beneficial. Mol. Med. 8:495–505.

Eschbach, J. W. 1989. The anemia of chronic renal failure: Pathophysiological and the effects of recombinant erythropoietin. Kidney Int. 35:134–148.

Eschbach, J. W. and Adamson, J. 1985. Anemia of end stage renal disease (ESRD). Kidney Int. 28:1–5.

Fan, Q., Leuther, K. K., Holmes, C. P., Fong, K. L., Zhang, J., Velkovska, S., Chen, M. J., Mortensen, R. B., Leu, K., Green, J. M., Schatz, P. J., and Woodburn, K. W. 2006. Preclinical evaluation of Hematide, a novel erythropoiesis stimulating agent, for the treatment of anemia. Exp. Hematol. 34:1303–1311.

Foley, F. N., Parfrey, P. S., Harnett, J. D., Kent, G. M., Murray, D. C., and Barre, P. E. 1996. The impact of anemia on cardiomyopathy, morbidity and mortality in end stage renal disease. Am. J. Kidney Dis. 28:53–61.

Gross, J., Moller, R., Henke, W., and Hoesel, W. 2006. Detection of anti-EPO antibodies in human sera by a bridging ELISA is much more sensitive when coating biotinylated rhEPO to streptavidin rather than using direct coating of rhEPO. J. Immunol. Method. 313:176–182.

Hoesel, W., Gross, J., Moller, R., Kanne, B., Wessner, A., Muller, G., Muller, A., Gromnica-Ihle, E., Fromme, M., Bischoff, S., and Haselbeck, A. 2004. Development and evaluation of a new ELISA for the detection and quantification of antierythropoietin antibodies in human sera. J. Immunol. Method. 294:101–110.

Jelkmann, W. 2007. Erythropoietin after a century of research: younger than ever. Eur. J. Haematol. 78:183–205.

Kaufman, J. S., Reda, D. J., Fye, C. L., Goldfarb, D. S., Henderson, W. G., Kleinman, J. G., and Vaamonde, C. A. 1998. Subcutaneous compared with intravenous epoetin in patients receiving hemodialysis. N. Engl. J. Med. 339:578–583.

Kelley, M., Cooper, C., Matticoli, A., and Greway, A. 2005. The detection of anti-erythropoietin antibodies in human serum and plasma: part II. Validation of a semi-quantitative 3H-thymidine uptake assay for neutralizing antibodies J. Immunol. Method. 300:179–191.

Kessler, M., Goldsmith, D., and Schellekens, H. 2006. Immunogenicity of biopharmaceuticals. Nephrol. Dial. Transplant. 21(Suppl. 5):9–12.

Kientsch-Engel, R., Hallermayer, K., Dessauer, A., and Wieczorek, L. 1990. New enzyme-linked immunosorbent assay methods for measurement of serum erythropoietin levels and erythropoietin antibodies. Blood Purif. 8:255–259.

Krantz, S. B. 1974. Pure red cell aplasia. N. Engl. J. Med. 291:345–350.

Kromminga, A. and Schellekens, H. 2005. Antibodies against erythropoietin and other protein-based therapeutics: an overview. Ann. N.Y. Acad. Sci. 1050:257–265.

Kuhlmann, M. and Covic, A. 2006. The protein science of biosimilars. Nephrol. Dial. Transplant. 21(Suppl. 5):4–8.

Locatelli, F., Aljama, P., Barany, P., Canaud, B., Carrera, F., Eckardt, K. U., Hörl, W. H., Mac Dougall, I. C., Macleod, A., Wiecek, A., and Cameron, S. 2004. Revised European best practice guidelines for the management of anaemia in patients with chronic renal failure. Nephrol. Dial. Transpl. 19(Suppl. 2):ii1–ii47.

Mac Dougall, I. C. 2002. Optimizing the use of erythropoietic agents. Pharmacokinetic and pharmacodynamic considerations. Nephrol. Dial. Transplant. 17(Suppl. 5): 66–70.

Mac Dougall, I. C. 2005. Adverse event issue management: What have we learnt from pure red cell aplasia (PRCA)? Nephrol. Dial. Transplant. 20(Suppl. 8):18–21.

Marti, H. H., Bernaudin, M., Petit, E., and Bauer, C. 2000. Neuroprotection and Angiogenesis: Dual Role of Erythropoietin in Brain Ischemia. News Physiol. Sci. 15:225–229.

Mason, S., La, S., Mytych, D., Swanson, S. J., and Ferbas, J. 2003. Validation of the BIACORE 3000 platform for detection of antibodies against erythropoietic agents in human serum samples. Curr. Med. Res. Opin. 19:651–659.

NKF-K/DOQI. 2001. Clinical practice guidelines for anemia of chronic kidney disease. Am. J. Kidney Dis. 37:S182–S238.

Sasaki, H., Ochi, N., Dell, A., and Fukuda, M. 1988. Site-specific glycosylation of human recombinant erythropoietin: analysis of glycopeptides or peptides at each glycosylation site by fast atom bombardment mass spectrometry. Biochemistry 27:8618–8626.

Schellekens, H. 2002. Bioequivalence and the immunogenicity of biopharmaceuticals. Nat. Rev. Drug Discov. 1:457–462.

Schellekens, H. 2005. Follow-on biologics: challenges of the "next generation". Nephrol. Dial. Transplant. 20(Suppl. 4):31–36.

Schett, G., Firbas, U., Fureder, W., Hiesberger, H., Winkler, S., Wachauer, D., Koller, M., Kapiotis, S., and Smolen, J. 2001. Decreased serum erythropoietin and its relation to anti-erythropoietin antibodies in anaemia of systemic lupus erythematosus. Rheumatology (Oxford) 40:424–431.

Singh, A. K., Szczech, L., Tang, K. L., Barnhart, H., Sapp, S., Wolfson, M., and Reddan, D. 2006. Correction of anemia with epoetin alfa in chronic kidney disease. N. Engl. J. Med. 355:2085–2098.

Sipsas, N. V., Kokori, S. I., Ioannidis, J. P., Kyriaki, D., Tzioufas, A. G., and Kordossis, T. 1999. Circulating autoantibodies to erythropoietin are associated with human immunodeficiency virus type 1-related anemia. J. Infect. Dis. 180: 2044–2047.

Stoffel, M. P., Haverkamp, H., Kromminga, A., Lauterbach, K. W., and Baldamus, C. A. 2007. Prevalence of anti-erythropoietin antibodies in hemodialysis patients without clinical signs of pure red cell aplasia. Comparison between hypo- and normoresponsive patients treated with epoetins for renal anemia. Nephron. Clin. Pract. 105:c90–c98.

Stravitz, R. T., Chung, H., Sterling, R. K., Luketic, V. A., Sanyal, A. J., Price, A. S., Purrington, A., and Shiffman, M. L. 2005. Antibody-mediated pure red cell aplasia due to epoetin alfa during antiviral therapy of chronic hepatitis C. Am. J. Gastroenterol. 100:1415–1419.

Swanson, S. J., Ferbas, J., Mayeux, P., and Casadevall, N. 2004. Evaluation of methods to detect and characterize antibodies against recombinant human erythropoietin. Nephron. Clin. Pract. 96:c88–c95.

Tacey, R., Greway, A., Smiell, J., Power, D., Kromminga, A., Daha, M., Casadevall, N., and Kelley, M. 2003. The detection of anti-erythropoietin antibodies in human serum and plasma. Part I. Validation of the protocol for a radioimmunoprecipitation assay. J. Immunol. Methods. 283:317–329.

Thorpe, R. and Swanson, S. J. 2005. Assays for detecting and diagnosing antibody-mediated pure red cell aplasia (PRCA): an assessment of available procedures. Nephrol. Dial. Transplant. 20(Suppl. 4):16–22.

Tzioufas, A. G., Kokori, S. I., Petrovas, C. I., and Moutsopoulos, H. M. 1997. Autoantibodies to human recombinant erythropoietin in patients with systemic lupus erythematosus: correlation with anemia. Arthritis Rheum. 40:2212–2216.

Urra, J. M., Torre, M., Alcazar, R., and Peces, R. 1997. Rapid method for detection of anti-recombinant human erythropoietin antibodies as a new form of erythropoietin resistance. Clin. Chem. 43:848–849.

Verhelst, D., Rossert, J., Casadevall, N., Kruger, A., Eckardt, K. U., and Macdougall, I. C. 2004. Treatment of erythropoietin induced pure red cell aplasia: a retrospective study. Lancet 363:1768–1771.

Weber, G., Gross, J., Kromminga, A., Loew, H. H., and Eckardt, K. U. 2002. Allergic skin and systemic reactions in a patient with pure red cell aplasia and anti-erythropoietin antibodies challenged with different epoetins. J. Am. Soc. Nephrol. 13:2381–2383.

Wiecek, A. and Mikhail, A. 2006. European regulatory guidelines for biosimilars. Nephrol. Dial. Transplant. 21(Suppl. 5):17–20.

Winearls, C. G., Oliver, D. O., Pippard, M. J., Reid, C., Downing, M. R., and Cotes, P. M. 1986. Effect of human erythropoietin derived from recombinant DNA on the anemia of patients maintained by chronic haemodialysis. Lancet 2: 1175–1178.

Case Study: Immunogenicity of Interferon-Beta

Klaus Bendtzen and Arno Kromminga

7.1. Abstract

While autoantibodies (autoAbs) to IFN-beta are rarely found in humans, antibodies (Abs) to IFN-beta are frequently seen in patients receiving prolonged therapies with recombinant human IFN-beta. As autoAbs, they neutralize wild-type IFN-beta, they cross-react with both currently used IFN-beta biopharmaceuticals, but not IFN-alpha, and they interfere with biological and immunometric assays for IFN-beta in vitro and in vivo. Although anti-IFN-beta Abs usually neutralize IFN-beta in vivo, making further therapies useless, there is experimental support for the idea that some anti-IFN-beta Abs, at least early during 'immunization', may function as enhancers and paradoxically prolong and amplify the activities of IFN-beta in vivo. There are significant difficulties in obtaining reliable methods for monitoring patients on prolonged IFN-beta therapies. These include IFN-beta analyses in blood required for optimal and individualized therapies, and Ab detection induced during therapy. In an effort to assess the clinical relevance of in vitro Ab measurements, many investigators distinguish between 'binding' Abs (BAbs) and in vitro 'neutralizing' Abs (NAbs) even though such a distinction may not be justified in real terms. For example, the so-called non-neutralizing BAbs may affect drug bioavailability and drug clearance, while NAbs may not necessarily neutralize circulating IFN-beta in vivo. Moreover, anti-IFN-beta Abs may cause serious complications and theoretically initiate autoimmune reactions whether or not they neutralize in vivo. Regular screening for NAbs and discontinuation of therapy in multiple sclerosis patients with sustained high-level NAbs are now generally recommended.

7.2. Introduction

Interferon (IFN) is a group of natural proteins produced by many cell types in response to challenge by infectious agents, primarily viruses, but also bacteria and parasites. Natural, partly purified IFN preparations have been used for many years, primarily as therapies against viral infections and certain cancers. From the 1980s, recombinant gene technologies allowed mass cultivation and purification from bacterial and mammalian cell cultures. This paved the way for use of IFN in many diseases, including the use of human recombinant IFN-beta in patients with multiple myeloma and multiple sclerosis (MS). Hence, IFN-beta is the first-line treatment of patients with relapsing-remitting MS, as it has been shown to reduce the progression of disability and suppress signs and severity of the disease.

It took more than 10 years to fully realize the problem of immunogenicity of human recombinant IFN-beta preparations. This delay was mostly due to the belief that the immune system is tolerant to biopharmaceuticals with peptide sequences identical or almost identical to naturally occurring counterparts, but recognition of the problem was also delayed by the relapsing-remitting nature of MS and the use of inappropriate tests for anti-IFN-beta antibodies (Ab) (Schellekens 2002, Bendtzen 2003). It is now well known that up to 90% of treated MS patients may develop binding Abs (BAbs) and neutralizing Abs (NAbs) against IFN-beta (Ross et al. 2000). However, the frequency and the clinical relevance of the induced Abs depend on the nature of the IFN-beta preparation as well as on treatment characteristics such as dosage and mode of administration. Furthermore, the assay format for Ab detection greatly influences the frequency of Ab-positives.

7.3. Description of the IFN Biopharmaceuticals

7.3.1. Structure and Function

Type 1 IFNs, consisting of IFN-alpha (previously termed leukocyte IFN), IFN-beta (previously termed fibroblast IFN), IFN-delta, IFN-epsilon, IFN-kappa, IFN-tau, IFN-omega and IFN-zeta or limitin, are a group of related glycoproteins that are involved primarily in the regulation of antiviral and antiproliferative responses of the immune system. All subgroups of type 1 IFNs share the same receptor complex called IFN-alpha receptor (IFNAR) that consists of IFNAR1 and IFNAR2 chains (Figure 7.1). Activation of the complex starts intracellular signaling through IFNAR1, and this leads to activation in the nucleus of IFN-stimulated regulatory elements (ISRE), which govern transcription of more than 100 genes. Several of these genes have been used for development of tests for type 1 IFN activity and anti-IFN NAbs.

Type 1 IFNs, mainly IFN-alpha, have been used as therapy for patients with viral infections, including hepatitis B and C virus, as well as patients with malignant conditions. Composed of a group of at least 23 subtypes of 19–26 kDa (glyco)proteins, IFN-alpha is produced primarily by virus-infected leukocytes but also by many other cell types.

IFN-beta is produced primarily by virus-infected fibroblasts and consists of a group of at least two members of 23–42 kDa glycoproteins called IFN-beta1 and IFN-beta3 (IFN-beta2, also known as interleukin-6, does not belong to this group). In contrast to IFN-alpha, IFN-beta is strictly species specific in that IFN-beta of other species is inactive in human cells. Both IFN-alpha and IFN-beta interfere with replication of many viruses in almost all cell types and, in addition, have antiproliferative and immunomodulatory functions.

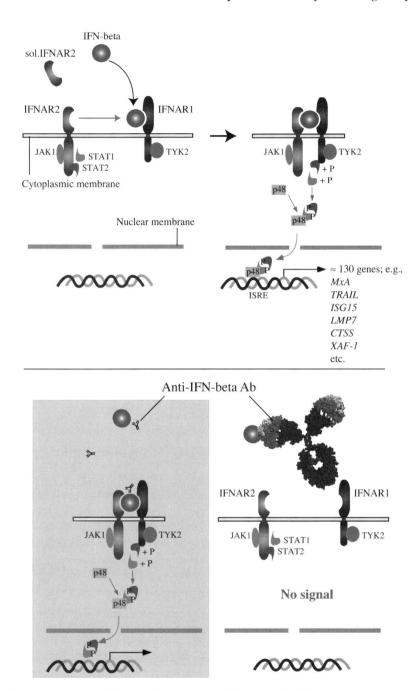

Figure 7.1 Type 1 IFN signaling and anti-IFN-beta BAb/Nabs.
The example shows IFN-beta signaling through IFN-alpha receptors 1 and 2 (IFNAR1 and IFNAR2). The *upper panel* shows ligand–receptor binding, association of the two receptor chains and intracellular signaling and activation of genes through IFN-stimulated regulatory elements (ISRE). The *left lower panel* shows anti-IFN-beta BAbs (non-neutralizing) as they are often depicted. The *right lower panel* shows the correct size relations. (*See* Color Plate 1)

7.3.2. Manufacturers of Recombinant Human IFN-Beta

There are currently two main therapeutic preparations of recombinant IFN-beta:

IFN-beta-1b is produced by Berlex Laboratories (Montville, NJ, USA) and Bayer-Schering (Berlin, Germany) under the trade names Betaseron® and Betaferon® and was the first in use in MS patients. It is produced in *Escherichia coli* and is therefore non-glycosylated, unlike its natural counterpart. In addition, IFN-beta-1b differs from wild-type IFN-beta in that it lacks the N-terminal amino acid (methionine) and that one amino acid in position 17 is different (cysteine substituted with serine). IFN-beta-1a is produced by Biogen (Cambridge, MA, USA) under the trade name Avonex® and by Serono Inc. (Rockland, MA, USA) under the trade name Rebif®. IFN-beta-1a preparations are produced in mammalian Chinese hamster ovary cells. The amino acid sequence is identical to native IFN-beta, and it is glycosylated, although not exactly equal to the wild-type human IFN-beta.

7.4. Immune Reactions Against IFN-Beta

Naturally occurring autoAbs to IFN-beta have been reported, but the frequency is low (less than 0.1% of healthy individuals) and their clinical relevance is unknown. In contrast, patients treated with human recombinant IFN-beta frequently develop anti-IFN-beta Abs. The reported frequencies and titers vary considerably depending on diseases, IFN preparations and administration, and the types of assays being used. However, Ab-mediated decrease in bioactivity of IFN, a condition in which the clinical effect of continued injection of IFN-beta is minimized or abrogated, is now generally recognized (Pachner 2003).

Not surprisingly, the risk appears to be greatest for *E. coli*-derived IFN-beta-1b and lowest for mammalian IFN-beta-1a. We have found that BAbs and NAbs develop in 30–90% of MS patients treated with IFN-beta-1a and IFN-beta-1b, respectively, and regular testings for NAbs and discontinuation of therapy in MS patients with sustained high-level NAbs are now recommended (Bendtzen 2003, Pachner 2003, Ann Marrie and Rudick 2006, Gilli et al. 2006). A recently developed mouse model, transgenic for the human IFN-beta gene, reflects the differences in the immunogenic potential of the different IFN-beta preparations (Hermeling et al. 2005).

Apart from neutralizing the effects of continued IFN-beta therapy, it is theoretically possible that NAbs as well as BAbs may trigger host autoimmune processes, for example, through antibody-dependent cell-mediated injury or complement-mediated attack initiated by Ab binding to IFN-beta associated to cells producing or responding to the cytokine. Though this appears to be rare, de novo production of antithyroid, antinuclear and other autoAbs has been reported in connection with IFN-beta-1b therapy, as has clinical manifestations of autoimmunity after IFN-beta therapies (Borg and Isenberg 2007). It is noteworthy that autoimmune phenomena, for example, systemic lupus and autoimmunity involving the thyroid gland, liver and joints have been reported much more frequently in patients treated with IFN-alpha (Selmi et al. 2006).

7.5. Methods of Detection

The need for clinically useful, inexpensive and standardized screening assays is obvious, but attempts in this direction have failed despite the recommendation of WHO to use biological assays, where antiviral neutralization is expressed as a titer, defined as the reciprocal of the serum dilution that reduces the IFN potency from 10 to 1 LU/ml; 1 laboratory unit (LU)/ml is the level of IFN inducing 50% protection against challenge virus in a given assay (Grossberg 2003). A major reason for the lack of standardization is the inconvenience and high cost of carrying out elaborate bioassays and the fact that many assays have not been validated with regard to clinical relevance and therefore may provide little useful information to the clinician.

7.5.1. BAbs and NAbs

There is some controversy whether the development of anti-IFN-beta Abs always leads to response failure. Some investigators distinguish between BAbs (in vitro binding Abs) and NAbs (in vitro neutralizing Abs) and argue that only the latter have clinical importance. This may not always be the case, however (Bendtzen 2003). First, the discrimination between BAbs and NAbs may reflect a quantitative rather than a qualitative difference in the Abs because of different assay sensitivities and because development of Abs in vivo is a dynamic process, where initially produced NAbs may not yet present as such, simply because of their low level. Though not yet detectable in NAb assays, they may be detected in a sensitive BAb assay. And though not yet having a major effect on therapeutic efficacy, they may neutralize portions of the administered drug and cause local or systemic side effects at any time point. They also signal further induction of NAbs if therapy/immunization continues, especially because Ab maturation and increased polyclonality contribute to neutralization. Second, the determination of false positive BAbs, often seen with the use of solid-phase assays (see below), would be interpreted as 'non-neutralizing' BAbs, especially if NAbs are tested by insufficiently sensitive assays. Third, if 'non-neutralizing' BAbs exist *sui generis* in IFN-beta-treated patients (Figure 7.1), they may still have clinically important pharmacological effects. BAbs may, for example, inhibit absorption of IFN-beta from s.c. and i.m. sites (decreasing bioavailability), and BAbs may reduce the half-life of the drug in the circulation and/or prevent IFN-beta from reaching pathologically affected sites, for example in the brain. Finally, immune complexes containing BAbs and possibly complement may cause side effects whether or not IFN-beta bioactivity is neutralized.

7.5.2. Binding Assays for BAbs

Methods for the detection of BAbs to IFN-beta include direct and sandwich-type ELISAs, blotting techniques and radioligand assays (Brickelmaier et al. 1999, Ross et al. 2000, Pachner 2003). Since BAbs bind to both conformational and sequence-restricted (linear) epitopes on proteins, immunometric assays and immunoblotting techniques using a more or less denatured cytokine in the capture phase may hamper detection of BAbs restricted to the native conformation of the molecules (Bendtzen 2003). These techniques may also reveal BAbs even in cases where Abs affinity is low. As this binding is often non-saturable and hence non-specific, such Abs cannot be categorized as true BAbs. Although these techniques can be used for screening purposes, demonstration of ligand binding to the Fab fragments of the immunoglobulins, combined with saturation binding analysis and fluid phase demonstration of cross-binding to the drug, is necessary to verify the presence of specific BAb to IFN-beta.

Another approach for the determination of BAbs is the use of a bridging type of ELISA. This format uses immobilized IFN-beta as catching reagent and a labeled IFN-beta as detecting antigen. BAbs in patient samples recognize both immobilized and dissolved antigen due to their bivalent binding characteristics. A bridging ELISA therefore combines the high throughput need of a screening assay and the specificity of a liquid-phase assay. It should be noted, however, that a bridging type of ELISA fails to detect monovalent BAbs against IFN-beta, for example, Abs of the IgG4 isotype. This may be a significant disadvantage, as IgG4 Abs may neutralize IFN-beta binding to IFNAR1 and IFNAR2, increase drug clearance and/or prevent the drug from reaching affected tissues.

Because of the above-mentioned problems with solid-phase assays, a fluid-phase radioimmunoassay (RIA) for direct binding to ^{125}I-labeled IFN-beta may be beneficial. There are several reasons for this: The tracer preserves as closely as possible the natural configuration of IFN-beta and allows detection of BAbs directed against conformational epitopes; it can be validated and tested for retained bioactivity; it allows high assay sensitivity, and the specificity, kinetics, avidity and capacity of the IFN-beta–BAb binding may be assessed, as can cross-binding to non-Ab factors in serum. However, denaturation may occur when iodinating proteins, and one should therefore always purify the tracer and validate for specific activity, stability and immunoreactivity before use. Steps should also be included to control for saturability of binding and for factors other than BAbs that may interfere with IgG binding. Indeed, it is important to note that many serum proteins may influence BAb assays, for example, soluble receptors (Figure 7.1) and preexisting IFN-alpha and IFN-beta. BAbs in immune complexes may also escape detection because of a low exchange rate between BAb-bound unlabeled IFN-beta and ^{125}I-IFN-beta during incubation. This may also occur if the tracer and the BAbs form complexes with high dissociation rates allowing them to dissociate during the (brief) time it takes to separate bound from free tracer.

Surface plasmon resonance analysis of BAbs is a well-established method for further Ab characterization (Thorpe and Swanson 2005). The determination of binding kinetics as well as the isotyping and subclassing of the Abs enables a more detailed view into the mechanism of the immune reaction. Though the method of choice for characterization of the nature of the antigen–antibody interaction, this method is unsuited as a screening assay due to low throughput and low sensitivity.

7.5.3. Bioassays for NAbs

These include antiviral neutralization assays measured in a cytopathic effect (CPE) setup and tests for inhibition of cellular effects induced by IFN-beta, for example, induction of myxovirus resistance protein A (MxA). Recently, reporter-gene assays offer interesting possibilities for monitoring anti-IFN-beta NAbs.

The *CPE assay* (Figure 7.2) is the currently recommended assay for IFN-beta NAbs, as this assay has been used for several years and is clinically validated in MS patients (Ross et al. 2000, Grossberg 2003, Pachner et al. 2005, Ross et al. 2006). The test is usually carried out in one of two modifications: (1) neutralization capacity assay and (2) an assay yielding a titer calculated as the serum dilution that reduces IFN potency from 10 to 1 LU/ml.

The *neutralization capacity assay* yields semiquantitative data on the ability of NAb-containing serum samples to counteract the protective effect of IFN-beta when an IFN-beta-sensitive cell line is exposed to a cytopathic virus. The test directly measures the capacity of an NAb-containing test sample to inhibit the antiviral activity of IFN-beta. There are several advantages of this test compared to titer determinations (see below). A practical one is that it eliminates the need for measurements of serially diluted samples and thus is better suited for economical screening of large numbers of patients. More importantly, however, this test is closer to the in vivo situation, where a certain level of NAbs is set to neutralize a fixed amount of IFN-beta at the site of injection or a relatively fixed level in the circulation.

The *10 to 1 LU/ml neutralization assay*, often called Kawade assay (Kawade 1980), is also a semiquantitative test for NAbs against type 1 IFN, where serially diluted serum samples are tested for IFN-beta neutralization in an otherwise similar setup. The most important advantage of this test is the ability to more accurately measure NAbs at very high levels and, thus, the ability to follow changes in NAb titers over time which may have prognostic value. A potential problem with titer determinations of NAbs is that the antigen–antibody complexes are formed in a scenario far from the clinical setting. In patients with high-titered NAbs, immune complexes would form in vivo in the presence of relatively high levels of Abs at the injection site(s), and even in Ab excess in the circulation, whereas the in vitro testings would take place in antigen excess. This is because NAbs are diluted excessively in the assay, frequently several thousand times, while the IFN-beta level is fixed at 10 LU/ml. This artificial situation has an impact on both size and solubility of the IFN-beta–Ab complexes. To what extent this concern affects the interpretation of NAb levels in vivo, and hence the clinical relevance of this method, has not been addressed.

MxA assays are carried out in two major modifications (Figure 7.3) (Pachner et al. 2005). One assay makes use of an IFN-sensitive cell line and measures change in MxA expression in the presence of NAbs. In the second format, the MxA expression rate or the concentration of the MxA protein is analyzed in whole blood.

The principle underlying *reporter-gene assays* is to replace an IFN-sensitive gene with one that is easy to measure. As shown in Figure 7.1 (*upper panel*), IFN-beta signaling through IFNAR involves activation of ISRE which then induces a host of genes governing antiviral, immune and proliferative responses. Using genetic engineering techniques, MxA or other indigenous genes specifically activated through this pathway can be replaced with a gene which, under control of a relevant promoter, may be used as a reporter gene yielding quantitative responses in IFNAR-bearing cell lines. This may be used for easy assessments of type 1 IFN activities, and since NAbs

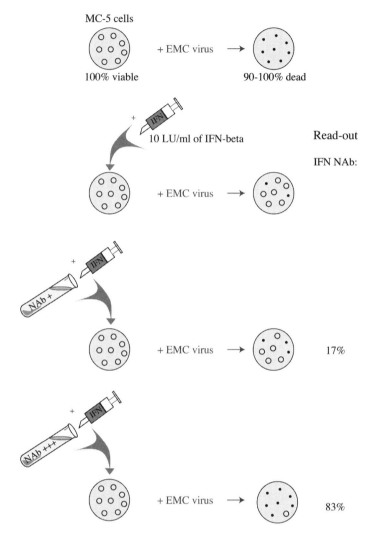

Figure 7.2 Basic principle for CPE assays for NAbs.
Example of an *NAb neutralization capacity assay* (Ross et al. 2000, Bendtzen 2003): A pre-titrated dose of encephalo-myocarditis (EMC) virus is added to an IFN-beta-sensitive cell line (e.g., MC-5 cells, a subclone of A549 human lung carcinoma cells) so that 90–100% of the cells die (*upper panel*). When 10 LU/ml of human recombinant IFN-beta is added to the cells prior to EMC virus, most of the cells survive (*second panel*). If the same amount of IFN-beta is preincubated in patient serum containing a small amount (+) of anti-IFN-beta NAbs, the protective effect of IFN-beta is only minimally affected (*third panel*). However, if the same amount of IFN-beta is preincubated in patient serum containing a large amount (+++) of anti-IFN-beta NAbs, the protective effect of IFN-beta is lost, resulting in substantial cell death (*lower panel*).
The *10 to 1 LU/ml neutralization assay* utilizes the same type of assay except that the NAb-containing sera are serially diluted until the endpoint 50% protection is reached (the definition of 1 LU/ml of IFN-beta) (Kawade 1980, Grossberg 2003).

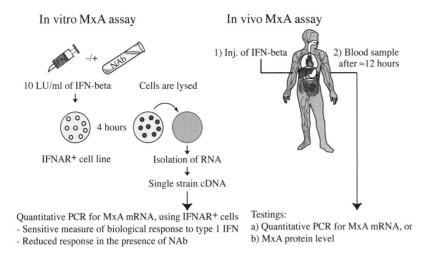

Figure 7.3 Two types of MxA assays for IFN-beta bioactivity and Nabs.

interfere with IFN-beta binding to IFNAR, appropriately modified reporter-gene assays may also be used to detect IFN-beta NAbs. These assays are now available for routine use in patients treated with IFN-beta, and results of preliminary investigations show promise in terms of reproducibility, accuracy, specificity and insensitivity to interfering serum factors (toxic and antiviral) which may interfere with both CPE and MxA assays. It is noteworthy that biological NAb assays often vary significantly in specificity and precision. For example, misinterpretations of CPE assays are likely, if they are carried out without controls for sample toxicity and endogenous antiviral activity, and in vivo MxA NAb assays may be misinterpreted if patients have ongoing infections (viral) or if they receive therapies that affect MxA gene expression.

7.6. Clinical Relevance and Therapeutic Consequences

MS is a chronic, inflammatory autoimmune disease that affects the central nervous system. The disease may lead to a variety of symptoms, including changes in sensation and vision, muscle weakness, depression, difficulties with coordination and speech, severe fatigue, cognitive impairment, problems with balance and pain. The disease causes gradual destruction of myelin (demyelination) and transection of neuronal axons in patches throughout the brain and spinal cord.

The signs and symptoms of MS can be treated by the administration of human IFN-beta. The exact pathomechanism behind the beneficial function(s) of IFN-beta is unknown. Patients are not cured by this form of therapy, but IFN-beta reduces attack frequency and severity. Treatment with both IFN-beta species is therefore long-lasting, usually years, unless anti-IFN-beta Ab induction inhibits drug efficacy or causes side effects. Because up to half the patients treated with IFN-beta may develop NAbs during prolonged therapies, it makes sense to monitor at regular intervals for development of NAbs to IFN-beta; see also Chapter 2 for further information.

References

Ann Marrie, R. and Rudick, R. A. 2006. Drug Insight: interferon treatment in multiple sclerosis. Nat. Clin. Pract. Neurol. 2:34–44.

Bendtzen, K. 2003. Anti-IFN BAb and NAb antibodies: A minireview. Neurology 61(Suppl. 5):S6–S10.

Borg, F. A. and Isenberg, D. A. 2007. Syndromes and complications of interferon therapy. Curr. Opin. Rheumatol. 19:61–66.

Brickelmaier, M., Hochman, P. S., Baciu, R., Chao, B., Cuervo, J. H., and Whitty, A. 1999. ELISA methods for the analysis of antibody responses induced in multiple sclerosis patients treated with recombinant interferon-beta. J. Immunol. Methods 227:121–135.

Gilli, F., Marnetto, F., Caldano, M., Sala, A., Malucchi, S., Capobianco, M., and Bertolotto, A. 2006. Biological markers of interferon-beta therapy: comparison among interferon-stimulated genes MxA, TRAIL and XAF-1. Mult. Scler. 12: 47–57.

Grossberg, S. E. 2003. Perspectives on the neutralization of interferons by antibody. Neurology 61:S21–S23.

Hermeling, S., Jiskoot, W., Crommelin, D., Bornaes, C., and Schellekens, H. 2005. Development of a transgenic mouse model immune tolerant for human interferon beta. Pharm. Res. 22:847–851.

Kawade, Y. 1980. An analysis of neutralization reaction of interferon by antibody: a proposal on the expression of neutralization titer. J. Interferon Res. 1:61–70.

Pachner, A. R. 2003. Anti-IFNb antibodies in IFNb-treated MS patients. Neurology 61(Suppl. 5):S1–S5.

Pachner, A. R., Dail, D., Pak, E., and Narayan, K. 2005. The importance of measuring IFNbeta bioactivity: monitoring in MS patients and the effect of anti-IFNbeta antibodies. J. Neuroimmunol. 166:180–188.

Ross, C., Clemmesen, K. M., Svenson, M., Sorensen, P. S., Koch-Henriksen, N., Skovgaard, G. L., and Bendtzen, K. 2000. Immunogenicity of interferon-b in multiple sclerosis patients: influence of preparation, dosage, dose frequency, and route of administration. Danish Multiple Sclerosis Study Group. Ann. Neurol. 48:706–712.

Ross, C., Svenson, M., Clemmesen, K. M., Sorensen, P. S., Koch-Henriksen, N., and Bendtzen, K. 2006. Measuring and evaluating interferon-beta-induced antibodies in patients with multiple sclerosis. Mult. Scler. 12:39–46.

Schellekens, H. 2002. Immunogenicity of therapeutic proteins: clinical implications and future prospects. Clin. Ther. 24:1720–1740.

Selmi, C., Lleo, A., Zuin, M., Podda, M., Rossaro, L., and Gershwin, M. E. 2006. Interferon alpha and its contribution to autoimmunity. Curr. Opin. Investig. Drugs 7:451–456.

Thorpe, R. and Swanson, S. J. 2005. Current methods for detecting antibodies against erythropoietin and other recombinant proteins. Clin. Diagn. Lab. Immunol. 12: 28–39.

8

Case Study: Immunogenicity of Insulin

Henriette Mersebach, Fannie Smith, Thomas Sparre and Lisbeth Bjerring Jensen

8.1. Introduction to Diabetes Mellitus and Insulin

Diabetes mellitus is an important endocrine disorder characterised by abnormal metabolism and in particular abnormal glucose homeostasis as well as an increased risk of developing microvascular and macrovascular complications such as neuropathy, retinopathy, nephropathy and atherosclerosis. Type 1 diabetes is characterised by absolute insulin deficiency. The cause of type 1 diabetes is considered to be an autoimmune destruction of the insulin-producing beta cells in the pancreas. Type 2 diabetes is characterised by insufficient insulin secretion and/or decreased insulin sensitivity leading to insufficient insulin action.

The overall goal for treatment of both type 1 and type 2 diabetes is normalisation of the blood glucose concentration in order to minimise the development and progression of micro- and macrovascular long-term complications. Insulin treatment is the cornerstone and a prerequisite in the diabetes treatment. The majority of patients with type 1 diabetes are treated with multiple daily injections (MDI) of insulin or continuous subcutaneous insulin infusion (CSII). In contrast, treatment of patients with type 2 diabetes includes lifestyle modifications (diet and exercise), oral antidiabetic drugs (OADs) and insulin treatment. Treatment of type 2 diabetes has primarily focused on controlling fasting plasma glucose levels with OADs and/or basal insulin without postprandial coverage. Such regimens may fail to achieve the current standards of good glycaemic control leading to progressive deterioration of diabetes control. Large intervention studies in patients with both type 1 diabetes (DCCT 1993) and type 2 diabetes (UKPDS 1998) have shown that strict blood glucose control with intensive insulin treatment reduces the risk of developing the micro- and macrovascular complications associated with hyperglycaemia.

Insulin is a small protein, containing 51 amino acids arranged in two chains (A and B) linked by disulphide bridges. Insulin is synthesised from pro-insulin (a long single-chain protein molecule) by hydrolysis, which in addition to insulin generates the residual connecting segment, or C-peptide, by removal of four amino acids.

The normal, physiological insulin profile is essentially composed of two components: a constant, low-level, background basal supply and large but transitory insulin peaks that occur at mealtimes. Continued efforts to carefully imitate this physiologic profile prompted the development of insulin products with improved physicochemical properties based on analogues of human insulin (HI). The advancement in protein engineering offers targeted development of insulin analogues. These analogues display either faster absorption kinetics or longer time–action profiles compared with HI and, therefore, more closely replicate endogenous insulin secretion. Insulin preparations can be categorised by duration of action: short-acting insulin, intermediate-acting insulin, long-acting insulin and mixed preparations of short-acting and intermediate-acting insulins (Table 8.1). Three genetically engineered short-acting insulin analogues are currently available. All are designed to have a rapid onset and short duration of action when injected subcutaneously:

Humalog® (Eli Lilly Nederland B.V., The Netherlands), NovoRapid® (Novo Nordisk A/S, Denmark) and Apidra® (Sanofi-Aventis Deutschland GmbH, Germany). With the exception of the amino acid modifications, these rapid-acting insulin analogues are homologous to regular HI. Similar to the rapid-acting insulin analogues, two long-acting analogues of HI have been manufactured by protein engineering: Lantus® (Sanofi-Aventis Deutschland GmbH, Germany) and Levemir® (NovoNordisk A/S, Denmark). Finally, two premixed insulin preparations containing a mixture of a rapid-acting insulin analogue and a protamine-crystallised insulin analogue are marketed: HumalogMix® (Eli Lilly Nederland B.V., The Netherlands) and NovoMix® (Novo Nordisk A/S, Denmark). Both premixed analogues have been formulated to exploit the advantage of a rapid-acting insulin analogue (targeting meal-related hyperglycaemia), whereas the protamine-crystallised component has an extended duration of action, like that of neutral protamine Hagedorn (NPH) insulin (intermediate acting HI), and can address basal insulin needs.

Table 8.1 Overview of the most frequently used insulin formulations.

Rapid-acting insulin	Insulin aspart (analogue)	Asp^{B28}
	Insulin glulisine (analogue)	Lys^{B3}, Glu^{B29}
	Insulin lispro (analogue)	Lys^{B28}, Pro^{B29}
Short-acting insulin	Regular human insulin (soluble)	
Intermediate-acting insulin	Neutral protamine Hagedorn (NPH) insulin (isophane)	Complex with protamine
Long-acting insulin	Insulin glargine (analogue)	Gly^{A21}, Arg^{B31}, Arg^{B32}
	Insulin detemir (analogue)	$desThr^{B30}$, myristic acid bound to Lys^{B29}
Premixed insulin	50% NPH insulin, 50% regular human insulin	
	70% NPH insulin, 30% regular human insulin	
	70% insulin aspart protamine suspension, 30% insulin aspart	
	70% insulin lispro protamine suspension, 30% insulin lispro	

8.2. Immunogenicity of Subcutaneously Administered Insulin

Immunological complications of insulin therapy were recognised already when insulin became available for the treatment of diabetes mellitus in 1922. Insulin antibodies of the immunoglobulin G (IgG) and immunoglobulin E (IgE) type can develop (Schernthaner 1993), and anti-insulin antibodies are common in patients with diabetes treated with subcutaneous HI (Marshall et al. 1988; Velcovsky and Federlin 1982): Marshall and co-workers (Marshall et al. 1988) have reported that as many as 80% of patients treated with subcutaneous insulin may develop anti-insulin antibodies.

Following administration of exogenous insulin, the formation of anti-insulin antibodies may affect the pharmacokinetic and pharmacodynamic profiles, and thereby the clinical effects, of the insulin. Glycaemic control may worsen if insulin antibodies neutralise insulin, or hypoglycaemic events may become more frequent if insulin antibodies serve as a carrier to prolong the glucose reducing effect of the insulin (Bolli et al. 1983; Bolli et al. 1984). Insulin antibodies have also been associated with insulin resistance and allergic reactions (Schernthaner 1993).

It is generally agreed that the purity of the insulin preparation influences the level of insulin antibodies generated in patients with diabetes. Also, it is recognised that bovine insulin is more immunogenic than porcine insulin given in the same formulation (Heding et al. 1984). Much attention has been directed to the lower immunogenicity and allergenicity of highly purified recombinant HI preparations. And while the proportion of patients who develop insulin antibodies after exogenous insulin administration can be high (Marshall et al. 1988), the introduction of highly purified recombinant HI and HI analogues has meant that actual immune-mediated reactions to insulin are now less frequent (Schernthaner 1993; Lapolla, Dalfra, and Fedele 2005).

8.3. Immunogenicity of Insulin Treatment with Insulin Analogues

Data from studies in patients with both type 1 and type 2 diabetes have demonstrated that rapid-acting insulin analogues generate similar low levels of insulin antibodies as recombinant HI, with no correlations to dose, glycaemic control or adverse events (Fineberg et al. 1996; Lindholm et al. 2002; Fineberg et al. 2003). As the rapid-acting analogues are homologous to HI except for minor changes in the amino acid sequence, the majority of antibodies will be cross-reacting.

The immunogenicity of Humalog® versus regular HI was studied in four open-label, 1-year-long randomised trials involving patients with both type 1 and type 2 diabetes, all previously treated with insulin (Fineberg et al. 1996). At baseline, insulin antibodies specific to HI or insulin lispro were absent in most patients, whereas 41–45% of patients with type 1 diabetes and 23–27% of patients with type 2 diabetes had cross-reacting antibodies. Within studies, no significant differences were noted over time. Patients with type 1 diabetes were more likely to develop or maintain cross-reacting antibody levels than patients with type 2 diabetes. There was no evidence that insulin lispro differs in immunogenicity from HI in previously treated patients.

In a pooled analysis of four multinational, open, parallel group studies comprising a total of 2420 patients with diabetes, treatment with NovoRapid® or NovoMix® was associated with an initial increase in cross-reacting insulin antibodies after three months of exposure, followed by a decrease towards baseline values over the first year of treatment (Lindholm et al. 2002). However, clinical efficacy (HbA$_{1c}$ and insulin dose) and safety (hypoglycaemia) outcomes were not correlated with any changes in insulin antibody levels, and therefore the clinical relevance of these observations was considered to be trivial. Only few patients developed antibodies specific to HI or insulin aspart during the 6- to 12-month study periods, whereas more than half of the patients had antibodies cross-reacting between HI and insulin aspart when entering the studies (mean levels $\sim$ 10–17%). Baseline levels of cross-reacting insulin antibodies of zero are only to be expected in insulin-naive patients never exposed to exogenous insulin. Antibody levels showed similar changes in patients with type 1 and type 2 diabetes, and there was no consistent relationship between antibody formation and glycaemic control or between antibody formation and safety in terms of adverse events. Data on the immunogenicity of long-acting insulin analogues are sparse, but both Lantus® and Levemir® appear to be comparable to human NPH insulin in terms of immunogenicity. New data from a 2-year-long, multinational, multicentre, parallel trial in patients with type 1 diabetes randomised 2:1 to treatment with Levemir® or NPH insulin, both in combination with NovoRapid® at mealtime, address the long-term immunogenicity of combined treatment with rapid-acting and long-acting insulin analogues (Bartley et al. 2007). Results on antibodies cross-reacting between insulin detemir and insulin aspart showed maximum antibody binding after 1 year of treatment, followed by a small but significant decline at end of trial after two years of exposure. Insulin detemir-specific or insulin aspart-specific antibody levels showed a modest increase after one year. All analyses confirmed that the antibody formation stabilised and tended to reduce after about one year. The antibody samples were obtained after transfer of patients from insulin detemir to NPH insulin for 4–8 days prior to blood sampling to ensure minimum interference of insulin detemir in the samples during analysis of insulin antibodies.

8.4. Immunogenicity of Insulin in Special Populations

8.4.1. Immunogenicity of Insulin Treatment of Children and Adolescents with Diabetes

The immunogenicity of insulin has mainly been studied in adult patients with diabetes. Long-term immunogenicity in children and adolescents was studied in a 30-month study including 72 insulin-naive children and adolescents with newly diagnosed type 1 diabetes. The patients were allocated to treatment with NovoRapid® or HI both in combination with NPH insulin from diagnosis of type 1 diabetes (Holmberg et al. 2007). The results showed that the level of insulin aspart-specific antibodies remained low throughout the study. After 9 months of treatment, the level of cross-reacting antibodies was increased from a low baseline level to a mean level of 40–50% and remained elevated.

It was concluded that treatment with NovoRapid® and with HI was associated with an increase in cross-reacting insulin antibodies in insulin-naive children, but with no measurable impact on the efficacy or safety of the treatment.

8.4.2. Immunogenicity of Insulin Treatment of Pregnant Women with Diabetes

A few studies have addressed the antibody response to insulin in pregnant women, but the results are currently inconclusive and sparse (Menon et al. 1990, Weiss, Kainer and Haas 1998; Lindsay et al. 2004). A possible link between neonatal complications and transfer of insulin antibodies across the placenta has been investigated, but not confirmed (Menon et al. 1990; Weiss, Kainer and Haas 1998; Lindsay et al. 2004). There is data to support that insulin antibodies can cross the placenta. In a study of 138 pregnant women with type 1 diabetes, insulin antibodies were detected in the cord blood of 95% of the offspring at birth (Lindsay et al. 2004). Recently, these results have been confirmed by McCance (McCance et al. 2007) in a subset of pregnant women with type 1 diabetes participating in a randomised, controlled trial comparing NovoRapid® with HI (Mathiesen et al. 2007). There was a significant positive correlation between the level of cross-reacting insulin antibodies assessed in the pregnant women and in the umbilical cord blood in the offspring, indicating a transfer of maternal cross-reacting insulin antibodies across the placental barrier.

In the same study, serial assessments of insulin antibody levels during pregnancy demonstrated that insulin antibody levels in pregnant women with type 1 diabetes treated with the NovoRapid® do not differ from insulin antibody levels in those treated with HI (McCance et al. 2007). This result is reassuring and is comparable to results in previous studies involving non-pregnant patients with type 1 and type 2 diabetes or those with gestational diabetes mellitus (Jovanovic et al. 1999; Jovanovic et al. 2005). In the present trial, the baseline levels of cross-reacting insulin antibodies agree with previous observations in non-naive patients previously exposed to exogenous insulin (Lindholm et al. 2002). However, unlike the Lindholm study, there was no increase in cross-reacting insulin antibody levels throughout pregnancy in those women treated with NovoRapid®. This suggests that insulin antibodies do not develop further during pregnancy, even though high insulin doses were administered in the latter part of pregnancy. In general, levels of cross-reacting insulin antibodies appear to decrease during pregnancy, perhaps similar to the drops in insulin antibody levels seen after some months of treatment (Lindholm et al. 2002; Hamalainen et al. 2000; Exon, Dixon and Malins 1974; Spellacy and Goetz 1963) or similar to reductions seen with other types of antibodies during pregnancy, for example, serum antithyroglobulin antibodies (D'Armiento et al. 1980).

8.5. Pulmonary Insulin

Non-invasive/needle-free delivery options for insulin are being investigated with increased efforts and interest. At present, the most promising alternative route to subcutaneous injections of insulin is by inhalation. Systemic insulin delivery to lower blood glucose via the lungs has been described in the medical literature as far back as 1924 (Heubner, De Jongh and Laquer 1924) and 1925 (Gänsslen 1925). Only recently has this mode of insulin administration been used for the registration of Exubera® (Pfizer Limited, UK) in the USA and EU for use in patients with diabetes.

The pulmonary alveoli have an estimated surface area of approximately 100 m^2 and this allows for rapid absorption of small peptides from the inhaled air to the blood (Agu et al. 2001), and thus the possibility of formation of neutralising antibodies or developing allergic immune responses via this route of administration arises. It is well known that exogenous insulin administration can elicit both local and systemic immunologic responses although allergic responses are rare (Schernthaner 1993).

8.5.1. Immunogenicity of Insulin Treatment with Pulmonary Insulin

All classes of antibodies (IgA, IgE, IgG and IgM) have been studied in patients using different inhaled insulins, but the results cannot be directly compared as different antibody assays have been utilised (Hermansen et al. 2004; Fineberg et al. 2005; Ceglia, Lau and Pittas 2006; Teeter and Riese 2006). In type 1 and type 2 diabetes patients using the AERx® iDMS (NovoNordisk A/S, Denmark), both total and IgG insulin antibody levels were higher for inhaled insulin than for subcutaneous insulin aspart or HI (Hermansen et al. 2004; Wollmer et al. 2007). In a long-term study in patients with type 1 diabetes, the levels increased for 3–6 months and plateaued from 6 to 12 months (Wollmer et al. 2007). Elevated IgE antibody levels were detected in a small number of type 2 patients, and no change was observed for IgA antibody levels (Hermansen et al. 2004). In Exubera® studies, the antibody titres cover a wide range of IgG levels, while IgM, IgA and IgE antibodies have been below the limits of quantification for the respective assays (Fineberg et al. 2005). The immune response after exposure to Exubera® inhalation consisted of a heterogeneous population of antibodies representing a range of binding affinities and binding capacities, as has been described for subcutaneous insulin (Heise et al. 2005). The rise in insulin antibody levels occurs rapidly after the onset of use of inhaled insulin and reaches a plateau after a period of 6–12 months in both patients with type 1 and 2 diabetes using Exubera®, as is the case with antibodies associated with subcutaneous insulin administration (Fineberg et al. 2005; Ceglia, Lau and Pittas 2006). Similar results have been reported showing an increase in insulin-specific antibody titres compared to subcutaneous insulin in patients with type 1 diabetes using HI inhalation powder (Eli Lilly) over 12 weeks (Garg et al. 2006).

The effects of inhaled insulin on the immune system have been observed to have a greater response in patients with type 1 diabetes and in islet cell antibody-positive type 2 diabetes patients compared to patients with type 2 diabetes (Fineberg et al. 2005; Ceglia, Lau and Pittas 2006). Furthermore, patients with type 2 diabetes who were initially insulin-naive had lower antibody responses than previously insulin-treated patients. This difference in immunogenicity between initially insulin-naive versus insulin-treated patients was maintained over 2 years of inhaled insulin exposure with Exubera® despite the addition of subcutaneous basal insulin and may reflect active suppression of the humoral insulin responses (Fineberg et al. 2005). The immune response has been studied in both powder- and liquid-based inhaled insulin formulations and does not appear to be related to excipients (Wollmer et al. 2007; Fabbri 2006; Quattrin et al. 2004).

In a 24-week study with 226 patients with type 1 diabetes randomised to inhaled insulin with Exubera® or subcutaneous insulin for 12 weeks followed by an antibody washout period of 12 weeks, the small lung function changes observed with inhaled insulin therapy were not mediated by the humoral immune response or associated with the acute decrements in lung function immediately after initiation of insulin inhalation (Heise et al. 2005). Furthermore, no effects were observed on the metabolic effects or action of insulin when examining the pharmacodynamic impact of the development of insulin antibodies after 24 weeks of therapy with Exubera®(Fabbri 2006); no correlation with low or high affinity binding insulin antibodies and postprandial glucose levels, fasting blood glucose, duration of insulin action or increased hypoglycaemic event rate as in other long-term clinical trials with Exubera® (Fabbri 2006). Similar results have been observed for AIR® (Lilly/Alkermes) and AERx® iDMS (Quattrin et al. 2004; Moses et al. 2006). Insulin antibody response was also measured in a long-term study comparing inhaled insulin via AERx® iDMS with subcutaneous NovoRapid® in patients with type 1 diabetes. Total and IgG insulin antibody levels were higher with inhaled insulin compared to subcutaneous NovoRapid® (Moses et al. 2006). Further analyses in a subgroup of patients treated for 23 months revealed no influence of elevated antibody levels on pharmacokinetic characteristics after a single inhalation or inhaled insulin or over three mealtime inhalations (Roberts et al. 2006).

Patients with type 2 diabetes treated with inhaled HI with the AERx® iDMS before meals for 12 weeks were compared to pre-meal injections of HI (Hermansen et al. 2004). Median total insulin antibody levels increased in the inhaled group from 6 to 35% tracer binding compared to no changes in the subcutaneous insulin-treated group, but no correlations were found between change in total insulin antibody level, metabolic control and insulin dose. IgG antibody levels showed a substantial increase in only five patients in the inhaled group, but median levels only increased slightly (Hermansen et al. 2004). A review of several trials in patients with type 2 diabetes using inhaled human insulin with Exubera®demonstrated similar results with no correlation of antibodies to $HbA1_c$, insulin dose, incidence of hypoglycaemia or pulmonary function (Fineberg et al. 2005). In trials where patients have been followed after discontinuation of the inhaled insulin, antibody levels start to decline towards the baseline values within the approximately 12 weeks (Teeter and Riese 2006).

8.6. Conclusions

Protein drugs such as insulin are immunogenic. The development of insulin antibodies with the use of subcutaneous or inhaled administration appears to be common, although the antibody level varies dependent on factors such as the preparation, route of administration and age of the patient. Despite initial increases in antibody formation, there appears to be no consistent relationship between antibody formation and glycaemic control or between antibody formation and safety in terms of adverse events.

References

Agu, R. U., Ugwoke, M. I., Armand, M., Kignet, R., and Verbaeke, N. 2001. The lung as a route for systemic delivery of therapeutic proteins and peptides. Respir. Res. 2:198–209.

Bartley, P. C., Bogoev, M., Larsen, J., and Philotheou, A. 2007. Long-term efficacy and safety of insulin detemir versus NPH insulin in subjects with type 1 diabetes using a treat-to-target basal-bolus regimen with insulin aspart at meals: A 2-year, randomized, controlled trial. Diabetic Medicine (in press).

Bolli, G., de Feo, P., Compagnucci, P., Cartechini, M. G., Angeletti, G., Santeusanio, F., Brunetti, P., and Gerich, J. E. 1983. Abnormal glucose counterregulation in insulin-dependent diabetes mellitus. Interaction of anti-insulin antibodies and impaired glucagon and epinephrine secretion. Diabetes 32:134–141.

Bolli, G. B., Dimitriadis, G. D., Pehling, G. B., Baker, B. A., Haymond, M. W., Cryer, P. E., and Gerich, J. E. 1984. Abnormal glucose counterregulation after subcutaneous insulin in insulin-dependent diabetes mellitus. N. Engl. J. Med. 310:1706–1711.

Ceglia, L., Lau, J., and Pittas, A. G. 2006. Meta-analysis: efficacy and safety of inhaled insulin therapy in adults with diabetes mellitus. Ann. Intern. Med. 145:665–675.

The Diabetes Control and Complications Trial Research Group. 1993. The effect of intensive treatment of diabetes on the development and progression of long-term complications in insulin-dependent diabetes mellitus. N. Eng. J. Med. 329:977–986.

D'Armiento, M., Salabé, H., Vetrano, G., Scucchia, M., and Pachi, A. 1980. Decrease of thyroid antibodies during pregnancy. J. Endocrin. Invest. 3:437–438.

Exon, P. D., Dixon, K., and Malins, J. M. 1974. Insulin antibodies in diabetic pregnancy. Lancet 2 (7873):126–128.

Fabbri L. 2006. Pulmonary safety of inhaled insulins: a review of the current data. Curr. Med. Res. Opin. 22 (Suppl 3):21–28.

Fineberg, N. S., Fineberg, S. E., Anderson, J. H., Birkett, M. A., Gibson, R. G., and Hufferd, S. 1996. Immunologic effects of insulin lispro (Lys (B28), Pro (B29) human insulin) in IDDM and NIDDM patients previously treated with insulin. Diabetes 45:1750–1754.

Fineberg, S. E., Huang, J., Brunelle, R., Gulliya, K. S., and Anderson, J. H. 2003. Effect of long-term exposure to insulin lispro on the induction of antibody response in patients with type 1 or type 2 diabetes. Diabetes Care 26:89–96.

Fineberg, S. E., Kawabata, T., Finco-Kent, D., Liu, C., and Krasner, A. 2005. Antibody response to inhaled insulin in patients with type 1 or type 2 diabetes. An analysis of initial phase II and III inhaled insulin (Exubera) trials and a two-year extension trial. J. Clin. Endocrinol. Metab. 90:3287–3294.

Garg, S., Rosenstock, J., Silverman, B. L., Sun, B., Konkoy, C. S., de la Pena, A., and Muchmore, D. B. 2006. Efficacy and safety of preprandial human insulin inhalation powder versus injectable insulin in patients with type 1 diabetes. Diabetologia 49:891–899.

Gänsslen, M. 1925. Über inhalation von insulin. Klin. Wochenschr. 4 (Jahrgang 2):71.

Hamalainen, A. M., Ronkainen, M. S., Akerblom, H. K., and Knip, M. 2000. Postnatal elimination of transplacentally acquired disease-associated antibodies in infants born to families with type 1 diabetes. The Finnish TRIGR Study group Trial to reduce IDDM in the genetically at risk. J. Clin. Endocrionol. Metab. 85: 4249–4253.

Heise, T., Bott, S., Tusek, C., Stephan, J.-A., Kawabata, T., Finco-Kent, D., Liu, C., and Krasner, A. 2005. The effect of insulin antibodies on the metabolic action of inhaled and subcutaneous insulin: a prospective randomized pharmacodynamic study. Diabetes Care 28:2161–2169.

Heding, L. G., Marshall, M. O., Persson, B., Dahlquist, G., Thalme, B., Lindgren, F., Åkerblom, H. K., Rilva, A., Knip, M., Ludvigsson, J., Stenhammar, L.,

Strömberg, L., Søvik, O., Bævre, H., Wefring, K., Vidnes, J., Kjærgård, J. J., Bro, P., and Kaad, P. H. 1984. Immunogenicity of monocomponent human and porcine insulin in newly diagnosed Type 1 (insulin-dependent) diabetic children. Diabetologia 27:96–98.

Hermansen, K., Rönnemaa, T., Petersen, A. H., Bellaire, S., and Adamson, U. 2004. Intensive therapy with inhaled insulin via the AERx insulin diabetes management system: a 12-week proof-of-concept trial in patients with type 2 diabetes. Diabetes Care 27:162–167.

Heubner, W., De Jongh, S. E., and Laquer, E. 1924. Über inhalation von insulin. Klin. Wochenschr. 3 (Jahrgang 51):2342–2343.

Holmberg, H., Mersebach, H., Kanc Hanzel, K., and Ludvigsson, J. 2007. Antibody response to insulin in children and adolescents with newly diagnosed type 1 diabetes. Diabetes 56 (Suppl 1):A476 (submitted for publication).

Jovanovic, L., Ilic, S., Pettitt, D. J., Hugo, K., Gutierrez, M., Bowsher, R. R., and Bastyr, E.J. 1999. Metabolic and immunologic effects of insulin lispro in gestational diabetes. Diabetes Care 22:1422–1427.

Jovanovic, L., Howard, C., Pettitt, D., Zisser, H., and Ospina P. 2005. Insulin aspart vs. regular human insulin in basal/bolus therapy for patients with gestational diabetes mellitus: safety and efficacy. Diabetologia 48 (Suppl 1):A317.

Lapolla, A., Dalfra, M. G., and Fedele, D. 2005. Insulin therapy in pregnancy complicated by diabetes: are insulin analogs a new tool? Diabetes Metab. Res. Rev. 21:241–52.

Lindholm, A., Jensen, L. B., Home, P. D., Raskin, P., Boehm, B. O., and Rastam, J. 2002. Immune responses to insulin aspart and biphasic insulin aspart in people with type 1 and type 2 diabetes. Diabetes Care 25:876–882.

Lindsay, R. S., Ziegler, A. G., Hamilton, B. A., Calder, A. A., Johnstone, F. D., and Walker, J. D. 2004. Type 1 diabetes-related antibodies in the fetal circulation: Prevalence and influence on cord insulin and birth weight in offspring of mothers with type 1 diabetes. J. Clin. Endocrinol. Metab. 89:3436–3439.

Marshall, M. O., Heding, L. G., Villumsen, J., Aakerblom, H. K., Baevre, H., Dahlquist, G., Kjaergaard, J. J., Knip, M., Lindgren, F., Ludvigsson, J., Persson, B., Stenhammar, L., Stromberg, L., Sovik, O., Thalme, B., Vidnes, J., and Wefring, K. 1988. Development of insulin antibodies, metabolic control and beta cell function in newly diagnosed insulin dependent diabetic children treated with monocomponent human insulin or monocomponent porcine insulin. Diabetes Res. 9:169–175.

Mathiesen, E., Kinsley, B., McCance, D., Duran, S., Heller, S., Bellaire, S., and Raben, A. 2007. Maternal Hypoglycemia and Glycemic Control in Pregnancy: A Randomized Trial Comparing Insulin Aspart with Human Insulin in 322 Subjects with Type 1 Diabetes. Diabetes Care 30:771–776.

McCance, D., Damm, P., Mathiesen, E., Kaaja, R., Dunne, F., Hod, M., Jensen, L.E., and Mersebach, H. 2007. No increase in insulin antibodies during pregnancy and no clear evidence of transfer of insulin aspart across the placenta in pregnant women with type 1 diabetes. Diabetes 56 (Suppl 1):A22 (submitted for publication).

Menon, R. K., Cohen, R. M., Sperling, M. A., Cutfield, W. S., Mimouni, F., and Khoury, J. C. 1990. Transplacental passage of insulin in pregnant women with insulin-dependent diabetes mellitus. Its role in fetal macrosomia. N. Engl. J. Med. 323:309–315.

Moses, R., Lunt, H., Bartley, P., O'Brien, R., Clauson, P., Vesterager, A., Wollmer, P., and Roberts, A. 2006. Periprandial inhaled human insulin via the AERx insulin Diabetes Management System (iDMS) vs. subcutaneous insulin aspart in type 1 diabetes. Diabetic Med. 23 (Suppl 4):338.

Roberts, A., Wilson, D., McElduff, A., Prins, J., Simpson, R., Haahr, H., Raastam, J., and Moses, R. 2006. Pharmacokinetics of inhaled human insulin via the AERx® insulin Diabetes Management System (iDMS) in subjects with type 1 diabetes, naïve and non-naïve to inhaled insulin. Diabetic Med. 23 (Suppl 4):343.

Schernthaner, G. 1993. Immunogenicity and allergenic potential of animal and human insulins. Diabetes Care 16:155–165.

Spellacy, W. N., and Goetz, F. C. 1963. Insulin antibodies in pregnancy. Lancet 2:222–224.

Teeter, J. G., and Riese, R. J. 2006. Dissociation of lung function changes with humoral immunity during inhaled human insulin therapy. Am. J. Respir. Crit. Care Med. 173:1194–2000.

UKPDS Group. 1998. Intensive blood-glucose control with sulphonylureas or insulin compared with conventional treatment and risk of complications in patients with type 2 diabetes (UKPDS 33). Lancet 352:837–853.

Quattrin, T., Berlanger, A., Bohannon, N. J., Schwartz, S. L., and Exubera Phase III Study Group. 2004. Efficacy and safety of inhaled insulin (Exubera) compared with subcutaneous insulin therapy in patients with type 1 diabetes: results of a 6-month, randomized, comparative trial. Diabetes Care 27:2622–2627.

Velcovsky, H. G., and Federlin, K. F. 1982. Insulin-specific IgG and IgE antibody response in type 1 diabetes subjects exclusively treated with human insulin (recombinant DNA). Diabetes Care 5 (Suppl 2):126–128.

Weiss, P. A., Kainer, F., and Haas J. 1998. Cord blood insulin to assess the quality of treatment in diabetic pregnancies. Early Hum. Dev. 51:187–195.

Wollmer, P., Peiber, T. R., Gall, M.-A., and Brunton, S. 2007. Delivering Needle-Free Insulin using AERx®iDMS (Insulin Diabetes Management System) Technology. Diabetes Technol. & Ther. 9 (Suppl 1):S57–64.

9

Case Study: Immunogenicity of Factor VIII

Silke Ehrenforth and Stephanie Seremetis

9.1. Introduction

Blood coagulation factor VIII (FVIII) is an essential component of blood coagulation. In this process, activated FVIII functions as a cofactor for the serine protease factor (F) IXa, and their membrane-bound complex (factor Xase) activates FX to FXa. Subsequently, FXa participates in activation of prothrombin to thrombin, the key enzyme of the coagulation cascade. Haemophilia A is a bleeding disorder caused by a functional absence, or reduced levels, of FVIII. In the developed world, treatment of acute bleeds and bleeding prevention are based on the infusion of virus-attenuated plasma-derived or recombinant clotting factor replacement. Such replacement therapy has substantially improved the quality of life of haemophiliacs by avoiding or rapidly resolving bleeding episodes, thus minimizing their long-term consequences, particularly in the joints. Alloantibodies (inhibitors) towards transfused FVIII represent the major complication in haemophilia care, as they render classical substitution therapy ineffective.

This chapter will address some basic characteristics of inhibitory antibodies to FVIII, risk factors predisposing or contributing to inhibitor development and the principle therapeutic management of haemophilia patients with FVIII inhibitors.

9.2. Blood Coagulation Factor VIII and Haemophilia A

Congenital haemophilia A is a rare X-linked inherited bleeding disorder, characterized by an increased bleeding tendency due to either a partial or complete deficiency of the essential blood clotting factor VIII. Approximately 1 in 5,000 males has haemophilia A and 1 in 25,000 has haemophilia B. While the birth incidence is constant in all ethnic groups, the prevalence of diagnosed haemophilia patients varies greatly as a function of haemophilia care in the region. According to the World Federation of Haemophilia (WFH, www.wfh.org), there are globally 250,000–300,000 haemophilia patients of which 90,000–100,000 receive some kind of haemophilia care.

Factor VIII, encoded by the FVIII gene on Xq28, is a large plasma glycoprotein synthesized as a single chain polypeptide consisting of six different domains (A1-A2-B-A3-C1-C2) and three short acidic segments. In vivo, it circulates as a heterodimer, consisting of a light chain (comprised of domains A3-C1-C2) associated with a heavy chain (comprised of domains A1-A2-B) through a non-covalent metal ion dependent linkage between the A1 and A3 domains. Upon proteolytic activation by thrombin or activated coagulation FX (FXa), activated FVIII (FVIIIa) participates in the formation of intrinsic Xase complex as a cofactor for activated coagulation FIX (FIXa). Intrinsic Xase complex is assembled on a phospholipid surface and converts coagulation FX to its activated form (FXa). In turn, FXa together with activated coagulation FV forms a prothrombinase complex that converts prothrombin to thrombin and leads to the formation of fibrin clot. In the bloodstream, FVIII circulates as a complex with von Willebrand factor (VWF), which protects and stabilizes FVIII. For further details on FVIII the reader is referred to the following papers: Vehar et al. 1984, Fay et al. 1986, Fay et al. 1996, Mann 1999, Saenko et al. 2002, Fay 2004.

In the context of a deficiency or absence of FVIII (haemophilia A) or FIX (haemophilia B), activation of FX becomes severely impaired, and consequently, the thrombin burst becomes delayed and insufficient for normal haemostasis. The haemostatic plug formed in these patients is therefore fragile and easily dissolved by normal fibrinolytic activity, leading to impaired haemostasis and prolonged bleeding episodes.

Haemophilia A is classified as "severe", "moderate" or "mild" based on the residual FVIII plasma activity. In mild haemophilia A, FVIII levels are >5% of normal, and bleeding usually only occurs after trauma or surgery. The clinical hallmark of moderate (FVIII levels are 1–5% of normal) or severe (FVIII levels are <1% of normal) haemophilia A is bleeding into joints and muscles. Persistent or repeated joint bleeding results in synovial inflammation and hypertrophy and predisposes to recurrent bleeding with progressive damage to the cartilage and subchondral bone. In the long term, inadequate treatment of joint bleeds may result in progressive severe arthropathy, which may be painful and disabling.

The therapeutic target in haemophilia care is to prevent bleeding, if possible, or to rapidly and definitively treat bleeding episodes when they do occur, in order to prevent joint damage and to secure a nearly normal lifestyle. The mainstay in treatment for haemophilia A patients is substitution therapy, i.e. replacement of the missing FVIII via repeated infusions of purified plasma-derived or recombinant FVIII products.

Treatment with coagulation factor concentrate may be given when bleeds occur (on-demand treatment) or to prevent bleeds occurring and thereby also prevent development of arthropathy (prophylaxis). For patients with a low bleeding tendency (i.e. mild or moderate haemophilia), on-demand treatment is the current standard therapy, while the preferred treatment modality for severely affected haemophilia patients without inhibitors is mostly routine prophylaxis using regular administration of FVIII concentrates (usually three times weekly) and supplemental on-demand treatment of bleeding episodes. Prophylactic treatment regimens enable patients to live a near-normal life, reduce the risk for developing life-and-limb-threatening bleeding episodes, reduce the severity of arthropathy, decrease pain and increase mobility and quality of life.

Despite the widespread availability of FVIII concentrates in developed countries since the early 1970s, there is surprisingly little solid evidence defining optimal levels of dosing, both in relation to treatment of joint and muscle bleeds and to prevent surgical bleeding (Bolton-Maggs, Stobart, and Smyth 2004). Rather, the dosing regimens for FVIII replacement therapy need to be adjusted for each patient and are primarily based on the various pharmacokinetic parameters of the particular factor, the minimal haemostatic factor level required to control the particular type and the severity of haemorrhage being treated. Detailed considerations and recommendations for the management of haemophilia and treatment regimens for various clinical settings can be taken from country-specific guidelines or those published by the World Federation of Haemophilia (WFH, www.wfh.org).

9.3. Coagulation Factor VIII Concentrates

A variety of concentrates are currently available for FVIII replacement therapy in patients with congenital haemophilia A. As summarized by Kessler (2005), these differ by several parameters: "(1) their source material, e.g., pooled normal plasma versus genetically engineered in 'perpetual' mammalian cell lines; (2) their degree of purity, e.g., calculated on the basis of their specific activity (International Units [IU] of specific clotting factor activity/mg of total protein); (3) the viral pathogen inactivation methods employed during manufacture, e.g. heat treatment, addition of solvent detergents, chromatographic separation steps, and nanofiltration, or combinations of the above; and finally (4) by the presence or absence of extraneous animal proteins or human albumin in the cell culture milieu as a nutrient source or in the final product as a stabilizer" (Kessler 2005).

9.3.1. Plasma-Derived Factor VIII Concentrates

Improved viral-depleting processes and donor screening practices have resulted in plasma-derived (pd) FVIII products that have greatly reduced risk for transmission of human immunodeficiency virus (HIV), hepatitis B (HBV) and C (HCV). No seroconversions to HIV, HBV or HCV have been reported with any of the pdFVIII products currently marketed in the United States, including products that are heated in aqueous solution (pasteurized), solvent-detergent treated and/or immunoaffinity purified (MASAC Recommendation #177, 2006). Thus, each of these methods appears to have greatly reduced the risk of viral transmission compared with older methods of viral inactivation. There remains, however, the possibility of viral and prion pathogen transmission with the use of currently marketed, viral-inactivated, plasma-derived products (MASAC Recommendation #177, 2006).

9.3.2. Recombinant Factor VIII Concentrates

Recombinant (r) FVIII is produced by well-established hamster cell lines that have been transfected with the gene for human FVIII (Addiego et al. 1992, Lusher et al. 1993, Bray et al. 1994). One rFVIII product has the B domain deleted (BDD) from the FVIII gene before it is inserted into Chinese hamster ovary cells (Sandberg et al. 2001). The development of BDD-rFVIII was initiated by the discovery that the B domain is dispensable for FVIII procoagulant function (Toole et al. 1986). The removal of the B domain, which comprises approximately 40% of the molecule, allowed for improvement of FVIII expression efficiency in mammalian expression systems due to a 10-fold to 20-fold increase in FVIII mRNA synthesis and a twofold increase in protein secretion into culture medium (Pittman et al. 1993). First-generation rFVIII contains animal and/or human plasma-derived proteins in the cell culture medium and in the final formulation vial. Second-generation rFVIII contains animal or human plasma proteins in the medium but not in the final formulation, while third-generation rFVIII does not contain any animal or human plasma-derived proteins in the culture medium or in the final formulation vial. The risk of human viral contamination associated with rFVIII is definitely much lower than for plasma-derived FVIII products. No seroconversions to HIV, HBV or HCV have been reported with any of the currently available products; thus rFVIII products are widely recommended as the treatment of choice for patients with haemophilia A (MASAC Recommendation #177, 2006).

9.3.3. Commercially Available FVIII Concentrates

In the United States, as an example, available FVIII concentrates derived from human plasma that contain vWF include Humate-P (ZLB Behring), Koate DVI (Talecris) and Alphanate SD (Grifols). Immunoaffinity-purified FVIII concentrates derived from human plasma include Monoclate P (ZLB Behring), Hemofil M (Baxter Hyland Immuno) and Monarc M (Baxter, from American Red Cross-collected plasma). Currently available first-, second- and third-generation rFVIII products include Recombinate (Baxter); Kogenate FS (Bayer), Helixate FS (Bayer, distributed by ZLB Behring) and B-domain-deleted ReFacto (Wyeth Genetics Institute); and Advate (Baxter), respectively. For detailed product informations please refer to MASAC Recommendation #177, 2006, www.hemophilia.org).

The choice of FVIII product usually depends on perception of safety with respect to pathogen transmission and/or inhibitor development, the patient's previous treatment history, the presence or absence of factor antibodies, product purity and cost, as well as personal preferences of the patient and the physician. It is generally accepted that all of the currently available FVIII replacement products have similar haemostatic efficacy for the treatment and prophylaxis of bleeding events (exclusive of inhibitors) (Kessler 2005). Furthermore, it is generally recognized that currently available products are virtually viral pathogen-free, although there is debate about the risk of transmission of parvovirus B19 and prion pathogens. Recombinant products generally are perceived as potentially safer than plasma-derived products and there is general consensus that previously untreated patients with haemophilia should receive recombinant clotting factor concentrates, if at all possible.

9.4. Development of Inhibitory Antibodies Against Factor VIII in Haemophilia A

Now that FVIII replacement products have attained a high level of safety and purity and the supply of these agents is no longer an issue, the development of anti-FVIII antibodies (FVIII inhibitors) which results in an inadequate response to FVIII infusion has emerged as the most serious and challenging complication of coagulation factor replacement therapy in haemophilia. Many patients have died from uncontrollable bleeds, and development of severe joint damage still presents a serious problem. Furthermore, surgery in patients with inhibitors presents a particular challenge to haemostasis management and, in the past, inhibitor patients were often denied elective surgical procedures.

Antibodies neutralizing the haemostatic effect of FVIII (FVIII inhibitors) arise in about 25–35% of patients with severe haemophilia A and a smaller proportion of patients with mild/moderate haemophilia (DiMichele 2000, Ananyeva et al. 2004, Key 2004, Hay 2006). Because they are genetically deficient in FVIII, the development of inhibitors in those with congenital haemophilia A represents an alloimmune response to the foreign protein administered to prevent or treat bleeding episodes. These alloantibodies are typically polyclonal, high-affinity IgG antibodies, of which the majority belong to the immunoglobulin (Ig)G4 subtype, although this IgG type only accounts for a few percent of the IgG fraction in normal plasma (Fulcher et al. 1987, Gilles et al. 1993). The FVIII antibodies are mainly directed against epitopes in FVIII (towards the A2, A3 and C2 domains) that are involved in the interaction of FVIII with other coagulation factors in the formation of the Xase complex (Astermark 2006).

Inhibitors predominantly occur during the initial phase of treatment with FVIII in early childhood (Ehrenforth et al. 1992), with a high-risk period for the development of inhibitors during the first 50 days of exposure to infused factor (Wight and Paisley 2003), and after a median of 9–12 exposures in studies of children with severe haemophilia A (Ehrenforth et al. 1992, Addiego et al. 1993, Lusher et al. 1993, Bray et al. 1994) and of 15 days in previously untreated patients (PUPs) (Kreuz et al. 2005a). Factor VIII inhibitors may, nevertheless, develop at any time in the patient's life (McMillan et al. 1988, Sultan 1992). The late-onset inhibitors occur in haemophiliacs who have accumulated hundreds of FVIII treatment days and often arise following an intensive treatment episode for bleeding or surgery (Hay 2006). It seems likely that these FVIII inhibitors have a different aetiology than the early-onset inhibitors. The development of an inhibitor after few FVIII exposure days is likely evidence of primary intolerance to a foreign antigen, whereas the late-onset of an inhibitor in a previously tolerant patient represents the breakdown of tolerance (Hay 2006).

9.4.1. Risk Factors Predisposing or Contributing to FVIII Inhibitor Formation

Although it is widely accepted that the driving force of inhibitor formation is the presentation of a novel or an immunologically altered FVIII antigen to the patient's immune system and that the development of inhibitors in a given haemophilia A patient is determined by a complex interaction of several genetic and non-genetic (environmental) variables, the pathophysiology of inhibitor formation has not been completely elucidated. It is still unclear (1) why any haemophiliacs develop inhibitors, (2) why not all haemophiliacs develop antibodies and (3) if it is possible to accurately predict which patients might most likely develop inhibitory antibodies.

Patient-related risk factors such as severity of haemophilia, FVIII gene mutation (Schwaab et al. 1995), ethnic origin (Aledort and DiMichele

1998), family history of inhibitors (Frommel and Allain 1977, Shapiro 1984, Astermark et al. 2001) and immunogenotypic differences such as HLA complex genotype (Frommel et al. 1981, Hay et al. 1997, Oldenburg et al. 1997) and IL-10 gene polymorphism (Astermark et al. 2006) combined with treatment-related variables such as age at first exposure (Lorenzo et al. 2001, van der Bom et al. 2003) and therapy regimen (Santagostino et al. 2005) may all play a role. Other host–environmental risk factors, such as concomitant infection and vaccination, are suspected to influence inhibitor development but have yet to be fully characterized.

9.4.1.1. Genetic Risk Factors

The early observations that the risk of inhibitor formation is influenced by disease severity, family history of inhibitor development amongst first-degree relatives and ethnicity pointed to the important role of genetics. The nature of the FVIII mutation, in particular, the severity and the localization of the factor gene defect, and genes involved in the immune response [e.g. major histocompatibility complex (MHC) and cytokine genes] have all been identified as factors determining the risk of inhibitor development (Oldenburg, El-Maarri, and Schwaab 2002, Oldenburg and Tuddenham 2002, Goodeve and Peake 2003).

In severe haemophilia A there is a well-established correlation between the FVIII genotypes and inhibitor development (Schwaab et al. 1995, Oldenburg et al. 2004). The relationship between major defects in the FVIII gene and inhibitor development is postulated to reflect the absence of circulating FVIII, which may affect the development of immune tolerance to FVIII in these patients (Oldenburg et al. 2004). Those mutations that result in the absence or severe truncation of the FVIII protein are associated with the highest risk for inhibitor formation, with a spectrum of inhibitor risks ranging from >75% for multidomain deletions through a 20–30% risk with the common intron 22 inversion mutation, to <10% with missense mutations and small FVIII deletions and insertions (Antonarakis et al. 1995, Schwaab et al. 1995, Goodeve et al. 2000, Goodeve and Peake 2003, Oldenburg et al. 2004, Oldenburg and Pavlova 2006).

In addition, there are almost certainly immunogenetic influences on the inhibitor risk, but linkage to specific HLA types has been difficult to document (Hay et al. 1997, Oldenburg et al. 1997). However, the recently described association between FVIII inhibitor development and polymorphisms in genes coding for cytokines [interleukin-10 (IL-10)] and other immunoregulatory factors [tumour necrosis factor-alpha (TNF-α)] confirms the likely complex involvement of genes regulating host immunity (Astermark et al. 2006, Berntorp and Lefvert 2006). Furthermore, the risk of FVIII inhibitor formation increases significantly in families with a history of inhibitors (Gill 1999, Astermark et al. 2001, Astermark et al. 2005). The discordant inhibitor status observed in monozygotic twins, amongst inhibitor families as well as in second- and third-degree haemophilic relatives (Gill 1999, Astermark et al. 2001, Astermark et al. 2005, Berntorp et al. 2005), suggests that constitutional factors outside the FVIII gene also affect inhibitor development. Differences in immunogenetic characteristics are most likely to account for this hereditary predisposition either to form or not to form inhibitors and are probably also responsible for a markedly higher incidence of inhibitors observed in African-Americans and Hispanic, Asian and Indian patients (Addiego et al.

1994, Scharrer, Bray, and Neutzling 1999, Astermark et al. 2001, Goudemand et al. 2006), although the common FVIII genotypes are similarly distributed in all racial groups.

All together, these observations indicate that the genetic component of inhibitor risk may well result from a complex interaction of multiple immune response gene polymorphisms in addition to the FVIII gene mutation (Hay 2006, Oldenburg and Pavlova 2006).

9.4.1.2. Non-genetic (Environmental) Risk Factors

While genetic factors constitute the imprinted and fixed individual genetic risk profile of a haemophilic patient, non-genetic (environmental) factors may increase or decrease the inhibitor risk in an individual patient. Non-inherited influences on inhibitor development that have been investigated include antenatal factors which might lead to fetomaternal blood exchange and FVIII exposure in utero, breast feeding and immune system challenges at the start of treatment, such as immunization, inflammation and trauma or surgery. The currently most debated variables, however, are treatment-related factors such as age at first FVIII replacement therapy, type of FVIII product used, product switching, treatment intensity and type and mode of administration.

Whether the actual age at onset of FVIII replacement therapy is important in determining inhibitor development has become a matter of debate, following initial reports from Spain and the Netherlands that early exposure to exogenous FVIII during the first 6 months of life may be associated with a higher incidence of inhibitor development (Lorenzo et al. 2001, van der Bom et al. 2003). A higher risk in patients, who were first treated with FVIII at a younger age than those first treated at a later age, was also observed in some subsequent studies (Goudemand et al. 2006, Chalmers et al. 2007, Gouw, van der Bom, and van den Berg 2007) but not in others (Fontes, Carvalho, and Amorim 2004, Santagostino et al. 2005). Among other potential explanations, it was suggested that the observed relationship between age at first treatment and inhibitor incidence could simply reflect the more severe genotype and therefore clinical phenotype in that patient. In a multivariate analysis of the retrospective concerted action on neutralizing antibodies in severe haemophilia A (CANAL study) the association between incidence of inhibitors and age at first treatment largely disappeared after adjustment for treatment intensity, which appears to be an independent risk factor for inhibitor development (Gouw, van der Bom, and van den Berg 2007). Intensive replacement therapy has already been shown to be a risk factor for inhibitor development in patients with mild/moderate haemophilia (Hay et al. 1998). Reports of FVIII inhibitor development in association with the use of continuous infusion in previously extensively treated patients and in patients with mild haemophilia have raised the question as to whether this mode of administration may have the potential to increase immunogenicity (Sharathkumar et al. 2003, von Auer et al. 2005). Theoretically this may be the case, due to the prolonged contact with plastic devices, prolonged storage and/or the continuous exposure of the immune system to the allogeneic factor over a longer period (Astermark 2006). However, these observations were uncontrolled, and as intensive replacement therapy for surgery is a risk factor for inhibitors in this group, it is likely that the mode of administration was irrelevant.

Finally, early, regular prophylaxis may have a protective effect against the development of inhibitors in patients with haemophilia (Santagostino et al. 2005, Morado et al. 2005, Gouw, van der Bom, and van den Berg 2007), but additional studies are required to confirm this association (Calvez and Laurian 2006, Santagostino and Mannucci 2006).

9.4.1.3. Type of FVIII Product and Incidence of FVIII Inhibitor Development

The interplay of quantitative and qualitative influences of clotting factor concentrates on inhibitor development has been extensively discussed, but it is still controversial whether presently available FVIII products have differential immunogenicity. While most studies indicate that recombinant FVIII products are no more immunogenic than their plasma-derived predecessors, there remains outstanding controversy regarding this issue.

In a systematic literature review of available data on inhibitor formation associated with the use of plasma-derived and recombinant FVIII products (Wight and Paisley 2003), the cumulative incidence of FVIII inhibitor formation in PUPs infused with more than one plasma-derived product of low or intermediate purity ranged from 20.3 to 33.0%. In contrast, for patients treated with a single plasma-derived concentrate, the cumulative FVIII inhibitor incidence ranged from 0 to 12.4%. The cumulative incidence for patients treated exclusively with a single recombinant product ranged from 36.0 to 38.7%. In common, comparative studies indicate a slightly lower FVIII inhibitor incidence in PUPs treated with a unique pdFVIII product (predominantly with high content of VWF) (Kreuz et al. 2005a, Goudemand et al. 2006).

When considering the various recombinant products together (Peerlinck and Hermans 2006), the observed FVIII inhibitor incidence across the pivotal trial programmes was in the range of 15–32% in PUPs and 0.9–2.9% in previously treated patients (PTPs) (Schwartz et al. 1990, Lusher et al. 1993, Bray et al. 1994, White et al. 1997, Seremetis et al. 1999, Abshire et al. 2000, Rothschild et al. 2000, Courter and Bedrosian 2001, Lusher et al. 2003, Lusher 2004, Tarantino et al. 2004, Lusher and Roth 2005, Kreuz et al. 2005b). High-titre inhibitors (peak >5 BU) were detected in 10–16% of PUPs and 0–2.3% of PTPs (Peerlinck and Hermans 2006). Notably, the inhibitor incidences reported from the various rFVIII pivotal trial programmes were of a similar magnitude, and in general, PUPs were approximately ten times more likely to experience inhibitors to rFVIII products than PTPs (Peerlinck and Hermans 2006).

Of interest are also the possible protective roles of von Willebrand factor (VWF) (Behrmann et al. 2002) and (co-purified) immunomodulatory proteins in the plasma-derived concentrates (Wight and Paisley 2003, Aledort 2004, Lusher 2004, Ettingshausen and Kreuz 2006, Goudemand et al. 2006, Hodge, Saxon, and Revesz 2006). A role for VWF as a chaperone molecule for procoagulant FVIII has been extensively documented (Lollar 1991, Vlot et al. 1998, Kaufman and Pipe 1999, Federici 2003). Under physiologic conditions, VWF binds to FVIII after its release in the circulation. VWF protects FVIII from proteolysis by lipid-bound proteases, stabilizes the FVIII heterodimeric

structure, modulates its activity by thrombin and further regulates its elimination by lipoprotein-related receptors (Lenting et al. 1999, Schwartz et al.
2000).

Supporting the hypothesis that plasma-derived FVIII concentrates
containing VWF are less immunogenic, several retrospective clinical studies
show a lower occurrence of inhibitors in patients treated with VWF-containing
FVIII products (Yee et al. 1997, Rokicka-Milewska et al. 1999, Kreuz et al.
2003, Wight and Paisley 2003, Ettingshausen and Kreuz 2005, Goudemand
et al. 2006) as compared with the historical cohorts of patients treated
with rFVIII. Among others, this observation may be influenced by the high
concentration of FVIII antigen (FVIII:Ag) and the reduced VWF-binding
capacity in the recombinant products (Lin et al. 2004). A preliminary evaluation of one large multicentre prospective study investigating the impact of
different variables on inhibitor development in PUPs with haemophilia A
or B (Kreuz et al. 2005a) revealed a small, but statistically insignificant,
difference in the incidence of inhibitors in relation to the type of concentrate
given (Ettingshausen and Kreuz 2006). The suggested cellular and molecular
underlying mechanisms range from a potential protective role of VWF for
some epitopes, or even for the whole tertiary structure of the FVIII molecule
(Behrmann et al. 2002), to a greater FVIII affinity in these concentrates
for VWF (Lin et al. 2004), which allows a faster and fuller binding of
this factor to endogenous plasma VWF and hence a shorter exposure to
antigen-presenting cells (Gringeri et al. 2006). The hypothesis that VWF
blocks access to antibody binding (particularly C2-domain-directed-epitopes),
thereby attenuating an expected "ramp-up" of neutralizing antibodies against
these highly antigenic epitopes (Hoots 2006), is consistent with some in vivo
immunological data (Behrmann et al. 2002, Berntorp 2003). In the absence
of prospectively designed studies, it is not possible to establish the inferred
reduced immunogenicity of plasma-derived FVIII products containing VWF,
but it is clearly possible to state that there is a body of evidence that the
immunogenicity of these products is low (Gringeri et al. 2006).

Furthermore, content of other immunomodulatory peptides (e.g. TNF-α,
transforming growth factor-β) may have immunomodulatory effects and thus
an impact on inhibitor development (Hodge, Flower, and Han 1999, Hodge,
Saxon, and Revesz 2006), which should be considered in the context of
analysing the immunomodulatory effect of different FVIII products (Ettingshausen and Kreuz 2006).

In general, however, making definitive comparisons of inhibitor data
reported from different studies is problematic, if not impossible, because
of the variability in the risk factors of enrolled patients and study designs
(Scharrer and Ehrlich 2004). As mentioned above, several patient risk factors
for FVIII inhibitors have been identified, including disease severity, FVIII
genotype, previous FVIII exposure, ethnicity and family history of inhibitor
development. Infections and immunizations around the time of FVIII infusion,
an inflammatory response to a haemorrhage, mode of infusion and frequent
large doses of FVIII for a severe bleeding episode or major surgery may also
play a predisposing role. Finally, inhibitor assay methodology and frequency
of inhibitor monitoring applied in different studies need careful considerations
(Peerlinck and Hermans 2006).

9.5. Clinical Features and Principles of Treatment in Haemophilia Patients with FVIII Inhibitors

By inducing a partial or complete refractoriness to conventional replacement therapy and thereby greatly increasing the risk of life-threatening bleeds, the presence of a FVIII inhibitor significantly influences the clinical care of the patient from two aspects: the requirement for alternative approaches to effect haemostasis through the use of bypassing agents and the need to initiate immunomodulatory therapy to induce immunological tolerance to FVIII.

For clinical purposes, the magnitude of the antibody response can be quantified through the performance of a functional inhibitor assay from which a Bethesda unit (BU) inhibitor titre can be reported (Kasper et al. 1975). The International Society on Thrombosis and Haemostasis' supported definition of high titre is >5 BU mL^{-1} and low titre between 0.5 and 5 BU mL^{-1} (White et al. 2001). Furthermore, patients can be categorized as low or high responders, depending on the immune (anaemnestic) response they exhibit when re-exposed to FVIII: low responders demonstrate lack of anaemnestic response on exposure to FVIII and can be treated with specific factor replacement, while high responders demonstrate a brisk anaemnestic response to FVIII and are not treatable with specific factor replacement. The pathophysiologic mechanisms explaining and determining the type of immune responses are not known, and it is not possible to predict which immune response will be encountered in individual patients.

High-titre inhibitor patients, in particular, have a different, and far more severe, disease course than the patient without inhibitors. Their treatment options and the potential complications, as well as the costs of treatment, all differ from those of the patient with haemophilia uncomplicated by inhibitors. Patients with haemophilia and high-titre inhibitors experience severe morbidities including multiple episodes of joint, muscle and deep tissue bleeding, which can be life- and/or limb-threatening (DiMichele 2002). In general, these patients have a considerable reduction in quality of life with high frequency of pain, hospital visits and numerous days absence from school and work (Barr et al. 2002, Dolan 2005).

9.5.1. Principles of Management in Haemophilia Patients with Inhibitors

The principles of management in haemophilia patients with inhibitors include: (a) prevention of bleeding episodes, the rapid and definitive treatment of bleeds that do occur and the provision of adequate haemostasis during surgery and other major challenges to haemostasis in the presence of an inhibitor with therapeutic options depending upon the severity of bleed, inhibitor titre and anaemnestic pattern; (b) inhibitor eradication using immune tolerance induction (ITI) therapy, which is generally accepted as the most preferred treatment option in patients with high-responding inhibitors (DiMichele 1998).

Low responders have inhibitor levels of less than 5 BU/ml and do not develop an anaemnestic response on further exposure to FVIII. In these patients, the preferred treatment of acute haemorrhage as well as haemostatic prophylaxis during surgery involves the infusion of higher and/or more frequent doses of FVIII, which saturates the existing inhibitor and provides excessive antigen (FVIII) for haemostasis in most cases. However, the majority of haemophilia patients with inhibitors develop high-titre/responding inhibitors. High responders have historical inhibitor titres greater than 5 BU/ml and demonstrate an anaemnestic rise in their inhibitor titre when re-exposed to FVIII. In these patients even frequent, high-dose FVIII substitution therapy becomes ineffective in controlling bleeding episodes as the infused coagulation factor products are neutralized by the inhibitor. To obtain haemostasis for bleeding events or to prevent bleeding in association with interventions, treatment must either bypass the requirement of FVIII for clot formation or remove sufficient antibody.

The choice of specific treatment regimen and product depends on multiple factors, including clinical bleeding severity, individual historical response to therapy, type and interval between bleed and therapy, potential for anaemnesis, the clinical response to the various products the patient has previously been exposed to and the current inhibitor titre, available venous access, parent/patient choice, product availability and cost.

Porcine FVIII, which is obtained from a colony of carefully maintained pigs that are screened frequently for several viruses, can be used in patients with inhibitors to human FVIII (MASAC Recommendation #177, 2006). There has been no documented transmission of porcine viruses, in particular porcine parvovirus, to individuals who have been treated with this product (Morrison, Ludlam, and Kessler 1993). Currently, use of this product is restricted to life- and limb-threatening emergencies, and it is available in selected countries by direct communication with the manufacturer only (MASAC Recommendation #177, 2006).

In haemophilic patients with high-responding inhibitors, the FVIII bypass strategy was and remains the mainstay of therapeutic practice. Two products are primarily utilized as bypassing agents: plasma-derived activated prothrombin complex concentrate (aPCC) (FEIBA®, manufactured by Baxter Bioscience, Austria) and the recombinant FVIIa concentrate (NovoSeven®, manufactured by Novo Nordisk, Denmark).

The active components of aPCC (FXa, prothrombin (FII) and trace amounts of activated factors IX and VII) are involved in the production of thrombin generated by FXa in a complex with activated FV (FVa), divalent calcium and procoagulant membrane (prothrombinase) (Turecek et al. 2004). Since aPCC also contains some trace amounts of FVIII (100 IU FVIII/1000-unit vial), an increase of the anti-FVIII antibody levels following the administration of aPCC is possible. Such an anaemnestic response is seen with an incidence of 20–32% when defined as an inhibitor increase of greater than 50% over pre-infusion level (Hilgartner et al. 1990, Negrier et al. 1997).

The use of aPCC for treatment of acute haemorrhages and bleeding prevention during minor and major surgeries has a documented efficacy of approximately 50–80% in several studies, of which the largest retrospective multicentre study from France documented 81.3% good or excellent efficacy (Hilgartner et al. 1990, Negrier et al. 1997, Ettingshausen et al. 2003, Hilgartner, Makipernaa, and DiMichele 2003, Luu and Ewenstein 2004, Leissinger 2004).

The adverse event profile of aPCC includes systemic reactions, failure to achieve haemostasis, thrombogenicity and, as mentioned above, anaemnesis of inhibitor titre (Ehrlich, Henzl, and Gomperts 2002). The safety issue associated with the risk of virus transmission characteristic of plasma-derived products, i.e. the risk of transmission of currently known pathogens, is very low, although not zero. A theoretical risk remains for the transmission of infectious agents that are either resistant to the viral inactivation process or currently unable to be tested for in donors, such as emerging pathogens. The main safety issue with the use of aPCCs is an increased risk of thrombosis, and observed thrombotic adverse events associated with the use of aPCC include disseminated intravascular coagulation, coronary artery thrombosis, myocardial wall infarct, deep vein thrombosis and pulmonary embolus (Lusher 1991, Green 1999, Ehrlich, Henzl, and Gomperts 2002). However, overall, thrombosis related to the use of aPCC is a rare event (Ehrlich, Henzl, and Gomperts 2002, Luu and Ewenstein 2004) and the thrombotic risk when using aPCC in haemophilic patients is thought to be equivalent to that of recombinant FVIIa, but this issue is unresolved.

Recombinant coagulation FVIIa (NovoSeven®), a vitamin K-dependent glycoprotein that is essentially identical to human plasma FVIIa, is expressed in a baby hamster kidney cell line with foetal calf serum as the media in which the cells are propagated (Jurlander et al. 2001). It is stabilized with mannitol (second-generation recombinant product). Thus, the risk of transmission of human viruses is essentially zero (Key et al. 1998). The adverse event profile of rFVIIa includes thrombosis, lack of efficacy and uncommon systemic reactions (Green 1999, Roberts, Monroe and Hoffman 2004). Anaemnesis of inhibitor titres does not occur with rFVIIa, as there is neither FVIII nor FIX in the product to stimulate such response (Brackmann et al. 2000).

The mechanism of action of rFVIIa includes the binding of FVIIa to exposed TF. This complex activates FIX into FIXa and FX into FXa, leading to the initial conversion of small amounts of prothrombin into thrombin. Thrombin leads to the activation of platelets and FV and FVIII at the site of injury and to the formation of the haemostatic plug by converting fibrinogen into fibrin. Pharmacological doses of rFVIIa activate FX directly on the surface of activated platelets, localized to the site of injury, independently of TF. This results in the conversion of prothrombin into large amounts of thrombin independently of TF. Accordingly, the pharmacodynamic effect of FVIIa gives rise to an increased local formation of FXa, thrombin and fibrin.

Both FVIII bypassing agents, aPCC and rFVIIa, have been successfully and safely used in a variety of challenging clinical situations, including muscular haemorrhage, haemarthroses, emergency treatment of acute bleeds, home treatment and the prevention of surgical bleeds (Lusher et al. 1980, Syamsoedin et al. 1981, Hilgartner et al. 1983, Hedner et al. 1988, Hilgartner et al. 1990, Arkin et al. 1998, Smith and Hann 1996, Negrier et al. 1997, Key et al. 1998, Lusher 1996, Lusher et al. 1998, Santagostino, Gringeri, and Mannucci 1999, Abshire and Kenet 2004). Inhibitor patients treated with rFVIIa can undergo major surgery with minimal risk of uncontrolled haemorrhage and complications (Ingerslev et al. 1996, Ingerslev et al. 1997, Shapiro et al. 1998). Overall, the successful clinical use of these FVIII bypassing agents has contributed to prolongation of patients' life expectancies and improvement in quality of life (Triemstra et al. 1995, Gringeri et al. 2003, U.K. Haemophilia Centre Doctors' Organisation 2004).

In many centres use of rFVIIa has become the treatment of choice for the management of surgery and acute life- or limb-threatening bleeding in patients with haemophilia and high-responding inhibitors, because of its recombinant status and favourable efficacy and safety profile (O'Connell et al. 2002, Smith 2002, Hay 2002, Hedner 2003, Levi, Peters, and Buller 2005). The same arguments for improved pathogen safety mentioned above for rFVIII concentrates apply to a consideration of rFVIIa versus the plasma-derived bypassing agent aPCC for treatment of patients with high-titre inhibitors. Furthermore, in contrast to the use of aPCC, administration of rFVIIa does not produce an anaemnestic response (which may complicate the achievement of adequate coagulation); the inhibitor level may even decrease (Johannessen, Andreasen, and Nordfang 2000) since patients are not exposed to the specific clotting factors that they have antibodies against. Furthermore, the efficacy of rFVIIa is not influenced by the level of inhibitors (Nicolaisen 1996).

A number of controlled clinical trials as well as compassionate and emergency use programmes have examined and established the safety and efficacy of rFVIIa in haemophilia A or B patients with inhibitors presenting with various types of bleeding manifestations. In prelicensure clinical trials of non-surgical bleeding, rFVIIa was effective in the treatment of 70–100% of joint, muscle, dental and central nervous system bleeds (Bech 1996, Lusher et al. 1998). In patients undergoing major surgery, including knee and shoulder joint arthroplasty, rFVIIa is an effective first-line option and has been shown to restore haemostasis in 80–100% of patients (Ingerslev et al. 1996, Shapiro et al. 1998). Furthermore, the home-treatment study indicated that a mean of 2.2 doses of 90 µg/kg infused every 3 h controlled bleeding with 93% efficacy regardless of bleed site, and with increased efficacy when treated within 8 h of bleed detection (Key et al. 1998).

The recommended dose of rFVIIa is 90–120 µg/kg^{--1} every 2–3 h until haemostasis is achieved. However, results from in vitro studies indicate that high doses of rFVIIa increase the activation of platelets and the size of the initial thrombin burst, resulting in a more stabile clot with higher resistance to fibrinolysis (Hoffman, Monroe, and Roberts 1998). In accordance, numerous clinical data from the literature clearly show that rFVIIa doses above those currently recommended are commonly used, and suggest increasing efficacy and the need for fewer infusions with increasing dose without compromising safety (Chuansumrit et al. 2001, Santagostino et al. 2001, Cooper et al. 2001, Smith 2002, Kenet et al. 2003, Quintana-Molina et al. 2004, Parameswaran et al. 2005, Santagostino et al. 2006, Kavakli et al. 2006). In a recently completed multicentre, randomized, cross-over, double-blind trial evaluating the efficacy and safety of two rFVIIa dose regimens for treating haemarthroses in a home-treatment setting, administration of rFVIIa as a single 270 µg/kg dose was at least as efficacious and safe as the 90 µg/kg × 3 regimen (Kavakli et al. 2006). This observation could have important implications for patients, their carers and clinicians since therapy consisting of a single dose could facilitate home treatment, which enables early intervention, and be of special benefit to children or other inhibitor patients with restricted venous access. Additional clinical data advocate for the administration of rFVIIa early in the course of haemorrhage to minimize the number of doses and to maximize response rate (Lusher 2000).

Importantly, the development of high-responding inhibitors has previously excluded these patients from prophylaxis (prevention of bleeding), since the

FVIII inhibitor renders it impossible to achieve even low levels of circulating FVIII. Recent reports, however, have indicated that patients with high-titre inhibitors may benefit from prophylaxis with FVIII bypassing agent therapy. Prophylaxis with twice-daily aPCC has been used as part of the Bonn immune tolerance protocol (Brackmann, Oldenburg, and Schwaab 1996), and available data suggest that aPCC prophylaxis, with or without concomitant immune tolerance therapy, reduces total bleeds as well as joint bleeds, but that it does not prevent joint disease progression when used in doses of 50–100 units/kg three to four times a week (Hilgartner, Makipernaa, and DiMichele 2003). A recently completed prospective, randomized, double-blind, uncontrolled study (Konkle et al. 2006b) showed that once-daily rFVIIa when used as secondary prophylaxis for a three-month period in patients with haemophilia A or B complicated by inhibitors significantly reduced the frequency of bleeding episodes, particularly spontaneous joint bleeds, compared with acute treatment only when a bleed occurred. The effect was shown to be safe and durable, with persistence of the effect during the 3-month post-treatment period. Furthermore, secondary prophylaxis with rFVIIa has shown to improve the quality of life of haemophilia patients with inhibitors and frequent bleeds (Konkle et al. 2006a). Secondary prophylaxis with rFVIIa was not associated with any unexpected safety concerns, and no thromboembolic events were reported during the study.

Given the inhibitor-associated morbidity resulting from limited treatment options, the standard intervention, if feasible, is immune tolerance induction (ITI) for long-term inhibitor eradication and achieving antigen-specific tolerance to FVIII. The therapeutic concept is based on long-term uninterrupted high exposure to FVIII in an effort to sufficiently "tolerize" the immune system. In that state, the clinical responsiveness to FVIII replacement therapy is restored. Dose (low dose versus high dose), dosing regimen (daily versus non-daily), product type (pdFVIII versus rFVIII) and the use of immunomodulation for optimal outcome remain subjects of controversy.

In many of haemophilia A patients who undergo ITI, failure to eradicate the inhibitor is observed (Mariani and Kroner 1999, Wight, Paisley, and Knight 2003). The duration of effect is unclear, but relapses appear to be infrequent, with a relapse rate of 15% at 15 years documented in The International Registry. In addition, ITI treatment is very expensive and many patients will never be offered the opportunity to attempt to induce tolerance. In these patients, in those waiting for ITI to start, as well as in those undergoing ITI, acute bleeding episodes are generally treated with FVIII bypassing agents. Unlike other bypassing agents, rFVIIa does not contain any FVIII antigen and does not produce an anaemnestic response (Smith 2002, Levi, Peters, and Buller 2005) and is therefore a preferred option to treat acute bleeding episodes prior to commencing or during an immune tolerance programme and to cover surgical procedures until the immune tolerance programme is successful or in ITI failure. The use of rFVIIa as a bypassing agent therefore allows inhibitor titres to reduce to levels acceptable for initiation of ITI (usually <5 BU) (Johannessen, Andreasen, and Nordfang 2000), making it an ideal pre-ITI therapy.

Clinicians generally aspire to optimize the safety and clinical efficacy of inhibitor therapy, despite the very high cost of treatment. However, cost is a major consideration when treating patients with haemophilia and the costs of care for the patient with a high-responding FVIII inhibitor are substantially greater than the costs of treating non-inhibitor patients. In this context, immune tolerance is particularly expensive but may be economically justifiable in the long term as, if successful, it reduces the lifetime costs of treating that patient.

9.6. Conclusion

Anti-FVIII inhibitory antibodies, which develop in approximately 20–35% of persons with severe haemophilia A and make the use of FVIII concentrates ineffective for the treatment of bleedings, have emerged as the most challenging complication in haemophilia care. Haemophilic patients who develop inhibitory antibodies remain at higher risk for morbidity and mortality associated with recurrent or uncontrolled bleeding events.

Risk factors predisposing or contributing to FVIII inhibitor formation in congenital haemophilia are not well understood and hence therapy remains suboptimal. Genetic risk factors are known to be of importance, whereas the impact of non-genetic factors is less clear. While the FVIII genotype and less well defined immunogenetic factors constitute the imprinted and fixed individual genetic risk profile of a haemophilic patient, modifiable environmental factors may increase or decrease the inhibitor risk in an individual patient. Putative environmental risk factors currently debated include age at the start of treatment, treatment in association with immune challenges, type of FVIII product used and treatment intensity, among others. Improved understanding of the complex interaction of several genetic and environmental variables that lead to FVIII inhibitor formation may provide the ability to predict and perhaps even prevent inhibitor development in haemophilia patients.

This severe complication of replacement therapy requires the use of alternative haemostatic agents to treat bleeding episodes. In high-responder patients, FVIII bypassing agents (plasma-derived aPCCs or recombinant FVIIa) represent the mainstay of treatment and prevention of bleeding, and a substantial body of literature exists to document efficacy and adverse event profiles for these two products. Because of its recombinant status and favourable efficacy and safety profile rFVIIa is widely recommended as the treatment of choice for the management of surgery and acute bleeding episodes. The ultimate goal of treatment, however, is to permanently eradicate the inhibitor by immune tolerance induction therapy, thereby making it possible for the patient to be treated routinely with replacement therapy.

References

Abshire, T. C., Brackmann, H. H., Scharrer, I., Hoots, K., Gazengel, C., Powell, J. S., Gorina, E., Kellermann, E., and Vosburgh, E. 2000. Sucrose formulated recombinant human antihemophilic factor VIII is safe and efficacious for treatment of hemophilia A in home therapy. Thromb. Haemost. 83:811–816.

Abshire, T. and Kenet, G. 2004. Recombinant factor VIIa: review of efficacy, dosing regimens and safety in patients with congenital and acquired factor VIII or IX inhibitors. J. Thromb. Haemost. 2:899–909.

Addiego, J. E. Jr., Gomperts, E., Liu, S.-L., Bailey, P., Courter, S. G., Lee, M. L., Neslund, G. G., Kingdon, H. S., and Griffith, M. J. 1992. Treatment of hemophilia A with a highly purified factor VIII concentrate prepared by anti-FVIII immunoaffinity chromatography. Thromb. Haemost. 67:19–27.

Addiego, J. E., Kasper, C., Abildgaard, C., Hilgartner, M., Lusher, J., Glader, B., and Aledort, L. 1993. Frequency of inhibitor development in haemophiliacs treated with low-purity factor VIII. Lancet 342:462–464.

Addiego, J. E., Kasper, C., Abildgaard, C., Lusher, J., Hilgartner, M., Glader, B., Aledort, L., Hurst, D., and Bray, G. 1994. Increased frequency of inhibitors in African American hemophilic patients. Blood 1:293a.

Aledort, L. M. 2004. Is the incidence and prevalence of inhibitors greater with recombinant products? Yes. J. Thromb. Haemost. 2:861–862.

Aledort, L. M. and DiMichele, D. M. 1998. Inhibitors occur more frequently in African-American and Latino haemophiliacs. Haemophilia 4:68.

Ananyeva, N. M., Lacroix-Desmazes, S., Hauser, C. A. Shima, M., Ovanesov, M. V., Khrenov, A. V., and Saenko, E. L. 2004. Inhibitors in hemophilia A: mechanisms of inhibition, management and perspectives. Blood Coagul. Fibrinolysis 15: 109–124.

Antonarakis, S. E., Kazazian, H. H., and Tuddenham, E. G. D. 1995. Molecular etiology of factor VIII deficiency in hemophilia A. Hum. Mutat. 5:1–22.

Arkin, S., Cooper, H. A., Hutter, J. J., Miller, S., Schmidt, M. L., Seibel, N. L., Shapiro, A., and Warrier, I. 1998. Activated recombinant human coagulation factor VII therapy for intracranial hemorrhage in patients with hemophilia A or B with inhibitors. Results of the NovoSeven emergency-use program. Haemostasis 28: 93–98.

Astermark, J. 2006. Basic aspects of inhibitors to factors VIII and IX and the influence of non-genetic risk factors. Haemophilia 12 (Suppl. 6):8–14.

Astermark, J., Berntorp, E., White, G. C., and Kroner, B. L. 2001. The Malmo International Brother Study (MIBS): further support for genetic predisposition to inhibitor development in hemophilia patients. Haemophilia 7:267–272.

Astermark, J., Oldenburg, J., Escobar, M., White G. C., Berntorp E., and the MIBS Study Group. 2005. The Malmo International Brother Study (MIBS). Genetic defects and inhibitor development in siblings with severe hemophilia A. Haematologica 90:924–931.

Astermark, J., Oldenburg, J., Pavlova, A., Berntorp, E., Lefvert, A. K., and the MIBS Study Group. 2006. Polymorphisms in the IL-10 but not in the IL-1ß and IL-4 genes are associated with inhibitor development in patients with haemophilia A. Blood 107:3167–3172.

Barr, R. D., Saleh, M., Furlong, W., Horsman, J., Sek, J., Pai, M., and Walker, I. 2002. Health status and health-related quality of life associated with hemophilia. Am. J. Hematol. 71:152–160.

Bech, R. M. 1996. Recombinant factor VIIa in joint and muscle bleeding episodes. Haemostasis 26:135–138.

Behrmann, M., Pasi, J., Saint-Remy, J. M., Kotitschke, R., and Kloft, M. 2002. Von Willebrand factor modulates factor VIII immunogenicity: comparative study of different factor VIII concentrates in a haemophilia A mouse model. Thromb. Haemost. 88:221–229.

Berntorp, E. 2003. Variation in factor VIII inhibitor reactivity with different commercial factor VIII preparations: is it of clinical importance? Haematologica 88:EREP03

Berntorp, E., Astermark, J., Donfield, S. M., Nelson, G. W., Oldenburg, J., Shapiro, A. D., DiMichele, D. M., Ewenstein, B. M., Gomperts, E. D., Winkler, C. A., and the Hemophilia Inhibitor Genetics Study. 2005. Haemophilia Inhibitor Genetics Study – evaluation of a model for studies of complex diseases using linkage and associated methods. Haemophilia 11:427–429.

Berntorp, E. and Lefvert, A. 2006. A bi-allelic polymorphism in the promoter region of the TNF alpha gene influences the risk of inhibitor development in patients with hemophilia A. Haemophilia 12:abstract 14FP36

Bolton-Maggs, P. H., Stobart, K., and Smyth, R. L. 2004. Evidence-based treatment of haemophilia. Haemophilia 10 (Suppl. 4):20–24.

Brackmann, H. H., Effenberger, E., Hess, L., Schwaab, R., and Oldenburg, L. 2000. NovoSeven in immune tolerance therapy. Blood Coagul. Fibrinolysis 11 (Suppl. 1):S39–S44.

Brackmann, H. H., Oldenburg, J., and Schwaab, R. 1996. Immune tolerance for the treatment of FVIII inhibitors-twenty years of the Bonn protocol, Vox Sang. 70 (Suppl. 1):30–35.

Bray, G. L., Gomperts, E. D., Courter, S., Gruppo, R., Gordon, E. M., Manco-Johnson, M., Shaprio, A., Scheibel, E., White, G. 3rd, and Lee, M. 1994. A multi-center study of recombinant factor VIII (recombinate): safety, efficacy and inhibitor risk in previously untreated patients with hemophilia A. Blood 83:2428–2435.

Calvez, T. and Laurian, Y. 2006. Protective effect of prophylaxis on inhibitor development in children with haemophilia A: more convincing studies are required. Br. J. Haematol. 132:798–799.

Chalmers, E. A., Brown, S. A., Keeling, D., Liesner, R., Richards, M., Stirling, D., Thomas, A., Vidler, V., Williams, M. D., and Young, D. on behalf of the Paediatric Working Party of UKHCDO, 2007. Early factor VIII exposure and subsequent inhibitor development in children with severe haemophilia A. Haemophilia 13: 149–155.

Chuansumrit, A., Sri-Udomporn, N., Srimuninnimit, V., and Juntarukha, R. 2001. A single high dose of recombinant factor VIIa combining adjuvant therapy for controlling bleeding episodes in haemophiliacs with inhibitors. Haemophilia 7: 532–534.

Cooper, H. A., Jones, C. P., Campion, E., Roberts, H. R., and Hedner, U. 2001. Rationale for the use of high dose rFVIIa in a high-titre inhibitor patient with haemophilia B during major orthopaedic procedures. Haemophilia 7:517–522.

Courter, S. G. and Bedrosian, C. L. 2001. Clinical evaluation of B-domain deleted recombinant factor VIII in previously untreated patients. Semin. Hematol. 38:529.

DiMichele, D. M. 1998. Immune tolerance: a synopsis of international experience. Haemophilia 4:568–573.

DiMichele, D. M. 2000. Inhibitors in haemophilia: a primer. Haemophilia 6 (Suppl. 1):38–40.

DiMichele, D. 2002. Inhibitors: resolving diagnostic and therapeutic dilemmas. Haemophilia 8:280–287.

Dolan, G. 2005. ESOS: A European study on the orthopaedic status of patients with haemophilia and inhibitors. Haemophilia 11 (Suppl. 1):24–25.

Ehrenforth, S., Kreuz, W., Scharrer, I., Linde, R., Funk, M., Güngör, T., Krackhardt, B., and Kornhuber, B. 1992. Incidence of development of factor VIII and factor IX inhibitors in haemophiliacs. Lancet 339:594–598.

Ehrlich, H. J., Henzl, M. J., and Gomperts, E. D. 2002. Safety of factor VIII inhibitor bypass activity (FEIBA): 10-year compilation of thrombotic adverse events. Haemophilia 8:83–90.

Ettingshausen, C. E., Martinez Saguer, I., Funk, M. B., Klarmann, D., Stoll, H., Biller, R., and Kreuz, W. 2003. Long-term prophylaxis with FEIBA in patients with high-responding inhibitors. J. Thromb. Haemost. 1 (Suppl. 1):abstract P1628.

Ettingshausen, C. E. and Kreuz, W. 2005. Role of von Willebrand factor in immune tolerance induction. Blood Coagul. Fibrinolysis 16 (Suppl. 1):S27–S31.

Ettingshausen, C. E. and Kreuz, W. 2006. Recombinant vs. plasma-derived products, especially those with intact VWF, regarding inhibitor development. Haemophilia 12 (Suppl. 6):102–106.

Fay, P. J. 2004. Activation of factor VIII and mechanisms of cofactor action. Blood Rev. 18:1–15.

Fay, P. J., Anderson, M. T., Chavin, S. I., and Marder, V. J. 1986. The size of human factor VIII heterodimers and the effects produced by thrombin. Biochim. Biophys. Acta 871:268–278.

Fay, P. J., Beattie, T. L., Regan, L. M., O'Brien, L. M., and Kaufman, R. J. 1996. Model for the factor VIIIa-dependent decay of the intrinsic factor Xase: role of subunit dissociation and factor IXa-catalyzed proteolysis. J. Biol. Chem. 271: 6027–6032.

Federici, A. B. 2003. The factor VIII/von Willebrand factor complex: basic and clinical issues. Haematologica 88:EREP02

Fontes, E., Carvalho, S., and Amorim, L. 2004. Age at the beginning of factor VIII replacement is not a risk factor for inhibitor development in hemophilia A. Haemophilia 10:55 abstract 12 OC 14.

Frommel, D., and Allain, J. P. 1977. Genetic predisposition to develop factor VIII antibody in classic hemophilia. Clin. Immunol. Immunopathol. 8:34–38.

Frommel, D., Allain, J. P., Saint-Paul, E., Bosser, C., Noël, B., Mannucci, P. M., Pannicucci, F., Blombäck, M., Prou-Wartelle, O., and Muller, J. Y. 1981. HLA antigens and factor VIII antibody in classic hemophilia. European study group of factor VIII antibody. Thromb. Haemost. 46:687–689.

Fulcher, C. A., de Graaf Mahoney, S., and Zimmerman, T. S. 1987. FVIII inhibitor IgG subclass and FVIII polypeptide specificity determined by immunoblotting. Blood 69:1475–1480.

Gill, J. C. 1999. The role of genetics in inhibitor formation. Thromb. Haemost. 82:500–504.

Gilles, J. G., Arnout, J., Vermylen, J., and Saint-Remy, J. M. 1993. Anti-factor VIII antibodies of hemophiliac patients are frequently directed towards nonfunctional determinants and do not exhibit isotypic restriction. Blood 82:2452–2461.

Goodeve, A. C., and Peake, I. R. 2003. The molecular basis of hemophilia A: genotype-phenotype relationships and inhibitor development. Seminars in Thrombosis and Hemostasis, 29:23–30.

Goodeve, A. C., Williams, I., Bray, G. L., and Peake, I. R. 2000. Relationship between factor VIII mutation type and inhibitor development in a cohort of previously untreated patients treated with recombinant factor VIII (recombinate). Recombinate PUP Study Group. Thromb. Haemost. 83:844–848.

Goudemand, J., Rothschild, C., Demiguel, V., Vinciguerrat, C., Lambert, T., Chambost, H., Borel-Derlon, A., Claeyssens, S., Laurian, Y., and Calvez, T. 2006. Influence of the type of factor VIII concentrate on the incidence of factor VIII inhibitors in previously untreated patients with severe haemophilia A. Blood 107:46–51.

Gouw, S. C., van der Bom, J. G., and van den Berg, H. M. 2007. Treatment-related risk factors of inhibitor development in previously untreated patients with hemophilia A: the CANAL Cohort Study. Blood 109:4693–4697.

Green, D. 1999. Complications associated with the treatment of haemophiliacs with inhibitors. Haemophilia 5 (Suppl. 3):11–17.

Gringeri, A., Mantovani, L., Scalone, L., Mannucci, P. M., and the COCIS Study Group. 2003. Cost of care and quality of life for patients with hemophilia complicated by inhibitors: the COCIS Study Group. Blood 102:2358–2363.

Gringeri, A., Monzini, M., Tagariello, G., Scaraggi, F. A., Mannucci, P. M., and the Emoclot 15 Study Members. 2006. Occurrence of inhibitors in previously untreated or minimally treated patients with haemophilia A after exposure to a plasma-derived solvent-detergent factor VIII concentrate. Haemophilia 12:128–132.

Hay, C. R. M. 2002. The 2000 United Kingdom Haemophilia Centre Doctors' Organisation (UKHCDO) inhibitor guidelines. Pathophysiol Haemost Thromb 32 (Suppl. 1):19–21.

Hay, C. R. M. 2006. The epidemiology of factor VIII inhibitors. Haemophilia 12 (Suppl. 6):23–29.

Hay, C. R., Ludlam, C. A., Colvin, B. T., Hill, F. G., Preston, F. E., Wasseem, N., Bagnall, R., Peake, I. R., Berntorp, E., Mauser Bunschoten, E. P., Fijnvandraat, K., Kasper, C. K., White, G., and Santagostino, E. 1998. Factor VIII inhibitors in mild and moderate-severity haemophilia A. UK Haemophilia Centre Directors Organisation. Thromb. Haemost. 79:762–766.

Hay, C. R., Ollier, W., Pepper, L. Cumming, A., Keeney, S., Goodeve, A. C., Colvin, B. T., Hill, F. G., Preston, F. E., and Peake, I. R. 1997. HLA class II profile: A weak determinant of factor VIII inhibitor development in severe haemophilia A. UKHCDO Inhibitor Working Party. Thromb. Haemost. 77:234–237.

Hedner, U. 2003. Potential role of recombinant factor VIIa as a hemostatic agent. Clin. Adv. Hematol. Oncol. 1:112–119.

Hedner, U., Glazer, S., Pingel, K. Alberts, K. A., Blombäck, M., Schulman, S., and Johnsson, H. 1988. Successful use of recombinant factor VIIa in patient with severe hemophilia A during synovectomy. Lancet 2:1193.

Hilgartner, M., Aledort, L., Andes, A., and Gill, J. 1990. Efficacy and safety of vapor-heated anti-inhibitor coagulant complex in hemophilia patients. FEIBA Study Group. Transfusion 30:626–630.

Hilgartner, M., Knatterud, G. L. and the FEIBA Study Group. 1983. The use of factor VIII by-passing activity (FEIBA Immuno) product for treatment of bleeding episodes in haemophiliacs with inhibitor. Blood 61:36–40.

Hilgartner, W., Makipernaa, A., and DiMichele, D. M. 2003. Long-term FEIBA prophylaxis does not prevent progression of existing joint disease. Haemophilia 9:261–268.

Hodge, G., Flower, R., and Han, P. 1999. Effect of factor VIII concentrate on leucocyte cytokine production: characterisation of TGF-beta as an immunomodulatory component in plasma derived factor VIII concentrate. Br. J. Haematol. 106:784–791.

Hodge, G., Saxon, B., and Revesz, T. 2006. Effect of factor VIII concentrate on leucocyte cytokine receptor expression in vitro: relevance to inhibitor formation and tolerance induction. Haemophilia 12:133–139.

Hoffman, M., Monroe, D. M. III, and Roberts, H. R. 1998. Activated factor VII activates factors IX and X on the surface of activated platelets: thoughts on the mechanism of action of high-dose activated factor VII. Blood Coagul. Fibrinolysis 9 (Suppl. 1):S61–S65.

Hoots, W. K. 2006. Urgent inhibitor issues: targets for expanded research. Haemophilia 12:107–113.

Ingerslev, J., Freidman, D., Gastineau, D., Gilchrist, G., Johnsson, H., Lucas, G., McPherson, J., Preston, E., Scheibel, E., and Shuman, M. 1996. Major surgery in haemophilic patients with inhibitors using recombinant factor VIIa. Haemostasis 26 (Suppl. 1):118–123.

Ingerslev, J., Knudsen, L., Hvid, I., Tange, M. R., Fredberg, U., and Sneppen, O. 1997. Use of recombinant factor VIIa in surgery in factor VII deficient patients. Haemophilia 3:215–218.

Johannessen, M., Andreasen, R., and Nordfang, O. 2000. Decline of factor VIII and factor IX inhibitors during long-term treatment with NovoSeven. Blood Coagul. Fbrinolysis 11:239–242.

Jurlander, B., Thim, L., Klausen, N. K., Persson, E., Kjalke, M., Rexen, P., Jorgensen, T. B., Ostergaard, P. B., Erhardtsen, E., and Bjorn, S. E. 2001. Recombinant activated factor VII (rFVIIa): characterization, manufacturing, and clinical development. Semin. Thromb. Hemost. 27:373–384.

Kasper, C. K., Aledort, L., Aronson, D., Counts, R., Edson, J. R., van Eys, J., Fratantoni, J., Green, D., Hampton, J., Hilgartner, M., Levine, P., Lazerson, J.,

McMillan, C., Penner, J., Shapiro, S, and Shulman, N. R. 1975. A more uniform measurement of factor VIII inhibitors. Proceedings: A more uniform measurement of factor VIII inhibitors. Thromb. Diath. Haemorrh. 34:612.

Kaufman, R. J. and Pipe, S. W. 1999. Regulation of factor VIII expression and activity by von Willebrand factor. Thromb. Haemost. 82:201–208.

Kavakli, K., Makris, M., Zulfikar, B., Abrams, Z., and Kenet, G. 2006. Home treatment of haemarthroses using a single dose regimen of recombinant activated factor VII in patients with haemophilia and inhibitors. A multi-centre, randomised, double-blind, cross-over trial. Thromb. Haemost. 95:600–605.

Kenet, G., Lubetsky, A., Luboshitz, J., and Martinowitz, U. 2003. A new approach to treatment of bleeding episodes in young hemophilia patients: a single bolus megadose of recombinant activated factor VII (NovoSeven). J. Thromb. Haemost. 1:450–455.

Kessler, C. M. 2005. New perspectives in hemophilia treatment. Hematology (Am. Soc. Hematol. Educ. Program) 1:429–435.

Key, N. S. 2004. Inhibitors in congenital coagulation disorders. Br. J. Haematol. 127:379–391.

Key, N. S., Aledort, L. M., Beardsley, D., Cooper, H. A., Davignon, G., Ewenstein, B. M., Gilchrist, G. S., Gill, J. C., Glader, B., Hoots, W. K., Kisker, C. T., Lusher, J. M., Rosenfield, C. G., Shapiro, A. D., Smith, H., and Taft, E. 1998. Home treatment of mild to moderate bleeding episodes using recombinant factor VIIa (NovoSeven) in haemophiliacs with inhibitors. Thromb. Haemost. 80:912–918.

Konkle, B. A., Ebbesen, L. S., Auerswald, G. K. H., Friedrich, U., Ljung, R. C. R., Roberts, H. R., and Hoots, W. K. 2006a. Secondary prophylaxis with rFVIIa improves quality of life of hemophilia patients with inhibitors and frequent bleeds. Abstract presented during the 48th Annual Meeting and Exposition of the American Society of Hematology (ASH), Orlando, Florida, USA, 9–12 December 2006 (abstract no. 766).

Konkle, B. A., Ebbesen, L. S., Friedrich, U., Bianco, R. P., Lissitchkov, T., Rusen, L., Serban, M. A. and the NovoSeven (F7Haem-1505) Investigators. 2006b. Randomized, prospective clinical trial of rFVIIa for secondary prophylaxis in hemophilia patients with inhibitors. Data presented during the 48th Annual Meeting and Exposition of the American Society of Hematology (ASH), Orlando, Florida, USA, 9–12 December 2006 (abstract no. 1028).

Kreuz, W., Ettingshausen, C. E., Auerswald, G., Saguer, I. M., Becker, S., Funk, M., Heller, C., Klarmann, D., Klingebiel, T., and the GTH PUP Study Group. 2003. Epidemiology of inhibitors and current treatment strategies. Haematologica 88:EREP04.

Kreuz, W., Auerswald, G., Budde, U., Lenk, H., and the GTH-PUP-Study Group. 2005a. In: I. Scharrer and W. Schramm, Editors, Inhibitor development in previously untreated patients (PUPs) with haemophilia A and B. A prospective multicentre study of the German, Swiss and Austrian Society of Thrombosis and Haemostasis Research (GTH). 35th Haemophilia Symposium, Springer Verlag, Hamburg 2004, 34–37.

Kreuz, W., Gill, J. C., Rothschild, C., Manco-Johnson, M. J., Lusher, J. M., Kellermann, E., Gorina, E., Larson, P. J., and the International Kogenate-FS Study Group. 2005b. Full-length sucrose-formulated recombinant factor VIII for treatment of previously untreated or minimally treated young children with severe haemophilia A. Results of an international clinical investigation. Thromb. Haemost. 93:457–467.

Leissinger, C. A. 2004. Prevention of bleeds in hemophilia patients with inhibitors: emerging data and clinical direction. Am. J. Hematol. 77:187–193.

Lenting, P., Neels, J., van den Berg, B., Clijsters, P. P., Meijerman, D. W., Pannekoek, H., van Mourik, J. A., Mertens, K., and van Zonneveld, A. J. 1999.

The light chain of factor VIII comprises a binding site for low density lipoprotein receptor-related protein. J. Biol. Chem. 274:23734–23739.

Levi, M., Peters, M., and Buller, H. R. 2005. Efficacy and safety of recombinant factor VIIa for treatment of severe bleeding: a systematic review. Crit. Care Med. 33:883–890.

Lin, Y., Yang, X., Chevrier, M. C. Craven, S., Barrowcliffe, T. W., Lemieux, R., and Ofosu, F. A. 2004. Relationships between factor VIII:Ag and factor VIII in recombinant and plasma derived factor VIII concentrates. Haemophilia 10:459–469.

Lollar, P. 1991. The association of factor VIII with von Willebrand factor. Mayo Clin. Proc. 66:524–534.

Lorenzo, J. I., Lopez, A., Altisent, C., and Aznar, J. A. 2001. Incidence of factor VIII inhibitors in severe haemophilia: the importance of age. Br. J. Haematol. 113:600–603.

Lusher, J. M. 1991. Thrombogenicity associated with factor IX complex concentrates. Semin. Hematol. 28 (3 Suppl. 6):3–5.

Lusher, J. M. 1996. Recombinant factor VIIa (NovoSeven) in the treatment of internal bleeding in patients with factor VIII and IX inhibitors. Haemostasis 26:124–130.

Lusher, J. M. 2000. Acute hemarthroses: the benefits of early versus late treatment with recombinant activated factor VII. Blood Coagul. Fibrinolysis 11 (Suppl. 1): S45–S49.

Lusher, J. M. 2004. Is the incidence and prevalence of inhibitors greater with recombinant products? No. J. Thromb. Haemost. 2:863–865.

Lusher, J. M., Arkin, S., Abildgaard, C. F., and Schwartz, R. S. 1993. Recombinant factor VIII for the treatment of previously untreated patients with hemophilia A – safety, efficacy, and development of inhibitors. N. Engl. J. Med. 328:453–459.

Lusher, J., Ingerslev, J., Roberts, H., and Hedner, U. 1998. Clinical experience with recombinant factor VIIa. Blood Coagul. Fibrinol. 9:119–128.

Lusher, J. M., Lee, C. A., Kessler, C. M., Bedrosian, C. L., and the ReFacto Phase 3 Study Group. 2003. The safety and efficacy of B-domain deleted recombinant factor VIII concentrate in patients with severe haemophilia A. Haemophilia 9:38–49.

Lusher, J. M., Roberts, H. R., Davignon, G., Joist, J. H., Smith, H., Shapiro, A., Laurian, Y., Kasper, C. K., and Mannucci, P. M. 1998. A randomized, double-blind comparison of two dosage levels of recombinant factor VIIa in the treatment of joint, muscle and mucocutaneous haemorrhages in persons with haemophilia A and B, with and without inhibitors. rFVIIa Study Group. Haemophilia 4:790–798.

Lusher, J. M. and Roth, D. A. 2005. The safety and efficacy of B-domain deleted recombinant factor VIII concentrates in patients with severe haemophilia A: an update. Haemophilia 11:292–293.

Lusher, J. M., Shapiro, S. S., Palascak, J. E., Rao, A. V., Levine, P. H., and Blatt, P. M. 1980. Efficacy of prothrombin-complex concentrates in hemophiliacs with antibodies to factor VIII: a multicenter therapeutic trial. N. Engl. J. Med. 303: 421–425.

Luu, H. and Ewenstein, B. 2004. FEIBA safety profile in multiple modes of clinical and home-therapy application. Haemophilia 10 (Suppl. 2):10–16.

Mann, K. G. 1999. Biochemistry and physiology of blood coagulation. Thromb. Haemost. 82:165–174.

Mariani, G. and Kroner, B. L. 1999. International Immunetolerance Registry 1997 update. Vox Sang. 77:25–27.

MASAC Recommendation #177, revised October 2006. Medical and Scientific Advisory Council (MASAC) of the National Hemophilia Foundation. Recommendations concerning the treatment of hemophilia and other bleeding disorders (www.hemophilia.org).

McMillan, C. W., Shapiro, S. S., Whitehurst, D., Hoyer, L. W., Rao, A. V., and Lazerson, J. 1988. The natural history of factor VIII: C inhibitors in patients with hemophilia A: a National Cooperative Study. II. Observations on the initial development of factor VIII: C inhibitors. Blood 71:344–348.

Morado, M., Villar, A., Jimenez-Yuste, V., Quintana, M., and Hernandez Navarro, F. 2005. Prophylactic treatment effects on inhibitor risk: experience in one centre. Haemophilia 11:79–83.

Morrison, A. E., Ludlam, C. A., and Kessler, C. 1993. Use of porcine factor VIII in the treatment of patients with acquired hemophilia. Blood 81:1513–1520.

Negrier, C., Goudemand, J., Sultan, Y., Bertrand, M., Rothschild, C., and Lauroua, P. 1997. Multicenter retrospective study on the utilization of FEIBA in France in patients with factor VIII and factor IX inhibitors. French FEIBA Study Group. factor eight bypassing activity. Thromb. Haemost. 77:1113–1119.

Nicolaisen, E. M. 1996. Clinical experience with NovoSeven: lack of antigenicity after repeated treatment with NovoSeven. Haemostasis 26 (Suppl. 1):98–101.

O'Connell, N., Mc Mahon, C., Smith, J., Khair, K., Hann, I., Liesner, R., and Smith O. P. 2002. Recombinant factor VIIa in the management of surgery and acute bleeding episodes in children with haemophilia and high responding inhibitors. Br. J. Haematol. 116:632–635.

Oldenburg, J., El-Maarri, O., and Schwaab, R. 2002. Inhibitor development in correlation to factor VIII genotypes. Haemophilia, 8 (Suppl. 2):23–29.

Oldenburg, J. and Pavlova, A. 2006. Genetic risk factors for inhibitors to factors VIII and IX. Haemophilia 12 (Suppl. 6):15–22.

Oldenburg, J., Picard, J. K., Schwaab, R. Brackmann, H. H., Tuddenham, E. G., and Simpson, E. 1997. HLA genotype of patients with severe haemophilia A due to intron 22 inversion with and without inhibitors of factor VIII. Thromb. Haemost. 77:238–242.

Oldenburg, J., Schroder, J., Brackmann, H. H., Müller-Reible, C., Schwaab, R., Tuddenham, E. 2004. Environmental and genetic factors influencing inhibitor development. Semin. Hematol. 41 (Suppl. 1):82–88.

Oldenburg, J., and Tuddenham, E. 2002. Genetic basis of inhibitor development in severe haemophilia A and B. In: E. C. Rodriguez-Merchan and C. A. Lee, Editors, Inhibitors in patients with haemophilia, Blackwell Publishing, Oxford, pp. 21–26.

Parameswaran, R., Shapiro, A. D., Gill, J. C., Kessler, C. M., and the HTRS Registry Investigators. 2005. Dose effect and efficacy of rFVIIa in the treatment of haemophilia patients with inhibitors: analysis from the Hemophilia and Thrombosis Research Society Registry. Haemophilia 11:100–106.

Peerlinck, K. and Hermans, C. 2006. Epidemiology of inhibitor formation with recombinant factor VIII replacement therapy. Haemophilia 12:579–590.

Pittman, D. D., Alderman, E. M., Tomkinson, K. N., Wang, J. H., Giles, A. R., and Kaufman, R. J. 1993. Biochemical, immunological, and in vivo functional characterization of B-domain-deleted factor VIII. Blood 81:2925–2935.

Quintana-Molina, M., Martinez-Bahamonde, F., Gonzalez, G., Romero-Garrido, J., Villar-Camacho, A., Jiménez-Yuste, V., Fernández-Bello, I., and Hernández-Navarro, F. 2004. Surgery in haemophilic patients with inhibitor: 20 years of experience. Haemophilia 10 (Suppl. 2): 30–40.

Roberts, H. R., Monroe, D. M. III, and Hoffman, M. 2004. Safety profile of recombinant factor VIIa. Semin. Hematol. 41 (Suppl. 1):101–108.

Rokicka-Milewska, R., Klukowska, A., Dreger, B., and Beer, H. J. 1999. Incidence of factor VIII inhibitor development in previously untreated hemophilia A patients after exposure to a double viral inactivated factor VIII concentrate. Ann. Hematol. 78 (Suppl. 1):1–7.

Rothschild, C., Gill, J., Scharrer, I., and Bray, G. 2000. Transient inhibitors in the Recombinate PUP Study. Thromb. Haemost. 84:145–146.

Saenko, E. L, Ananyeva, N., Kouiavskaia, D., Schwinn, H., Josic, D., Shima, M., Hauser, C.A., and Pipe, S. 2002. Molecular defects in coagulation factor VIII and their impact on factor VIII function. Vox Sang. 83:89–96.

Sandberg, H., Almstedt, A., Brandt, J., Gray, E., Holmquist, L., Oswaldsson, U., Sebring, S., and Mikaelsson, M. 2001. Structural and functional characteristics of the B-domain-deleted recombinant factor VIII protein, r-VIII SQ. Thromb. Haemost. 85:93–100.

Santagostino, E., Gringeri, A., and Mannucci, P. M. 1999. Home treatment with recombinant activated factor VII in patients with factor VIII inhibitors: the advantages of early intervention. Br. J. Haematol. 104:22–26.

Santagostino, E., Mancuso, M. E., Rocino, A., Mancuso, G., Mazzucconi, M. G., Tagliaferri, A., Messina, M., and Mannucci, P. M. 2005. Environmental risk factors for inhibitor development in children with haemophilia A: a Case-Control Study. Br. J. Haematol. 130:422–427.

Santagostino, E., Mancuso, M. E., Rocino, A., Mancuso, G., Scaragg, F., and Mannucci, P. M. 2006. A prospective randomized trial of high and standard dosages of recombinant factor VIIa for treatment of hemarthroses in hemophiliacs with inhibitors. J. Thromb. Haemost. 4:367–371.

Santagostino, E. and Mannucci, P. M. 2006. Protective effect of prophylaxis on inhibitor development in children with haemophilia A: more convincing studies are required. Response to Calvez and Laurian. Br. J. Haematol. 132:800–801.

Santagostino, E., Morfini, M., Rocino, A., Baudo, F, Scaraggi, F. A., and Gringeri, A. 2001. Relationship between factor VII activity and clinical efficacy of recombinant factor VIIa given by continuous infusion to patients with factor VIII inhibitors. Thromb. Haemost. 86:954–958.

Scharrer, I., Bray, G. L., and Neutzling, O. 1999. Incidence of inhibitors in haemophilia A patients – a review of recent studies of recombinant and plasma-derived factor VIII concentrates. Haemophilia 5:145–154.

Scharrer, I. and Ehrlich, H. J. 2004. Reported inhibitor incidence in FVIII PUP studies: comparing apples with oranges? Haemophilia 10:197–198.

Schwaab, R., Brackmann, H. H., Meyer, C., Seehafer, J., Kirchgesser, M., Haack, A., Olek, K., Tuddenham, E. G., and Oldenburg, J. 1995. Haemophilia A: mutation type determinates risk of inhibitor formation. Thromb. Haemost. 74:1402–1406.

Schwartz, R. S., Abildgaard, C. F., Aledort, L. M., Arkin, S., Bloom, A. L., Brackmann, H. H., Brettler, D. B., Fukui, H., Hilgartner, M. W., Inwood, M. J., et al. 1990. Human recombinant DNA-derived antihemophilic factor (factor VIII) in the treatment of hemophilia A. N. Engl. J. Med. 323:1800–1805.

Schwartz, H. P., Lenting, P. J., Binder, B., Mihaly, J., Denis, C., Dorner, F., and Turecek, P. L. 2000. Involvement of low-density lipoprotein receptor-related protein (LRP) in the clearance of factor VIII in von Willebrand factor-deficient mice. Blood 95:1703–1708.

Seremetis, S., Lusher, J. M., Abildgaard, C. F., Kasper, C. K., Allred, R., and Hurst, D. 1999. Human recombinant DNA-derived antihaemophilic factor (factor VIII) in the treatment of haemophilia A: conclusions of a 5-year study of home therapy. Haemophilia 5:9–16.

Shapiro, S. S. 1984. Genetic predisposition to inhibitor formation. Prog. Clin. Biol. Res. 150:45–55.

Shapiro, A. D., Gilchrist, G. S., Hoots, W. K., Cooper, H. A., and Gastineau, D. A. 1998. Prospective, randomised trial of two doses of rFVIIa (NovoSeven) in haemophilia patients with inhibitors undergoing surgery. Thromb. Haemost. 80:773–778.

Sharathkumar, A., Lillicrap, D., Blanchette, V. S., Kern, M., Leggo, J., Stain, A. M., Brooker, L, and Carcao, M. D. 2003. Intensive exposure to factor VIII is a risk factor for inhibitor development in mild haemophilia A. J. Thromb. Haemost. 1:1228–1236.

Smith, O. P. 2002. Recombinant factor VIIa in the management of surgery and acute bleeding episodes in children with haemophilia and high-responding inhibitors. Pathophysiol. Haemost. Thromb. 32 (Suppl. 1):22–25.

Smith, O. P. and Hann, I. M. 1996. RFVIIa therapy to secure haemostasis during central line insertion in children with high-responding FVIII inhibitors. Br. J. Haematol. 92:1002–1004.

Sultan, Y. 1992. Prevalence of inhibitors in a population of 3435 hemophilia patients in France. French Hemophilia Study Group. Thromb. Haemost. 67: 600–602.

Syamsoedin, L. J., Heijnen, L., Mauser-Bunschoten, E. P. van Geijlswijk J. L., van Houwelingen, H., van Asten, P., and Sixma, J. J. 1981. The effect of activated prothrombin-complex concentrate (FEIBA) on joint and muscle bleeding in patients with hemophilia A and antibodies to factor VIII. A double-blind clinical trial. N. Engl. J. Med. 305:717–721.

Tarantino, M. D., Collins, P. W., Hay, C. R., Shapiro, A. D., Gruppo, R. A., Berntorp, E., Bray, G. L., Tonetta, S. A., Schroth, P. C., Retzios, A. D., Rogy, S. S., Sensel, M. G., Ewenstein, B. M., and the RAHF-PFM Clinical Study Group. 2004. Clinical evaluation of an advanced category antihaemophilic factor prepared using a plasma/albumin-free method: pharmacokinetics, efficacy, and safety in previously treated patients with haemophilia A. Haemophilia 10:428–437.

Toole, J. J., Pittman, D. D., Orr, E. C., Murtha, P., Wasley, L. C., and Kaufman, R. J. 1986. A large region (approximately equal to 95 kDa) of human factor VIII is dispensable for in vitro procoagulant activity. Proc. Natl. Acad. Sci. USA 83: 5939–5942.

Triemstra, M., Rosendaal, F. R., Smit, C., van der Ploeg, H. M., and Briët, E. 1995. Mortality in patients with hemophilia. Changes in a Dutch population from 1986 to 1992 and 1973 to 1986. Ann. Intern. Med. 123:823–827.

Turecek, P. L., Varadi, K., Gritsch, H., and Schwarz, H. P. 2004. FEIBA: mode of action. Haemophilia 10 (Suppl. 2):3–9.

UK Haemophilia Centre Doctors' Organisation. 2004. The incidence of factor VIII and factor IX inhibitors in the hemophilia population of the UK and their effect on subsequent mortality, 1977–99. J. Thromb. Haemost. 2:1047–1054.

Van der Bom, J. G., Mauser-Bunschoten, E. P., Fischer, K., and van den Berg, H. M. 2003. Age at first treatment and immune tolerance to factor VIII in severe hemophilia. Thromb. Haemost. 89:475–479.

Vehar, G. A., Keyt, B., Eaton, D., Rodriguez, H., O'Brien, D. P., Rotblat, F., Oppermann, H., Keck, R., Wood, W. I., Harkins, R. N., Tuddenham, E. G. D., Lawn, R. M., and Capon, D. J. 1984. Structure of human factor VIII. Nature 312: 337–340.

Vlot, A. J., Koppelman, S. J., Bouma, B. N., and Sixma, J. J. 1998. Factor VIII and von Willebrand factor. Thromb. Haemost. 79:456–465.

Von Auer, C., Oldenburg, J., Von Depka, M., Escuriola-Ettinghausen, C., Kurnik, K., Lenk, H., and Scharrer, I. 2005. Inhibitor development in patients with hemophilia A after continuous infusion of factor VIII concentrates. Ann. NY Acad. Sci. 1051: 498–505.

White, G. C. II, Courter, S., Bray, G. L., Lee, M., and Gomperts, E. D. 1997. A multicenter study of recombinant factor VIII (RecombinateTM) in previously treated patients with hemophilia A. Thromb. Haemost. 77:660–667.

White, G. C. II, Rosendaal, F. R., Aledort, L. M., Lusher, J. M., Rothschild, C., Ingerslev, J., and the Factor VIII and Factor IX Subcommittee. 2001. Definitions in hemophilia. Recommendation of the scientific subcommittee on factor VIII and factor IX of the Scientific and Standardization Committee of the International Society on Thromb Haemostas. Thromb. Haemost. 85:560.

Wight, J. and Paisley, S. 2003. The epidemiology of inhibitors in haemophilia A: a systematic review. Haemophilia 9:418–435.

Wight, J., Paisley, S., and Knight, C. 2003. Immune tolerance induction in patients with hemophilia A with inhibitors: a systematic review. Haemophilia 9:436–463.

Yee, T. T., Williams, M. D., Hill, F. G., Lee, C. A., and Pasi, K. J. 1997. Absence of inhibitors in previously untreated patients with severe haemophilia A after exposure to a single intermediate purity factor VIII product. Thromb. Haemost. 78: 1027–1029.

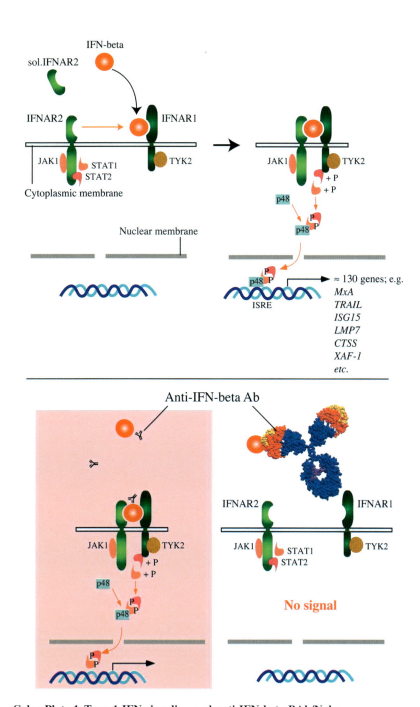

Color Plate 1 Type 1 IFN signaling and anti-IFN-beta BAb/Nabs.
The example shows IFN-beta signaling through IFN-alpha receptors 1 and 2 (IFNAR1 and IFNAR2). The *upper panel* shows ligand–receptor binding, association of the two receptor chains and intracellular signaling and activation of genes through IFN-stimulated regulatory elements (ISRE). The *left lower panel* shows anti-IFN-beta BAbs (non-neutralizing) as they are often depicted. The *right lower panel* shows the correct size relations.

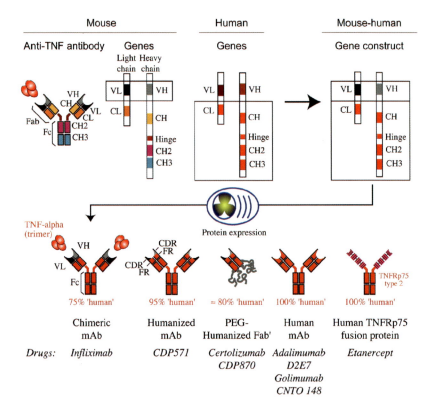

Color Plate 2 Genetically engineered anti-TNF antibody constructs.
The upper panel shows the light and heavy chain genes spliced together from TNF-alpha-immunized murine splenocytes (VL and VH segments) and from human IgG1 (CL, CH, Hinge, CH2, and CH3 segments). The chimeric protein, infliximab, is produced when the gene constructs are expressed in antibody-secreting immortalized myeloma cells.

Abbreviations: VL and VH: variable regions of IgG on light and heavy chains, respectively; CL, CH, CH2, and CH3: constant regions of IgG on light and heavy chains, respectively; Fab: fragment antigen binding, including the variable parts of IgG; Fc: human IgG1 Fc region; CDR: complementarity-determining regions; FR: framework regions; mAb: monoclonal antibody; PEG: polyethylene glycol; TNF: tumor necrosis factor; TNFRp75: tumor necrosis factor receptor type 2.

Case Study: Immunogenicity of Natalizumab

Meena Subramanyam

10.1. Introduction

Natalizumab (Tysabri®, Biogen Idec, Inc., and Elan Pharmaceuticals, Inc.), a recombinant antibody directed against α_4-integrin, belongs to a new class of drugs called selective adhesion molecule inhibitors. The agent was derived from a murine monoclonal antibody and humanized to form natalizumab by engineering the murine complementarity-determining regions into the most homologous naturally occurring heavy and light chains of immunoglobulin G4 (IgG_4) (Rudick and Sandrock 2004). Natalizumab is currently approved in the USA and in the European Union as a monotherapy for the treatment of relapsing forms of multiple sclerosis (MS) and is generally recommended for patients who do not respond to conventional therapies. Similar to the observations with other monoclonal antibody therapeutics (Schellekens 2002), antibodies to natalizumab developed during treatment resulting in increased drug clearance and diminished efficacy, likely due to the formation of drug:antibody complexes and blocking of the drug binding to the target α_4-integrin receptor.

Two randomized, double-blind, placebo-controlled studies (AFFIRM and SENTINEL) of patients with relapsing forms of MS were conducted using natalizumab. In the context of these studies, the antibodies that developed to natalizumab were analyzed with respect to both the incidence as well as the impact of the antibodies on the clinical effects of natalizumab treatment. Serum samples collected from patients enrolled in the trials were evaluated over a period of 2 years for the presence of "binding" antibodies against natalizumab using an enzyme-linked immunosorbent assay (ELISA) and for "neutralizing" or "blocking" activity using a flow cytometry-based assay. This chapter will discuss in detail the assays that were utilized for the assessments, the immunogenicity data from non-clinical and clinical studies and the correlation of presence of antibodies with clinical effects of natalizumab.

10.2. Mechanism of Action of Natalizumab in MS

Multiple sclerosis (MS) is a disease characterized by the intermittent development of inflammatory lesions in the brain and spinal cord, which cause episodes of sensory and motor dysfunctions, or relapses, and the progression of disability over time (Weinshenker et al. 1989, DeStefano et al. 1998). MS lesion formation is thought to involve the migration of lymphocytes across the blood–brain barrier of the central nervous system (CNS; ffrench-Constant 1994). The adhesion and migration of lymphocytes to areas of inflammation within the CNS is mediated in part by interactions between $\alpha_4\beta_1$-integrin, which is present on the surface of activated lymphocytes, and vascular cell adhesion molecule-1 (VCAM-1), which is present on the surface of vascular endothelial cells in the brain and spinal cord blood vessels (Elices et al. 1990, Baron et al. 1993, Lobb and Hemler 1994). VCAM-1 is the major ligand for $\alpha_4\beta_1$-integrin, and its expression is increased in active CNS plaques (Wolinsky 2003). Other ligands for $\alpha_4\beta_1$-integrin, including fibronectin (Mould et al. 1990) and osteopontin (Bayless et al. 1998), may modulate the survival, priming, and activation of leukocytes in the parenchyma of the CNS (Davis et al. 1990, Chan and Aruffo 1993, O'Regan et al. 1999, Chabas et al. 2001). Taken together, these findings suggest that α_4-integrin-dependent adhesion pathways may represent a critical intervention point in the treatment of inflammatory autoimmune disorders such as MS (Lobb and Hemler 1994).

Three specific modes of action have been proposed for the observed efficacy of natalizumab in MS (Rudick and Sandrock 2004). First, natalizumab is thought to prevent the migration of mononuclear leukocytes across the endothelium into the parenchyma by blocking interactions between α_4-integrin and endothelial cells, as well as extracellular matrix proteins. In doing so, the release of proinflammatory cytokines is subsequently reduced. Natalizumab has also been proposed to block T-cell effector function by blocking "antigen presenting cell-target T-cell" interaction in the CNS via its interactions with osteopontin and VCAM-1 on the surface of microglial cells and monocytes. In addition, natalizumab may induce apoptosis of activated effector T cells as a result of its ability to disrupt interactions between α_4-integrin-bearing leukocytes and extracellular matrix proteins. It is interesting to note that, based on these proposed mechanisms, natalizumab may possess multiple anti-inflammatory effects that include the inhibition of immune cell recruitment into inflamed tissue and the suppression of existing inflammatory activity at the disease site (Rudick and Sandrock 2004).

10.3. Prescribed Use

In 2006, the United States Food and Drug Administration and the European Union approved natalizumab as a monotherapy for patients with relapsing forms of MS to delay the accumulation of physical disability and reduce the number of clinical exacerbations (Tysabri PI 2006). The recommended dose of Tysabri is 300 mg via IV infusion once every 4 weeks. Natalizumab is generally reserved for patients who have had an inadequate response to or are unable to tolerate other therapies for MS because of the risk of progressive multifocal leukoencephalopathy (PML) associated with its use. PML is an opportunistic viral infection of the brain that often leads to permanent disability or death. A total of two patients with MS and one patient with Crohn's disease who received natalizumab in clinical studies developed PML (Kleinschmidt-DeMasters and Tyler 2005, Langer-Gould et al. 2005, Van Assche et al. 2005). Tysabri is available through a special restricted distribution program called TOUCH™ in the USA and is administered only to patients enrolled in this program.

10.4. Immunogenicity of Natalizumab

Most protein-based therapies have been associated with some level of immunogenicity. Two fundamental mechanisms that are involved in the induction of immunogenicity upon exposure to protein-based therapeutics are (1) the recognition of non-self, when proteins (or parts of the protein) are derived from non-human sources such as bacteria, plant or animal cells and (2) for humanized therapies, the break down or lack of self-tolerance to the protein, particularly in patients with innate deficiencies of the administered protein (Schellekens 2002). The clinical consequences of such a response may include hypersensitivity reactions, altered pharmacokinetics, and compromised or enhanced efficacy to the administered therapeutic (Freund et al. 1989, Giannelli et al. 1994, Meager 1994). Given that natalizumab is a monoclonal antibody therapeutic containing murine CDR sequences, treatment with this agent has the potential to elicit the development of antibodies, which can alter drug clearance or hinder drug binding to α_4-integrin, the target receptor. Therefore, anti-natalizumab antibodies were measured throughout clinical development of the product.

10.5. Bioanalytical Assays to Assess Immunogenicity

Two types of antibody assays were used to evaluate the presence of drug-specific antibodies during the clinical studies of natalizumab. An enzyme-linked immunosorbent assay (ELISA) was performed to detect the presence of antibodies capable of interacting with or binding to natalizumab. In addition, a cell-based flow cytometry assay was used to characterize the ability of the binding antibodies to block natalizumab from binding to cell-surface α_4-integrins.

10.5.1. Natalizumab Antibody Detection by ELISA

In pre-clinical animal studies and in clinical studies, a bridging ELISA method was used to assess the serum concentration of anti-natalizumab antibodies in treated subjects (Figure 10.1; Calabresi et al. 2007). A bridging format was selected for assay configuration as (a) it facilitated the use of the drug, a humanized monoclonal antibody, as the capture reagent without concerns of generating a high background in normal human serum, and (b) the same basic assay could be adapted for evaluation of anti-drug antibodies in other species and matrices. To perform this assay, microtiter plates were coated with natalizumab ($0.25\,\mu g/mL$) and subsequently blocked to reduce non-specific protein binding. A murine monoclonal antibody against natalizumab (12C4) was used for quality control and to generate a standard curve. Natalizumab antibodies present in the standard, control and serum samples (diluted 1:10) were captured by the natalizumab coated on the plates. During early clinical development, the bound natalizumab-specific antibodies were detected using biotinylated natalizumab and a streptavidin-alkaline phosphatase-fluorescent substrate. The sensitivity of this assay as defined using a monoclonal anti-natalizumab antibody (12C4) in whole serum was 5 $\mu g/mL$. In order to enhance the sensitivity of the assay for the pivotal trials, the substrate was changed and the assay revalidated. The anti-drug antibodies captured by

Bridging ELISA   Blocking Assay

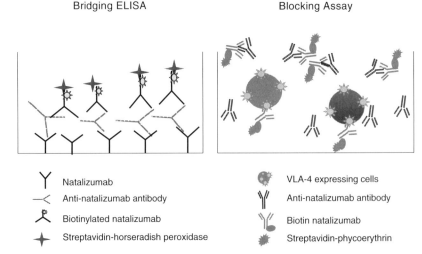

	Natalizumab		VLA-4 expressing cells
	Anti-natalizumab antibody		Anti-natalizumab antibody
	Biotinylated natalizumab		Biotin natalizumab
	Streptavidin-horseradish peroxidase		Streptavidin-phycoerythrin

Figure 10.1 Pictorial representation of the enzyme-linked immunosorbent bridging assay and FACS-based blocking assay utilized for the detection of anti-natalizumab binding antibodies.

natalizumab to the plate were detected using biotinylated natalizumab and a streptavidin-alkaline phosphatase colorimetric substrate. A *p*-nitrophenyl phosphate (*p*NPP) substrate was added to the reaction to generate a colored reaction product, and the optical density was measured at a wavelength of 405 nm using a plate reader. The sensitivity of the colorimetric assay to detect anti-natalizumab blocking antibodies as determined with the 12C4 monoclonal antibody is 0.5 µg/mL in neat serum.

The concentration of natalizumab antibodies in each quality control level was determined by interpolation from the standard curve that was generated by plotting the optical density of each standard point versus its concentration. Samples were deemed positive if they exhibited an optical density greater than or equal to the optical density of the minimum standard (50 ng/mL). Sera considered positive for antibodies in the initial screening were subsequently titrated in the assay (Calabresi et al. 2007).

10.5.2. Natalizumab Antibody Characterization in the Blocking Assay

During clinical studies of natalizumab, a cell-based assay was used to evaluate serum samples for the presence of blocking antibodies (Figure 10.1; Calabresi et al. 2007). The format of the flow cytometry-based blocking assay mimics the proposed mechanism of action of natalizumab to bind α_4-receptors. The blocking assay detects the ability of natalizumab-specific antibodies to block the binding of biotinylated natalizumab to α_4-receptor transfected K562 cells. Since the presence of drug (unlabeled natalizumab) in patients' sera will interfere with biotinylated natalizumab binding to produce a false-positive result in this assay, only those sera samples that were binding antibody–positive and shown to lack measurable circulating levels of natalizumab (<0.25 µg/mL) were evaluated in the blocking assay. The blocking assay included a screening and titration step. The screening assay used 1:10 diluted samples and the titration assay generally included samples serially diluted from 1:10 onward in normal human serum.

For the assay, biotinylated natalizumab was incubated with either positive quality control (normal human serum spiked with 12C4 antibody at the 50% inhibitory concentration level [IC50] and 100% inhibition levels) or negative (normal human serum) control or patient samples (Calabresi et al. 2007). K562 cells transfected to express $\alpha_4\beta_1$ were then added. Following incubation, cells were washed, resuspended, and then incubated with streptavidin phyco-erythrin conjugate. Cell-bound natalizumab conjugate was measured by flow cytometry. Samples were deemed positive for the presence of blocking antibodies if the binding of the fixed dose of biotin–natalizumab to $\alpha_4\beta_1$ receptors, as defined by the mean fluorescence intensity value (MFI), was decreased by 20% (mean fluorescence intensity -2 standard deviation of negative control sera). The sensitivity of the assay to detect anti-natalizumab blocking antibodies, as determined with the 12C4 monoclonal antibody, is 0.5 µg/mL in neat serum.

10.5.3. Limitations of Immunogenicity Assays

There are a number of limitations associated with the methodologies used to detect antibodies during clinical testing of protein therapeutics. It is recognized that natalizumab and anti-natalizumab antibodies in patient samples will mutually interfere in the respective detection assays, regardless of the assay technology employed, and could lead to an underestimation of the quantities of either analyte. The extent of this underestimation varies by sample and the type of immune response that is generated. The interference can be attributed at least partly to the formation of antigen/antibody complexes (immune complexes) when both analytes are present in the same sample. However, precise evaluation of the level of interference is complicated because the positive control antibodies used for this evaluation can be qualitatively different from the polyclonal immune response generated in patients, where varying isotypes, affinities, and epitope specificities can be expected between patients and within a patient over time.

The effect of free circulating drug in the natalizumab immunogenicity assay was evaluated, as it has the potential to interfere with the capture of anti-natalizumab antibodies and thereby cause a putative underestimation of relative levels of antibodies. For experimental demonstration, both pooled patient sera that tested positive for anti-natalizumab antibodies and a high-affinity anti-natalizumab monoclonal antibody (12C4) were utilized (Figure 10.2). The results showed that the concentration of free natalizumab that produced a false-negative result varied with the concentration of anti-natalizumab antibody added to the sample, with higher antibody levels requiring the presence of higher amount of drug to yield a false-negative result. As shown in Figure 10.2, when 20 µg/mL of 12C4 was spiked into serum in the presence of varying doses of natalizumab, interference was not detected until the drug concentration was $\sim$40 µg/mL for an antibody-to-drug ratio of 0.5 (10.2A), whereas when the antibody concentration was decreased to 0.1 µg/mL 12C4, interference by natalizumab was measured at an antibody-to-drug ratio of 2.5 (10.2B). With the polyclonal pooled patient sera containing approximately 2.5 µg/mL of antibody, interference by natalizumab was measured at

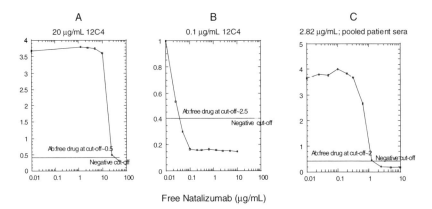

Figure 10.2 Characterization of free drug interference in natalizumab screening immunogenicity assay. Normal human serum was spiked with fixed concentrations of either 12C4 (20 μg/mL, 10 μg/mL, 1.0 μg/mL, and 0.1 μg/mL in neat serum) or pooled patient serum containing anti-natalizumab antibodies and with various concentrations of natalizumab. The samples were then evaluated in the bridging ELISA as described.

an antibody-to-drug ratio of 2 (10.2C). In general, therefore, drug interference in the anti-natalizumab antibody assay occurred when drug concentration was approximately two-fold above the anti-natalizumab antibody concentration. A similar effect of free drug was also observed in the flow cytometry-based blocking assay (Figure 10.3). In the clinical samples, therefore, it is likely that anti-drug antibodies were not detected when their concentration was lower than the trough drug concentration (10–20 μg/mL).

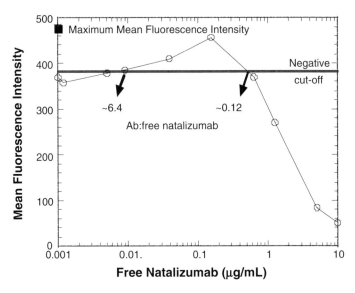

Figure 10.3 Characterization of free drug interference in natalizumab blocking assay. Normal human serum was spiked with fixed concentrations of an anti-natalizumab monoclonal antibody 12C4 (0.064 μg/mL) and with various concentrations of natalizumab. The samples were then evaluated in the blocking assay as described.

10.6. Immunogenicity Data from Preclinical Studies

Natalizumab, being a humanized IgG_4 molecule, was highly immunogenic in rodent studies and in non-human primate studies that were performed for the pharmacokinetic and toxicological evaluations. Based on species cross-reactivity of natalizumab, the primary species selected for toxicology evaluations were cynomolgus monkeys, rhesus monkeys, and guinea pigs. Mice were also used in some pre-clinical studies, even though natalizumab does not cross-react with the murine α_4-integrins. In general, immunogenicity of natalizumab varied according to animal species, natalizumab dose level, and dosing regimen used in pre-clinical studies.

Single-dose pharmacokinetic studies of natalizumab were conducted in mice, guinea pigs, and cynomolgus monkeys using doses from 0.3 to 30 mg/kg. In these studies, anti-natalizumab antibody analysis was performed only in cynomolgus monkeys. Drug-specific antibodies were detected in most cynomolgus monkeys from 14 to 17 days following the IV administration of a single 3-mg/kg dose (Biogen Idec, data on file). Overall, the detection of anti-natalizumab antibodies was associated with a rapid decrease in circulating natalizumab. There were no gender-related differences in immunogenicity observed in these animals.

Natalizumab pharmacokinetics were also evaluated in repeat-dose toxicity studies in mice, guinea pigs, cynomolgus monkeys, and rhesus monkeys at doses ranging from 0.06 to 60 mg/kg. Presence of anti-natalizumab antibodies was not analyzed following repeat dosing in mice. In guinea pigs, anti-natalizumab antibodies were detected at doses of 3 mg/kg and 10 mg/kg. In the 3-mg/kg dose group, approximately half of the animals with drug-specific antibodies had reduced circulating levels of drug. In the 6-month toxicity study in cynomolgus monkeys, anti-natalizumab antibodies were detected in one or more animals in all dose groups. In general, exposures were maintained throughout the dosing period in a majority of the animals at doses of 30 mg/kg or greater. Approximately 50% of the animals in the 30.0 and 60.0 mg/kg/week groups had detectable anti-natalizumab antibodies.

During weekly (juvenile and adult cynomolgus monkeys) or alternate-day (guineas pigs and pregnant cynomolgus monkeys) dosing, the development of anti-natalizumab antibodies was, in general, associated with a limited or decreased duration of drug exposure in some animals, particularly in the lower-dose groups (Biogen Idec, data on file). Gender-specific and species-related differences in immunogenicity were not observed during repeated dosing of cynomolgus or rhesus monkeys. Maternal studies of cynomolgus monkeys revealed the ability of anti-natalizumab antibodies to cross the placenta, and anti-natalizumab antibodies were identified in the cord blood of fetuses from antibody-positive dams.

10.7. Immunogenicity Data from Clinical Studies

The clinical immunogenicity data generated in the ELISA that detected binding antibodies and the flow cytometry assay that characterized the ability of antibodies to block natalizumab binding to the α_4-receptors were found to be highly concordant. Based on this, it is hypothesized that most if not all natalizumab-specific antibodies are anti-idiotypic and likely directed against the complementarity-determining regions (CDRs) of natalizumab. The reported incidence of anti-natalizumab antibodies in patients with MS from the pivotal phase 3 trials is therefore based on data from the ELISA only (Calabresi et al. 2007).

During early clinical studies, only a small percentage of patients treated with natalizumab developed drug-specific antibodies (Sheremata et al. 1999, Miller et al. 2003). The pivotal phase 3 trials consisted of two large, randomized, placebo-controlled studies over approximately 2 years in patients with relapsing MS; one study evaluated the use of natalizumab as monotherapy in 627 patients (AFFIRM), and the other evaluated the use of natalizumab as add-on therapy (SENTINEL) in 589 patients who were also receiving intramuscular (IM) interferon beta-1a (IFNβ-1a; Rudick et al. 2006, Polman et al. 2006). In both studies, the anti-natalizumab antibody status of patients was defined as follows: "antibody negative" (<0.5 μg/mL at all post-baseline visits); "transiently positive" (≥0.5 μg/mL at a single post-baseline visit prior to the final post-baseline visit); or "persistently positive" (≥0.5 μg/mL at ≥2 post-baseline visits that were at least 42 days apart, or a single time point with no follow-up samples; Calabresi et al. 2007).

At any time during the studies, 9% (57/625) of patients who received natalizumab monotherapy and 12% (70/585) of patients who received natalizumab plus IFNβ-1a tested positive for antibodies. Of the 57 patients with anti-natalizumab antibodies from the monotherapy study, 20 (3%) were transiently positive and 37 (6%) were persistently positive for antibodies. Similarly, of the 70 patients from the add-on therapy study with anti-natalizumab antibodies, 32 (5%) were transiently positive and 38 (6%) were persistently positive for antibodies.

Among those patients who developed anti-natalizumab antibodies, the timing of antibody development was consistent in both studies: most patients who developed antibodies at any time did so early in the treatment course. By

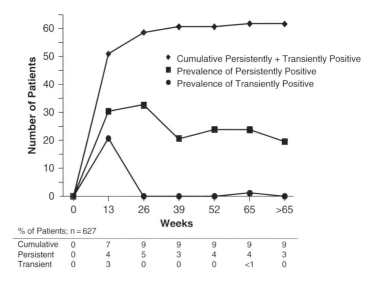

Figure 10.4 Time to development and prevalence of natalizumab antibodies in the monotherapy study.

week 12, antibodies were detected in 88% (50/57) of the antibody-positive group from the monotherapy study (Figure 10.4) and in 96% (67/70) of the antibody-positive group from the add-on therapy study (Calabresi et al. 2007). All patients with a one-time transient response tested antibody negative by the end of study. Furthermore, 53% (10/19) of persistently positive patients, treated for the full 2 years of the monotherapy study, reverted to antibody-negative status by the end of the study. Likewise, 42% (10/24) of persistently positive patients, treated for the full 2 years of the add-on therapy study, also reverted to antibody-negative status by study completion.

10.8. Correlation of Immunogenicity with Outcome Measures

10.8.1. Impact of Anti-drug Antibodies on Drug Binding to Target Receptor (Pharmacodynamics)

The relationship between anti-natalizumab antibodies and a reduction in the extent of α_4-integrin receptor saturation could not be determined in the monotherapy or add-on therapy studies. Although the presence of anti-natalizumab antibodies was correlated with a reduction in the extent of α_4-integrin receptor saturation, the number of patients on which these observations was made is small. In the monotherapy AFFIRM trial, only two patients in the intensive sampling cohort were antibody positive. At week 24, one antibody-positive patients had an α_4-integrin saturation level of approximately 2% prior to receiving the next dose, compared to over 88% in the antibody-negative patients. At week 48, another antibody-positive patients had an α_4-integrin saturation level of approximately 6% prior to receiving the next dose compared to approximately 68% in the antibody-negative patients. In the add-on therapy trial, only one patients in the intensive sampling cohort tested positive for presence of antibodies, and no data is available to assess the impact of antibodies on α_4-integrin receptor saturation in this patients.

10.8.2. Pharmacokinetics

The serum concentration of natalizumab was reduced or abolished in patients who developed anti-natalizumab antibodies, irrespective of the titer levels (Calabresi et al. 2007). During the course of the monotherapy study, serum trough concentrations of natalizumab (Table 10.1) were decreased slightly in transiently positive patients and were substantially reduced in those with persistent antibodies. The mean serum natalizumab concentration after 12 weeks of therapy was 14.9 µg/mL in antibody-negative patients compared with 1.3 µg/mL in antibody-positive patients. At this early time point, there were no differences identified in the serum levels of natalizumab between transiently positive and persistently positive patients. By week 36, mean natalizumab concentrations increased to 24.3 µg/mL in antibody-negative patients. In comparison, the natalizumab concentration was slightly lower (17.2 µg/mL) in transiently positive patients and substantially reduced (<2 µg/mL) in persistently positive patients. Natalizumab concentrations measured at all subsequent time points, up to week 120, were consistent with findings at week 36. The presence of persistent anti-drug antibodies increased natalizumab clearance approximately three-fold,

Table 10.1 Effect of anti-natalizumab antibodies on trough serum concentration of natalizumab in the monotherapy study.

Antibody status	Mean serum natalizumab concentration (µg/mL)			
	Week 12	Week 24	Week 36	Week 120
Persistently positive	1.3	BLQ*	1.4[‡]	2.9–7.9[§]
Transiently positive	1.3	6.4[†]	17.5	~20
Negative	14.9	21.2	24.3	~23

*Below limit of quantitation.
[†]2 out of 15 transiently antibody-positive subjects tested BLQ at week 24.
[‡]16 out of 20 persistently antibody-positive subjects tested BLQ at week 36.
[§]50–70% persistently antibody-positive subjects tested BLQ at week 120.

consistent with the reduced serum natalizumab concentrations observed in persistently antibody-positive subjects. The increase in detectable levels of natalizumab in some patients initially classified as persistently positive is likely due to the seroconversion of some of these patients (16/37) to antibody-negative status just prior to this time point (Calabresi et al. 2007).

10.8.3. Efficacy

During the phase 3 clinical studies of natalizumab, the effects of anti-natalizumab antibodies on the clinical efficacy of treatment were evaluated. Commonly assessed efficacy outcomes in clinical studies of MS therapies include disability progression, which is determined using the Expanded Disability Status Scale (EDSS) or the MS Functional Composite (MSFC); the incidence of relapse; and the formation of brain lesions as detected by magnetic resonance imaging (MRI; Lublin 2005).

In the clinical monotherapy study of natalizumab, the rate of sustained disability progression as determined by EDSS was two-fold higher in persistently positive patients (34%) compared with antibody-negative patients (17%; $p \leq 0.05$; Table 10.2; Calabresi et al. 2007). The difference between the two groups was apparent at approximately week 84 (month 18), when rates of disability progression were similar among persistently antibody-positive and placebo patients. However, patients who were transiently antibody positive did not experience a sustained loss of natalizumab efficacy. Over 2 years, the estimated proportion of patients with sustained disability progression was

Table 10.2 Cumulative probability of patients with sustained disability progression according to antibody status in the monotherapy study.

	Placebo	Antibody negative	Transiently antibody positive	Persistently antibody positive
Cumulative probability (%)	29	17	17	34*,[†]

*$p \leq 0.05$ vs. antibody-negative patients.
[†]$p = 0.66$ vs. placebo.

identical in the antibody-negative and transiently antibody-positive groups. In contrast to the findings in the monotherapy study, no differences were observed on disability progression between persistently positive patients and antibody-negative patients ($p = 0.503$) in the add-on therapy study (Calabresi et al. 2007). Over 2 years, the cumulative proportion of patients with sustained disability progression as measured by EDSS was 24% in antibody-negative patients, 19% in transiently positive patients, and 20% in persistently positive patients.

The results of the monotherapy study showed that persistently positive patients also had decreased efficacy compared with antibody-negative patients ($p < 0.001$) when disability was measured according to mean changes from baseline in the MSFC (Calabresi et al. 2007). No significant differences were found between transiently positive patients and antibody-negative patients in MSFC measures. Likewise, in the add-on therapy study, disability progression as measured by the MSFC worsened in persistently positive patients (–0.08) compared with antibody-negative patients (0.06, $p = 0.072$).

Patients with anti-natalizumab antibodies also demonstrated an increase in relapse rate in the phase 3 clinical program of natalizumab. During the course of the 2-year monotherapy study, persistently positive patients had a more than two-fold higher relapse rate (0.48) than transiently positive or antibody-negative patients (0.16 and 0.22, respectively; $p = 0.009$ vs antibody-negative patients). Likewise, in the add-on therapy study, the relapse rate was significantly higher in persistently positive patients compared with antibody-negative patients (0.65 vs 0.31, $p < 0.001$).

In the monotherapy study, persistently positive patients also experienced less favorable MRI outcomes than antibody-negative patients. There were significant differences in the numbers of gadolinium-enhancing (Gd+) lesions ($p < 0.001$), new or enlarging T2-hyperintense lesions ($p < 0.001$), and new T1-hypointense lesions ($p < 0.001$) between the groups in the monotherapy study (Calabresi et al. 2007). However, no significant differences in lesion numbers were found between transiently positive and antibody-negative patients. Similarly, persistently positive patients were more likely to develop Gd+ lesions ($p < 0.001$) and new or enlarging T2-hyperintense lesions ($p < 0.001$) compared with antibody-negative patients in the add-on therapy study, but no differences were found between these groups in the numbers of new T1-hypointense lesions ($p = 0.960$) (Calabresi et al. 2007).

Significant differences in lesion volume were also observed between antibody-positive and antibody-negative patients (Calabresi et al. 2007). For example, compared with baseline, T2-hyperintense lesion volume decreased by a median of 641.5 mm^3 in antibody-negative patients and 58.0 mm^3 in transiently antibody-positive patients ($p = 0.006$ vs antibody negative), and increased by a median of 569.0 mm^3 in persistently positive patients over 2 years ($p < 0.001$ vs antibody negative) in the monotherapy study. In the add-on therapy study, a significant difference in the median change in T2 lesion volume was found between the persistently positive group and the antibody-negative group (143.1 mm^3 vs –74.4 mm^3, $p = 0.029$).

10.8.4. Safety

In general, antibody status did not affect the incidence and types of adverse events reported during the clinical phase 3 studies of natalizumab

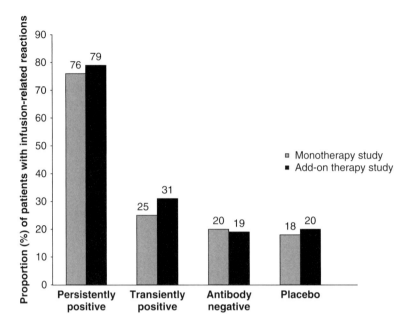

Figure 10.5 Incidence of infusion-related reactions by antibody status in phase 3 studies of natalizumab.

(Calabresi et al. 2007). However, persistently positive patients experienced higher rates of infusion-related (occurring within 2 hours of start of infusion) adverse events. In the 2-year monotherapy study, infusion-related reactions were reported in 76% (monotherapy study) of persistently antibody-positive patients compared to 20% of antibody-negative patients, 25% of transiently positive patients, and 18% of placebo-treated patients (Figure 10.5). The incidence of infusion-related adverse events according to antibody status was similar in the add-on study. In both studies, infusion-related reactions that commonly occurred more frequently in persistently positive patients included headache, flushing, nausea, discomfort, and rigors (Calabresi et al. 2007). Hypersensitivity reactions (urticaria, hypotension, dyspnea, chest pain) also occurred more frequently among persistently antibody-positive patients. In about 4% of natalizumab-treated individuals, acute hypersensitivity reactions were observed, which might be associated with the development of anti-natalizumab antibodies. In the monotherapy study, these reactions were identified in 17 (46%) persistently positive, 3 (15%) transiently positive, and 4 (0.7%) antibody-negative patients. Overall, 20/24 patients who experienced a hypersensitivity reaction had either transient or persistent antibodies. In the add-on therapy study, 8 (21%) persistently positive, 0 transiently positive, and 3 (0.6%) antibody-negative patients experienced hypersensitivity reactions (Calabresi et al. 2007).

10.9. Managing Immunogenicity Risk in Clinical Practice

Based on the finding that 94% of patients did not develop a persistent antibody response to natalizumab in the pivotal clinical studies, routine monitoring of antibody titers is not recommended during treatment with natalizumab

(Calabresi et al. 2007). Furthermore, a high proportion of patients who were antibody positive within the first 6 months of treatment became antibody negative later (Calabresi et al. 2007). However, given that persistence of anti-drug antibodies was associated with ongoing disease activity and infusion-related reactions, evaluating patients who exhibit such symptoms for antibody status during the course of treatment is recommended (Tysabri PI, 2006). If antibodies are detected upon testing, the results should be confirmed using sequential serum antibody tests. Repeat testing at 3 months after the initial positive result is recommended to confirm persistent antibody status (Tysabri PI 2006). At this time, the ELISA for the testing of anti-natalizumab antibodies is available through Focus Diagnostics, Inc. (Cypress, CA), Athena Diagnostics, Inc. (Worcester, MA), and IBT Laboratories (Lenexa, KS) in the USA. CIRION Biopharma Research, Inc. (Laval; Québec, Canada); and in key academic centers in the various EU countries.

10.10. Concluding Remarks

Natalizumab is a humanized antibody to the α_4-integrin and, like all protein therapeutics, has the potential to elicit immune responses in treated individuals. During clinical testing, ELISA and flow cytometry assays were used to assess the development of anti-natalizumab antibodies. Data in the ELISA and flow cytometry assays were highly concordant. The development of anti-natalizumab antibodies appeared to be dose-dependent based on dose range–finding non-clinical and early phase clinical studies. In non-clinical studies, the presence of antibodies was associated with a decrease in the amount of circulating natalizumab in treated animals. A similar observation was made in clinical studies of patients with MS. Patients who developed persistent antibodies experienced reduced efficacy as evidenced on a variety of clinical outcome measures. In contrast, the incidence of transient antibodies to natalizumab did not appear to compromise treatment efficacy. The risk of anti-natalizumab antibody development, albeit low, may be managed through the use of a commercially available ELISA test designed to detect the presence of antibodies in serum samples. Such testing should be reserved for patients with clinical signs or adverse events suggestive of persistent antibody development.

Acknowledgments. An Institutional Animal Use and Care Committee (IACUC) approved animal experiments described in this chapter. The author wishes to thank Drs. Susan Goelz, Paula Hochman, and Gordon Francis for critical review of the manuscript. Experimental data discussed in this chapter were derived from studies jointly sponsored by Biogen Idec, Cambridge, MA, and Elan Pharmaceuticals, San Francisco, CA. The author wishes to acknowledge the contributions of many individuals at Biogen Idec and at Elan in the design and execution of the studies and in the analysis of data. The contributions of Dr. Julie Taylor and the Bioanalytical Development group at Elan and of Michaela Lerner, Jeanine Keefe, Tatiana Plavina, Dr. Eric Wakshull, Dr. Jaya Goyal, Dr. Lakshmi Amaravadi, and the Clinical Science and Technology group at Biogen Idec in the development and validation of the bioanalytical methods and in clinical sample testing are acknowledged.

References

Baron, J. L., Madri, J. A., Ruddle, N. H., Hashim, G., and Janeway, C. A. Jr. 1993. Surface expression of α4 integrin by CD4 T cells is required for their entry into brain parenchyma. J. Exp. Med. 177:57–68.

Bayless, K. J., Meininger, G. A., Scholtz, J. M., and Davis, G. E. 1998. Osteopontin is a ligand for the α4β1 integrin. J. Cell Sci. 111:1165–1174.

Calabresi, P. A., Giovannoni, G., Confavreux, C., Galetta S. L, Havrdova E, Hutchinson M, Kappos L, Miller DH, O'Connor P. W, Phillips J. T, Polman C. H, Radue E. W, Rudick R. A, Stuart W. H, Lublin F. D, Wajgt A, Weinstock-Guttman B, Wynn D. R, Lynn F, Panzara M. A; AFFIRM and SENTINEL Investigators. 2007. The incidence and significance of anti-natalizumab antibodies: results from AFFIRM and SENTINEL. Neurology. 69:1391–1401.

Chabas, D., Baranzini, S. E., Mitchell, D., et al. 2001. The influence of the proinflammatory cytokine, osteopontin, on autoimmune demyelinating disease. Science 294:1731–1735.

Chan, P. Y. and Aruffo, A. 1993. VLA-4 integrin mediates lymphocyte migration on the inducible endothelial cell ligand VCAM-1 and the extracellular matrix ligand fibronectin. J. Biol. Chem. 268:24655–24664.

Davis, L. S., Oppenheimer-Marks, N., Bednarczyk, J. L., McIntyre, B. W., and Lipsky, P. E. 1990. Fibronectin promotes proliferation of naive and memory T cells by signaling through both the VLA-4 and VLA-5 integrin molecules. J. Immunol. 145:785–793.

DeStefano, N., Matthews, P. M., Fu, L., Narayanan, S., Stanley, J., Francis, G. S., Antel, J. P., and Arnold, D. L. 1998. Axonal damage correlates with disability in patients with relapsing-remitting multiple sclerosis. Results of a longitudinal magnetic resonance spectroscopy study. Brain 121:1469–1477.

Elices, M. J., Osborn, L., Takada, Y., Crouse, C., Luhowskyj, S., Hemler, M. E., and Lobb, R. R. 1990. VCAM-1 on activated endothelium interacts with the leukocyte integrin VLA-4 at a site distinct from the VLA-4/fibronectin binding site. Cell 60:577–584.

ffrench-Constant, C. 1994. Pathogenesis of multiple sclerosis. Lancet 343:271–275.

Freund, M., von Wussow, P., Diedrich, H., Eisert, R., Link, H., Wilke, H., Buchholz, F., Leblanc, S., Fonatsch, C., Deicher, H., and Poliwada, H. 1989. Recombinant human interferon (IFN) alpha-2b in chronic myelogenous leukaemia: dose dependency of response and frequency of neutralizing anti-interferon antibodies. Br. J. Haematol. 72:350–356.

Giannelli, G., Antonelli, G., Fera, G., Del Vecchio, S., Riva, E., Broccia, C., Schiraldi, O., and Dianzani, F. 1994. Biological and clinical significance of neutralizing and binding antibodies to interferon-alpha (IFN-α) during therapy for chronic hepatitis C. Clin. Exp. Immunol. 97:4–9.

Kleinschmidt-DeMasters, B. K. and Tyler, K. L. 2005. Progressive multifocal leukoencephalopathy complicating treatment with natalizumab and interferon beta-1a for multiple sclerosis. N. Engl. J. Med. 353:369–374.

Langer-Gould, A., Atlas, S. W., Green, A. J., Bollen, A. W., and Pelletier, D. 2005. Progressive multifocal leukoencephalopathy in a patient treated with natalizumab. N. Engl. J. Med. 353:375–381.

Lobb, R. R. and Hemler, M. E. 1994. The pathophysiologic role of alpha 4 integrins in vivo. J. Clin. Invest. 94:1722–1728.

Lublin, F. D. 2005. Multiple sclerosis trial designs for the 21st century: building on recent lessons. J. Neurol. 252(Suppl. 5):46–53.

Meager, A. 1994. Human antibodies to insulin in diabetes. J. Interferon Res. 14: 181–182.

Miller, D. H., Khan, O. A., Sheremata, W. A,. Blumhardt, L. D., Rice, G. P., Libonati, M. A., Willmer-Hulme, A.J., Dalton, C. M., Miszkiel, K. A., and O'

Connor, P. W. 2003. A controlled trial of natalizumab for relapsing multiple sclerosis. N. Engl. J. Med. 348:15–23.

Mould, A. P., Wheldon, L. A., Komoriya, A., Wayner, E. A., Yamada, K. M., and Humphries, M. J. 1990. Affinity chromatographic isolation of the melanoma adhesion receptor for the IIICS region of fibronectin and its identification as the integrin alpha 4 beta 1. J. Biol. Chem. 265:4020–4024.

O'Regan, A. W., Chupp, G. L., Lowry, J.A., Goetschkes M., Mulligan, N., and Berman, J. S. 1999. Osteopontin is associated wit T cells in sarcoid granulomas and has T cell adhesive and cytokine-like properties in vitro. J. Immunol. 162: 1024–1031.

Polman, C. H., O'Connor, P. W., Havrdova, E., Hutchinson, M., Kappos, L., Miller, D. H., Phillips, J. T., Lublin, F. D., Giovannoni, G., Wajgt, A., Toal, M., Lynn, F., Panzara, M. A., and Sandrock, A. W. 2006. A randomized, placebo-controlled trial of natalizumab for relapsing multiple sclerosis. N. Engl. J. Med. 354:899–910.

Rudick, R. A., Stuart, W. H., Calabresi, P.A., Confavreux, C., Galetta, S. L., Radue, E. W., Lublin, F. D., Weinstock-Guttman, B., Wynn, D. R., Lynn, F., Panzara, M. A., and Sandrock, A. W. 2006. Natalizumab plus interferon beta-1 for relapsing multiple sclerosis. N. Engl. J. Med. 354:911–923.

Rudick, R. A. and Sandrock A. 2004. Natalizumab: α_4-integrin antagonist selective adhesion molecule inhibitors for MS. Expert Rev. Neurotherapeutics 4:571–580.

Schellekens, H. 2002 Bioequivalence and the immunogenicity of biopharmaceuticals. Nat. Rev. 1:457–462.

Sheremata, W. A., Vollmer, T. L., Stone, L. A., Willmer-Hulme, A. J., and Koller, M. A. 1999. A safety and pharmacokinetic study of intravenous natalizumab in patients with MS. Neurology 52:1072–1074.

Tysabri Product Information. 2006. Biogen Idec Inc, Cambridge, MA.

Van Assche, G., Van Ranst, M., Sciot, R., Dubois, B., Vermeire, S., Noman, M., Verbeeck, J., Geboes, K., Robberecht, W., and Rutgeerts, P. 2005. Progressive multifocal leukoencephalopathy after natalizumab therapy for Crohn's disease. N. Engl. J. Med. 353:362–368.

Weinshenker, B. G., Bass, B., Rice, G. P. A., Noseworthy, J., Carriere, W., Baskerville, J., and Ebers, G. C. 1989. The natural history of multiple sclerosis: a geographically based study. I. Clinical course and disability. Brain 112:133–146.

Wolinsky, J. S. 2003. Rational therapy for relapsing multiple sclerosis. Lancet Neurol. 2:271–272.

11

Case Study: Immunogenicity of Anti-TNF Antibodies

Klaus Bendtzen

Abstract

Anti-tumor necrosis factor (TNF) therapy has become an important alternative in the management of several chronic immunoinflammatory diseases. Three recombinant anti-TNF drugs are currently approved for clinical use in patients with various chronic inflammatory diseases such as rheumatoid arthritis, Crohn's diseases, and severe psoriasis: (1) Remicade™ (infliximab), a mouse-human IgG1-kappa anti-TNF-alpha monoclonal antibody, (2) Enbrel™ (etanercept), a fusion protein of human TNF receptor 2 and human IgG1, and (3) Humira™ (adalimumab), a fully human IgG1-kappa anti-TNF-alpha monoclonal antibody. Two other anti-TNF-alpha antibody constructs have shown promise in pivotal phase III trials in patients with some of the same diseases: (4) Cimzia™ CDP870 (certolizumab pegol), a PEGylated Fab fragment of a humanized anti-TNF-alpha monoclonal antibody, and (5) CNTO 148 (golimumab), a fully human IgG1-kappa anti-TNF-alpha monoclonal antibody. All these proteins dramatically lower disease activity and, in some patients, may induce remission. Unfortunately, however, not all patients respond favorably to anti-TNF antibodies. Some patients either do not respond at all (primary response failure) or they respond initially but have later relapses (secondary response failure) despite increased dosage and/or more frequent administration of the drugs. The reason(s) for these response failures is(are) not entirely clear, but interindividual and even intraindividual differences in bioavailability and pharmacokinetics may contribute to the problem. Furthermore, immunogenicity of the drugs causing patients to develop anti-antibodies is a problem now recognized by many investigators, drug-controlling agencies, health insurance companies, and drug manufacturers. Monitoring of patients for circulating levels of functional anti-TNF drugs and anti-antibody development is therefore warranted so that administration can be tailored to the individual patient and so that prolonged therapies can be provided effectively and economically with little or no risk to the patients.

11.1. Historical Notes

With the appreciation of the central role of tumor necrosis factor (TNF)-alpha in the pathogenesis of many immunoinflammatory diseases, specific inhibition of the activities of this pleiotropic cytokine has been a major advance in the treatment of patients with rheumatoid arthritis (RA), juvenile idiopathic arthritis, ankylosing spondylitis (Bechterew's disease), inflammatory bowel diseases (Crohn's diseases and ulcerative colitis), severe psoriasis, chronic uveitis, sarcoidosis, Wegener's granulomatosis, and other diseases with inflammation as a central feature (Maini 2004, Moreland 2004, Vilcek and Feldmann 2004, Haraoui 2005, Smolen et al. 2005, Sandborn 2006, Scott and Kingsley 2006). The first of these specific inhibitors, infliximab, a chimeric human–mouse monoclonal antibody comprising human IgG1-kappa constant regions and mouse variable heavy and light chain domains directed against

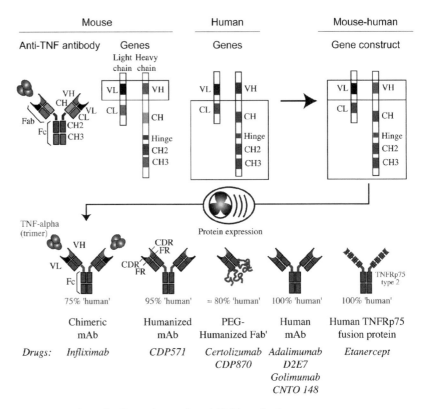

Figure 11.1 Genetically engineered anti-TNF antibody constructs.
The upper panel shows the light and heavy chain genes spliced together from TNF-alpha-immunized murine splenocytes (VL and VH segments) and from human IgG1 (CL, CH, Hinge, CH2, and CH3 segments). The chimeric protein, infliximab, is produced when the gene constructs are expressed in antibody-secreting immortalized myeloma cells.
Abbreviations: VL and VH: variable regions of IgG on light and heavy chains, respectively; CL, CH, CH2, and CH3: constant regions of IgG on light and heavy chains, respectively; Fab: fragment antigen binding, including the variable parts of IgG; Fc: human IgG1 Fc region; CDR: complementarity-determining regions; FR: framework regions; mAb: monoclonal antibody; PEG: polyethylene glycol; TNF: tumor necrosis factor; TNFRp75: tumor necrosis factor receptor type 2. (*See* Color Plate 2)

TNF-alpha, has been used for more than a dozen years. More recently, several human IgG constructs have been developed, including 'humanized' and so-called fully human monoclonal antibodies, Fab fragments of monoclonal antibodies, and TNF receptor (TNFR) constructs (Figure 11.1).

While treatment with TNF blockers dramatically lowers disease activity in many patients suffering from a range of immunoinflammatory diseases, the long-term response is largely uncharted. For example, TNF affects responses to infection and neoplastic growth, and preventing TNF activity may therefore precipitate side-effects due to TNF deficiency (Bongartz et al. 2006). In addition, the issue of immunogenicity of these protein drugs has in recent years caused concern (Han and Cohen 2004, Tangri et al. 2005). Many clinicians (and drug manufacturers) have previously paid little attention to this problem even though the recommended drug delivery resembles otherwise effective vaccination procedures, i.e., repeated and with some formulations subcutaneous administration of more or less aggregated proteins. Although the awareness of the problem is rising, with scattered evidence that anti-antibody responses may jeopardize treatment, it is still not generally recommended to monitor patients for development of anti-antibodies.

11.2. Anti-TNF Antibody Constructs

The five anti-TNF-alpha biopharmaceuticals currently in use are shown in Figure 11.1. Remicade™ (infliximab) is a mouse–human IgG1-kappa anti-TNF-alpha monoclonal antibody, Enbrel™ (etanercept) is a fusion protein of human TNFR type 2 and human IgG1, Humira™ (adalimumab) is a fully human IgG1-kappa anti-TNF-alpha monoclonal antibody, Cimzia™ CDP870 (certolizumab pegol) is a PEGylated Fab fragment of a 'humanized' anti-TNF-alpha monoclonal antibody where the complementarity-derived variable regions from a mouse monoclonal antibody against human TNF-alpha have been grafted into a human IgG1 Fab fragment, and CNTO 148 (golimumab) is a fully human IgG1-kappa anti-TNF-alpha monoclonal antibody. They all target both the soluble and membrane-bound forms of TNF-alpha (etanercept also targets TNF-beta/lymphotoxin-alpha), thus inhibiting TNF-alpha from triggering membrane TNFRs. In addition, infliximab and adalimumab and, possibly, golimumab have the potential to injure cells carrying membrane-bound TNF-alpha through complement activation and/or through binding to Fc-gamma receptors and antibody-dependent cell cytotoxicity.

Apart from infliximab, which is administered intravenously, the drugs are formulated also for self-administration (subcutaneously or intramuscularly). They are all used at standard dosages to patients with similar diseases. The dose regimes generally recommended by the manufacturers have been established on the basis of pivotal clinical trials using large cohorts of patients of both sexes, with differences in age, co-morbidities, and concurrent therapies. In clinical practice, however, individual patients may differ considerably from the average patient involved in randomized clinical trials (Flendrie et al. 2003). Despite this, the concept of individualized therapy is usually considered only when standard regimens fail. Furthermore, despite the considerable costs of these therapies, monitoring individuals for compliance, drug bioavailability, and pharmacokinetics is rarely part of current therapeutic regimens.

11.3. Monitoring Patients Receiving Anti-TNF Antibody Constructs for Compliance, Drug Bioavailability, and Pharmacodynamics

A number of studies have reported a concentration–effect relationship of therapeutic proteins directed against TNF-alpha in patients with RA and Crohn's disease (Maini et al. 1998, Clair et al. 2002, Baert et al. 2003, Wolbink et al. 2005, Bendtzen et al. 2006). Thus, high serum concentrations of anti-TNF antibody constructs just before an infusion, i.e., high trough levels, are associated with clinical improvement, whereas low trough levels are associated with poor clinical response. Several different methods have been used to assess circulating levels of anti-TNF biopharmaceuticals. Most of these are based on enzyme immunoassays (EIA), where the IgG construct, bound to TNF-alpha immobilized on plastic beads or wells, is detected with rabbit or goat anti-human IgG-Fc antibody (Figure 11.2A) (Baert et al. 2003, Gudbrandsdottir et al. 2004).

There is at present little information on the clinical potential of these assays, for example, concerning sensitivity, specificity, ease of use, and cost effectiveness. To alleviate these problems, we have developed a radioimmunoassay (RIA) for serum infliximab levels, quantified as the levels of infliximab in serum affording similar ^{125}I-TNF-alpha binding as the one observed in the test sample (Figure 11.2B) (Bendtzen et al. 2006, Svenson et al. 2007). There are several advantages of this assay: (1) It is functional in that it shows the capacity of the drug to bind TNF-alpha rather than disclosing a protein which may or may not be functional. (2) It is a fluid-phase assay resembling the in vivo situation better than solid-phase assays. (3) It may be easily modified to monitor other antibody constructs targeting TNF-alpha, including adalimumab and etanercept and the recently developed golimumab.

We have used this assay to study a cohort of 106 randomly selected RA patients receiving infliximab and followed for up to 18 months after start of therapy. Patient sera were examined with a RIA for ^{125}I-TNF-alpha binding to serum (Figure 11.2) and a RIA for anti-antibodies as discussed below, and data were obtained for bioavailability, relation between trough levels of infliximab and anti-antibody development, effects of disease activity and methotrexate therapy on these variables, and the ability to predict response failure and infusion-related side-effects. The data are detailed in Bendtzen et al. (2006) and will be summarized below in relation to tests for infliximab immunogenicity. A subgroup of 43 RA patients was evaluated separately. The results are detailed in Svenson et al. (2007), and some of the data are summarized in Figure 11.3.

Both studies showed that trough serum infliximab levels after intravenous infusions of 3 mg infliximab/kg varied considerably between patients (Figure 11.3). At an early stage, i.e., 1.5 months after start of therapy and after only two injections of infliximab, 13% were already positive for anti-antibodies, and the lowest drug levels were found in these sera with the median drug level below detection. As expected, low infliximab levels at this early time point predicted anti-antibody responses and later therapeutic failure. Pronounced baseline disease activity, judged both biochemically (high pre-treatment plasma C-reactive protein levels) and clinically (disease activity scores, DAS28), was associated with low early infliximab levels, possibly

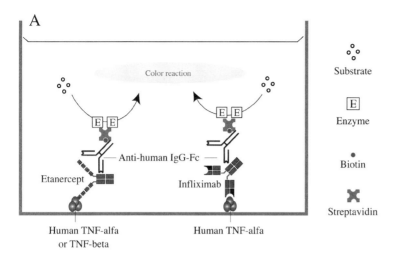

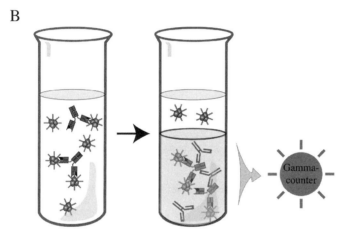

Figure 11.2 Measurements of anti-TNF antibody constructs.
A: Examples of enzyme-linked immunosorbent assays (ELISAs) for etanercept and infliximab using wells coated with TNF-alpha or, in case of etanercept, TNF-alpha or TNF-beta.
B: Fluid-phase RIA for ^{125}I-TNF-alpha-binding capacity (Bendtzen et al. 2006, Svenson et al. 2007). In this example, patient serum containing infliximab is incubated with ^{125}I-TNF-alpha followed by addition of rabbit anti-human IgG-Fc antibody. Bound and free ^{125}I-TNF-alpha are separated by centrifugation, and the pelleted radioactivity is counted and compared with a similar setup using the same amount of normal serum and known amounts of infliximab. This assay gives functional data on the TNF-alpha-binding capacity afforded by infliximab in patient sera. Similar tests can be carried out for all the other TNF-alpha antibody constructs, except certolizumab.

because these patients are in need of more anti-TNF drug than the average patient in the pivotal trials used to lay down the general dose recommendations (Bendtzen et al. 2006).

In contrast to infliximab, which is administered by intravenous infusions, etanercept, adalimumab, and golimumab are administered subcutaneously, possibly with formation of aggregates at the injection sites. The bioavailability issues are therefore likely to be even more problematic with the use of these anti-TNF drugs, and the problem would be expected to worsen if

Serum infliximab (µg/ml)

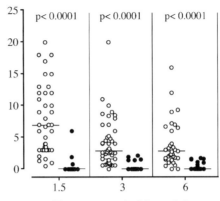

Treatment period (months)

Figure 11.3 Trough levels of functional infliximab in sera negative or positive for anti-infliximab antibodies.
Open circles: Patients without anti-antibodies (against infliximab).Closed circles: Patients with anti-antibodies.
Medians are shown, and P values were calculated by the Mann–Whitney rank sum test. Sera were collected from 43 RA patients at the indicated time points after start of infliximab therapy. Serum infliximab levels were measured by fluid-phase RIA detecting ^{125}I-TNF binding, and anti-antibodies were measured by fluid-phase RIA detecting ^{125}I-infliximab in complex with lambda light-chain-positive antibodies, as outlined below. The trough serum infliximab levels were distributed in a highly scattered fashion with the lowest levels found in sera positive for anti-antibodies (medians below detection at all three time points). When stratifying the data at time point 1.5 months into low and high infliximab levels (split by the median value), those with low levels had a significantly higher incidence of anti-antibody-positives at 3 months: 9 of 26 (35%) versus 2 of 26 (8%), $p = 0.04$ (Fisher's exact test). Adapted from Svenson et al. (2007).

anti-antibodies develop and cause immune complexes to accumulate at the injection sites (Figure 11.4).

In light of the above findings, it appears reasonable to conclude that early monitoring of RA patients on infliximab, and possibly other anti-TNF drugs, may help optimize dose regimens, diminish side-effects, and prevent prolonged use of inadequate (or uneconomical) therapy of individual patients.

11.4. Immunogenicity of Anti-TNF Antibody Constructs

Both product- and host-related factors have documented impact on the human immune response to protein therapeutics, including anti-TNF drugs, but many factors are still unknown (Han and Cohen 2004, Schellekens and Casadevall 2004, Tangri et al. 2005, Teillaud 2005). Direct clinical evidence for anti-antibody responses has been seen in a number of patients receiving anti-TNF drugs (Figure 11.4), but the extent of the problem has most likely not yet been fully realized (Watier 2005).

It is readily understandable that anti-antibody responses may be triggered in patients receiving repeated injections of antibody constructs containing aminoacid sequences originating from other species, as in the case of chimeric

Clinical evidence for anti-antibody development

Dose creep, i.e., more and more drug is needed to control disease
(eventually complete response failure)

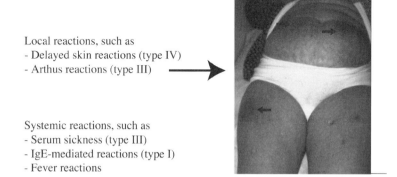

Local reactions, such as
- Delayed skin reactions (type IV)
- Arthus reactions (type III)

Systemic reactions, such as
- Serum sickness (type III)
- IgE-mediated reactions (type I)
- Fever reactions

Figure 11.4 The photo, kindly provided by Dr. Henning Bliddal, Copenhagen, shows an RA patient treated with etanercept. The third subcutaneous injection of the drug has resulted in acute Arthus reactions at the present and previous injection sites. This shows (a) that the patient has developed anti-etanercept antibodies during 'immunization', and (b) that residual drug is still present at the former injection sites, in this case up to 6 weeks after injection. Apart from revealing the immunogenicity of the drug, the phenomenon suggests that bioavailability of subcutaneously injected protein thera- peutics may vary from patient to patient, and it strongly suggests that antibody devel- opment may considerably diminish bioavailability through immune complex formation and, possibly, enzymatic degradation.

anti-TNF drugs (Figure 11.5). However, even so-called fully humanized antibodies may be immunogenic as well. For example, all antibody constructs consisting of human IgG-Fc and/or kappa light chains may provoke anti- allotypic antibody responses. IgG allotypes are minor differences in the primary aminoacid sequence between molecules of one IgG subclass that occur throughout a species. These allotypic determinants (allotopes) are polymorphic and inherited in a Mendelian pattern. Different allelic forms are expressed among individuals, and patients receiving an antibody construct containing a 'foreign' allotype may therefore respond with anti-antibody formation. At present, IgG1 can be typed for four different allotypes located on the heavy chain, G1m(a, x, f, z), also termed G1m(1, 2, 3, 17), and the kappa light chain can be typed for three different allotypes, Km(1, 2, 3); there are no known lambda light-chain allotypes. As shown in Figure 11.5, IgG1 constructs containing constant parts of the human IgG1 heavy chain and the human kappa light chain, including certolizumab consisting solely of the Fab fragment, may evoke production of anti-allotypic antibodies. Infliximab, for example, has been typed for the G1m(a) and G1m(x) allotypes (Svenson et al. 2007). Etanercept, which is a 'fully human' fusion protein consisting of IgG1-Fc coupled to two human TNFR type 2, may also provoke anti-allotypic responses. Additionally, even though etanercept consists of 100% human sequences, T- and B-lymphocytes may recognize peptide fragments overlapping the region between the two human parts as non- self and therefore raise specific immune responses to the drug (Figure 11.5). Finally, as anti-TNF-alpha antibodies are not normally part of our antibody repertoire, anti-idiotypic antibodies may theoretically be induced by all human

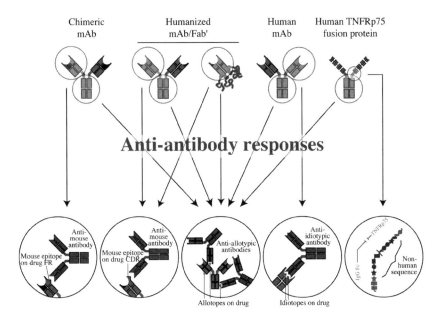

Figure 11.5 Possible mechanisms of immunogenicity of anti-TNF antibody constructs.
Anti-antibodies may be induced against mouse epitopes on the variable regions of chimeric anti-TNF antibody constructs, both the framework regions (FR) and the complementarity-derived regions (CDR). Anti-antibodies may also be induced against IgG allotypes. For example, patients not endowed with G1m(a) and G1m(x) allotypes may generate anti-antibodies against these allotypes on infliximab, which may or may not neutralize infliximab's binding to TNF-alpha. Idiotopes on 'fully human' antibody constructs may induce anti-idiotypic antibodies. Finally, 'fully human' fusion proteins, e.g., etanercept consisting of an IgG1-Fc moiety coupled to two human TNFR type 2 (TNFRp75), may provoke anti-allotypic responses as well as T- and B-cell responses against the non-human peptide fragments spanning the splicing region of the construct.

antibody constructs that bind to TNF-alpha through the variable parts of their heavy and light chains (Figure 11.5).

11.4.1. Monitoring Antibodies to Anti-TNF Antibody Constructs (Anti-antibodies)

Several different methods have been used to measure circulating antibodies against anti-TNF antibody constructs. Most of these have been based on ELISA technology using specific antibodies both for capture and detection, but competitive-type ELISAs and other techniques have been used as well (Figure 11.6A) (Maini et al. 1998, Baert et al. 2003). Unfortunately, commonly encountered problems with insufficient sensitivities, non-specific binding, and interference by rheumatoid factors reduce the usefulness of ELISAs. We have tried to overcome these shortcomings by developing fluid-phase RIAs for antibodies to infliximab, etanercept, and adalimumab (Figure 11.6B). These techniques presumably better reflect the in vivo situation as they are not influenced by artifacts induced by solid-phase adsorption of proteins (Bendtzen et al. 2006, Svenson et al. 2007).

As infliximab, adalimumab and golimumab are human IgG1-kappa constructs, which do not react with anti-human lambda light-chain antibodies,

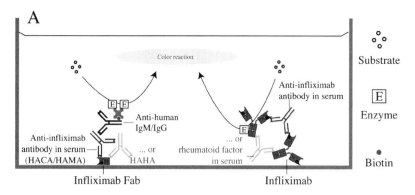

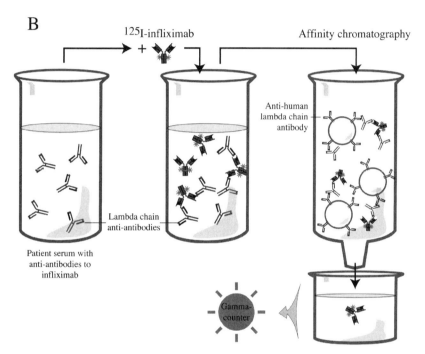

Figure 11.6 Measurements of human antibodies against anti-TNF antibody constructs.

A: Two examples of how to measure anti-antibodies by solid-phase ELISA, in this case antibodies directed against infliximab. The left part shows the detection of so-called human anti-chimeric antibodies (HACA), sometimes called human anti-mouse antibodies (HAMA), using wells coated with Fab fragments of the drug. As anti-antibodies in this setup may recognize human epitopes in the Fab fragments, being anti-human antibodies (HAHA), the terms HACA/HAMA may in some cases be misleading. The right part shows another ELISA for anti-antibodies against infliximab. Note that sera with rheumatoid factor are likely to cause false-positive results in this assay.

B: Fluid-phase RIA measuring anti-antibodies (all isotypes) from patients treated with infliximab (Bendtzen et al. 2006, Svenson et al. 2007). In this example, patient serum containing antibodies against infliximab is incubated overnight with purified ^{125}I-infliximab. Free and immunoglobulin-bound tracer are separated by affinity chromatography using matrix-bound anti-human lambda-chain antibody.

the RIAs are capable of monitoring antibodies to these antibody constructs using binding of radiolabeled drug to an anti-lambda light-chain affinity matrix (as etanercept does not contain light chains, both anti-lambda and -kappa light-chain antibodies may be used when measuring anti-etanercept antibodies). These assays reveal the traced drugs in complexes with lambda light-chain antibodies of all isotypes, including IgM and IgE.

We have compared the RIA for anti-infliximab antibodies with a more cumbersome assay using molecular size separation of unbound and Ig-bound infliximab with and without depletion of serum IgG (Svenson et al. 2007). We found that IgG is the single most important binding factor in serum of RA patients treated with infliximab and that about 50% of bound infliximab was in complex with lambda light-chain-containing IgG antibodies in these sera. The anti-lambda light-chain RIA was comparable in sensitivity to the molecular size separation RIA. Furthermore, the stability of the complexes was similar in the two tests, suggesting that equal binding avidity is expressed by kappa- and lambda-positive anti-infliximab IgG antibodies. The immune complexes generally consisted of ^{125}I-infliximab coupled to maximum three anti-infliximab IgG antibodies. Interestingly, more than 1/3 of the induced anti-antibodies were IgG4, a subclass known to form small complexes with low complement-activating capacity and with lower avidity to Fc-gamma receptors than the three other IgG subclasses. The B-cell epitopes of infliximab were mainly or solely located on the Fab parts of the drug, i.e., the parts containing murine aminoacid sequences (Svenson et al. 2007). We also found that a RIA where infliximab was fixed to ELISA plastic plates yielded fewer sera positive for anti-antibodies than the fluid-phase RIA shown in Figure 11.6 (Svenson et al. 2007). On the other hand, 40% of the sera found positive in the solid-phase RIA were negative in the fluid-phase RIA. Moreover, sera containing rheumatoid factor always gave false-positive findings in the solid-phase RIA, while never interfering with the fluid-phase RIA.

It is important to realize that the levels of both drug and anti-antibodies may be higher than estimated in patients with anti-antibodies, and such sera may also have reduced recoveries of functional anti-TNF drug. Underestimating the number of sera with anti-antibodies may also occur if the immune complexes consist solely of kappa light-chain antibodies. Although this may occur, it is probably a rare event as we have no evidence of 'hidden' antibody complexes when using size-chromatography instead of anti-lambda light-chain antibodies.

In summary:

- The fluid-phase RIA for antibodies to infliximab, and most likely other anti-TNF antibody constructs, is more sensitive than EIA (up to several hundred-fold).
- The fluid-phase RIA is unaffected by rheumatoid factor.
- Patients with RA frequently express antibodies against IgG allotypes, often in association with rheumatoid factor activity and most commonly against G1m types (and therefore potentially binding to IgG1 anti-TNF constructs) (Grubb et al. 1999).
- The fluid-phase RIAs also detect antibodies that are functionally monovalent. Functional multivalency is mandatory for a positive reaction in the solid-phase cross-binding assay. Thus, a standard double-antigen ELISA, such as the one shown to the right in Figure 11.6A, would

not detect functionally monovalent antibodies, for example IgG4, which might nevertheless neutralize TNF-alpha binding, increase drug clearance, and/or prevent the drug from reaching affected tissues in the recipients; as mentioned above, IgG4 constitutes a considerable amount of the anti-infliximab antibodies found in RA patients treated for 3–6 months (Svenson et al. 2007).

- Fluid-phase RIAs generally utilize ligands with highly conserved conformations. These techniques are therefore less sensitive to artifacts caused by neo-epitope formation or loss of epitopes which are known to occur when proteins are fixed to solid matrices (Svenson et al. 1995, Hennig et al. 2000, Bendtzen 2003).
- Fluid-phase RIAs do not favor detection of low-avidity antibodies.

11.4.2. Clinical Relevance of Anti-antibodies

Some investigators believe that the development of anti-antibodies is of limited importance, because there is not always readily observable clinical consequences of antibody development. This belief has unfortunately arisen from clinical experience where several factors may contribute to erroneous interpretations. The use of tests that yield false-positive anti-antibody results contributes to the problem, as it does in all cases where antibodies are induced by protein therapeutics (Bendtzen 2003). Also, clinicians may not realize that anti-antibodies are the cause of side-effects or loss of therapeutic efficacy if patients are not monitored routinely for anti-antibody development. On the other hand, patients in clinical remission may seem to have benefit from continued anti-TNF therapy even though they have developed anti-antibodies. Rather than continuing a costly therapy, and further immunizing the patient, it would probably be better to halt therapy in such patients.

Some investigators also believe that only anti-antibodies with a neutralizing effect in in vitro assays for TNF activities are of clinical significance. This is not necessarily correct, because in vitro non-neutralizing anti-antibodies may 'neutralize' drug effects in vivo as they may adversely affect bioavailability and pharmacokinetics of antibody constructs (Lobo et al. 2004). For example, immune complex formation at injection sites might impair absorption of drugs administered by the subcutaneous or intramuscular routes, whether or not the anti-antibodies prevent TNF binding to the drug. In vitro non-neutralizing anti-antibodies may also decrease the half-life of anti-TNF drugs by formation of immune complexes that are rapidly cleared from the circulation. Finally, anti-antibodies may prevent the drugs from reaching affected tissues whether or not they inhibit binding to TNF-alpha.

Our own experience shows that 1 of 106 (1%) randomly selected RA patients were positive in RIA for anti-antibodies before receiving infliximab. After only two drug infusions (1.5 months after start of therapy), 13% were antibody-positive, and with subsequent infusions, the percentage rose to 30 and 44% (3 and 6 months, respectively). As shown in Figure 11.7, the development of anti-antibodies was accompanied by diminished trough levels of infliximab. Indeed, low infliximab levels at 1.5 months predicted development of anti-antibodies and later therapeutic failure (within the observation period of 18 months). There were also highly significant correlations between high levels of anti-antibodies and later dose increases, side-effects such as

S-infliximab (μg/ml)

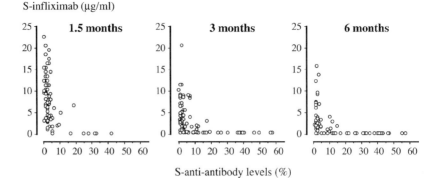

Figure 11.7 Early development of anti-antibodies in RA patients receiving infliximab and association with trough level TNF-alpha binding afforded by infliximab.

Antibodies against infliximab as well as drug levels were measured in sera from 106 RA patients beginning immediately before start of therapy, before the third drug infusion (1.5 months after start) and before infusions at time points 3 and 6 months, respectively. Modified from a figure first published in Arthritis & Rheumatism (Bendtzen et al. 2006).

infusion reactions, and cessation of therapy. Furthermore, pronounced baseline disease activity, judged by high pre-treatment plasma levels of C-reactive protein and disease activity score (DAS28), was associated with low early infliximab levels and later development of anti-antibodies. Co-treatment with methotrexate resulted in only slightly lower levels of anti-antibodies after 6 months; other disease-modifying antirheumatic drugs and prednisolone had no effect. We concluded that development of anti-antibodies, heralded by low pre-infusion serum infliximab levels, was associated with increased risk of infusion reactions and treatment failure and that early monitoring should help optimize dose regimens to individual patients, diminish side-effects, and prevent prolonged use of inadequate infliximab therapy.

It is clinically interesting that anti-antibodies invoked during infliximab therapy generally failed to react with the two other, currently approved anti-TNF-alpha IgG1 constructs, etanercept and adalimumab. Although this does not rule out that cross-reacting antibodies may appear after more prolonged infliximab therapy, it might explain why a shift to other anti-TNF-alpha drugs is effective in some patients with therapeutic failure or drug intolerance (Ang and Helfgott 2003, van Vollenhoven et al. 2003, Hansen et al. 2004, Haraoui et al. 2004, Solau-Gervais et al. 2006).

11.5. Conclusions

An increasingly recognized problem with prolonged use of biopharmaceuticals, including anti-TNF-alpha antibody constructs, is the induction of antibodies against the therapeutic proteins. Even though this is an area of increased interest, it is still unclear whether anti-antibodies measured by the most commonly used techniques (mostly solid-phase ELISA) yield clinically reliable data; for example whether ELISAs are sufficiently sensitive to reveal all in vivo 'functional' anti-antibodies and whether they relate to clinical manifestations such as infusion reactions and reduction of therapeutic efficacy (Cheifetz and Mayer 2005). This, and the fact that treatment with anti-TNF-alpha antibodies are a major and very expensive part of current medical therapies of a large number of patients with chronic immunoinflammatory diseases, calls for increased pharmacovigilance. Indeed, the growing realization of inadequate long-term therapies with anti-TNF-alpha drugs have raised concern as to whether it is justified to 'inoculate' patients for extended periods of time with anti-TNF antibodies without monitoring for anti-antibody responses, or whether it is ethically correct to deprive patients of other (effective) therapies while treatment is continued in patients harboring drug-neutralizing antibodies.

Acknowledgments. The author wishes to thank Morten Svenson, Marianna Thomsen, Pierre Geborek, Tore Saxne, Lotta Larsson, and Meliha Kapetanovic for their invaluable contributions. Financial support for this paper was from the Danish Biotechnology Programme.

References

Ang, H. T., and Helfgott, S. 2003. Do the clinical responses and complications following etanercept or infliximab therapy predict similar outcomes with the other tumor necrosis factor-alpha antagonists in patients with rheumatoid arthritis? J. Rheumatol. 30:2315–2318.

Baert, F., Noman, M., Vermeire, S., Van Assche, G., D' Haens, G., Carbonez, A., and Rutgeerts, P. 2003. Influence of immunogenicity on the long-term efficacy of infliximab in Crohn's disease. N. Engl. J. Med. 348:601–608.

Bendtzen, K. 2003. Anti-IFN BAb and NAb antibodies: A minireview. Neurology 61 (Suppl. 5):S6–S10.

Bendtzen, K., Geborek, P., Svenson, M., Larsson, L., Kapetanovic, M. C., and Saxne, T. 2006. Individualized monitoring of drug bioavailability and immunogenicity in rheumatoid arthritis patients treated with the tumor necrosis factor alpha inhibitor Infliximab. Arthrit. Rheum. 54:3782–3789.

Bongartz, T., Sutton, A. J., Sweeting, M. J., Buchan, I., Matteson, E. L., and Montori, V. 2006. Anti-TNF antibody therapy in rheumatoid arthritis and the risk of serious infections and malignancies: systematic review and meta-analysis of rare harmful effects in randomized controlled trials. JAMA 295:2275–2285.

Cheifetz, A., and Mayer, L. 2005. Monoclonal antibodies, immunogenicity, and associated infusion reactions. Mt. Sinai J. Med. 72:250–256.

Clair, E. W., St., Wagner, C. L., Fasanmade, A. A., Wang, B., Schaible, T., Kavanaugh, A., and Keystone, E. C. 2002. The relationship of serum infliximab concentrations to clinical improvement in rheumatoid arthritis. Results from ATTRACT, a multicenter, randomized, double-blind, placebo-controlled trial. Arthritis Rheum. 46:1451–1459.

Flendrie, M., Creemers, M. C., Welsing, P. M., den Broeder, A. A., and van Riel, P. L. 2003. Survival during treatment with tumour necrosis factor blocking agents in rheumatoid arthritis. Ann. Rheum. Dis. 62 (Suppl. 2):ii30–ii33.

Grubb, R., Grubb, A., Kjellen, L., Lycke, E., and Åman, P. 1999. Rheumatoid arthritis–a gene transfer disease. Exp. Clin. Immunogenet. 16:1–7.

Gudbrandsdottir, S., Larsen, R., Sorensen, L. K., Nielsen, S., Hansen, M. B., Svenson, M., Bendtzen, K., and Müller, K. 2004. TNF and LT binding capacities in the plasma of arthritis patients: effect of etanercept treatment in juvenile idiopathic arthritis. Clin. Exp. Rheumatol. 22:118–124.

Han, P. D., and Cohen, R. D. 2004. Managing immunogenic responses to infliximab: treatment implications for patients with Crohn's disease. Drugs 64:1767–1777.

Hansen, K. E., Hildebrand, J. P., Genovese, M. C., Cush, J. J., Patel, S., Cooley, D. A., Cohen, S. B., Gangnon, R. E., and Schiff, M. H. 2004. The efficacy of switching from etanercept to infliximab in patients with rheumatoid arthritis. J. Rheumatol. 31:1098–1102.

Haraoui, B. 2005. Differentiating the efficacy of tumor necrosis factor inhibitors. J. Rheumatol. Suppl. 74:3–7.

Haraoui, B., Keystone, E. C., Thorne, J. C., Pope, J. E., Chen, I., Asare, C. G., and Leff, J. A. 2004. Clinical outcomes of patients with rheumatoid arthritis after switching from infliximab to etanercept. J. Rheumatol. 31:2356–2359.

Hennig, C., Rink, L., Fagin, U., Jabs, W. J., and Kirchner, H. 2000. The influence of naturally occurring heterophilic anti-immunoglobulin antibodies on direct measurement of serum proteins using sandwich ELISAs. J. Immunol. Methods 235:71–80.

Lobo, E. D., Hansen, R. J., and Balthasar, J. P. 2004. Antibody pharmacokinetics and pharmacodynamics. J. Pharm. Sci. 93:2645–2668.

Maini, R. N., Breedveld, F. C., Kalden, J. R., Smolen, J. S., Davis, D., Macfarlane, J. D., Antoni, C., Leeb, B., Elliott, M. J., Woody, J. N., Schaible, T. F., and Feldmann, M. 1998. Therapeutic efficacy of multiple intravenous infusions of anti-tumor necrosis factor a monoclonal antibody combined with low-dose weekly methotrexate in rheumatoid arthritis. Arthrit. Rheum. 41:1552–1563.

Maini, S. R. 2004. Infliximab treatment of rheumatoid arthritis. Rheum. Dis. Clin. North Am. 30:329–347, vii.

Moreland, L. W. 2004. Drugs that block tumour necrosis factor: experience in patients with rheumatoid arthritis. Pharmacoeconomics 22:39–53.

Sandborn, W. J. 2006. What's new: innovative concepts in inflammatory bowel disease. Colorectal Dis. 8 (Suppl. 1):3–9.

Schellekens, H., and Casadevall, N. 2004. Immunogenicity of recombinant human proteins: causes and consequences. J. Neurol. 251 (Suppl. 2):II4–II9.

Scott, D. L., and Kingsley, G. H. 2006. Tumor necrosis factor inhibitors for rheumatoid arthritis. N. Engl. J. Med. 355:704–712.

Smolen, J. S., Redlich, K., Zwerina, J., Aletaha, D., Steiner, G., and Schett, G. 2005. Pro-inflammatory cytokines in rheumatoid arthritis: pathogenetic and therapeutic aspects. Clin. Rev. Allergy Immunol. 28:239–248.

Solau-Gervais, E., Laxenaire, N., Cortet, B., Dubucquoi, S., Duquesnoy, B., and Flipo, R. M. 2006. Lack of efficacy of a third tumour necrosis factor alpha antagonist after failure of a soluble receptor and a monoclonal antibody. Rheumatology (Oxford) 45:1121–1124.

Svenson, M., Geborek, P., Saxne, T., and Bendtzen, K. 2007. Monitoring patients treated with anti-TNF-alpha biopharmaceuticals – assessing serum infliximab and anti-infliximab antibodies. Rheumatology 46:1828–1834.

Svenson, M., Nedergaard, S., Heegaard, P. M. H., Whisenand, T. D., Arend, W. P., and Bendtzen, K. 1995. Differential binding of human interleukin-1 (IL-1) receptor antagonist to natural and recombinant soluble and cellular IL-1 type I receptors. Eur. J. Immunol. 25:2842–2850.

Tangri, S., Mothe, B. R., Eisenbraun, J., Sidney, J., Southwood, S., Briggs, K., Zinckgraf, J., Bilsel, P., Newman, M., Chesnut, R., Licalsi, C., and Sette, A. 2005. Rationally engineered therapeutic proteins with reduced immunogenicity. J. Immunol. 174:3187–3196.

Teillaud, J. L. 2005. Engineering of monoclonal antibodies and antibody-based fusion proteins: successes and challenges. Expert Opin. Biol. Ther. 5 (Suppl. 1):S15–27.

van Vollenhoven, R., Harju, A., Brannemark, S., and Klareskog, L. 2003. Treatment with infliximab (Remicade) when etanercept (Enbrel) has failed or vice versa: data from the STURE registry showing that switching tumour necrosis factor alpha blockers can make sense. Ann. Rheum. Dis. 62:1195–1198.

Vilcek, J., and Feldmann, M. 2004. Historical review: Cytokines as therapeutics and targets of therapeutics. Trends Pharmacol. Sci. 25:201–209.

Watier, H. 2005. Variability factors in the clinical response to recombinant antibodies and IgG Fc-containing fusion proteins. Expert Opin. Biol. Ther. 5 (Suppl. 1): S29–36.

Wolbink, G. J., Voskuyl, A. E., Lems, W. F., de Groot, E., Nurmohamed, M. T., Tak, P. P., Dijkmans, B. A., and Aarden, L. 2005. Relationship between serum trough infliximab levels, pretreatment C reactive protein levels, and clinical response to infliximab treatment in patients with rheumatoid arthritis. Ann. Rheum. Dis. 64:704–707.

12

Heparin-Induced Thrombocytopenia

Carmel A. Celestin and John R. Bartholomew

Abstract

Heparin-induced thrombocytopenia (HIT) is a devastating complication of either unfractionated heparin or any of the low molecular weight heparin (LMWH) preparations. This immune-mediated process generally develops within 5–14 days of administration, although it may occur more rapidly if there has been a recent exposure, or even days to weeks after either preparation has been discontinued. Although once considered necessary for the diagnosis of HIT, thrombocytopenia is no longer essential. A 50% reduction in the platelet count from pre-heparin treatment levels is now considered a more specific finding. Immediate cessation of heparin or LMWH is recommended once the diagnosis is suspected and alternative therapy with a non-heparin anticoagulant advised due to the potential for new thrombosis, amputation or even death.

12.1. Introduction

Unfractionated heparin, an anticoagulant that was discovered over 90 years ago, has been used by clinicians for approximately 70 years. It was first discovered by Jay McLean, a medical student at Johns Hopkins University, in 1916 while working with William H. Howell, a physiologist with an interest in coagulation (Ancalmo and Ochsner 1990). McLean was given the task of extracting the clot-promoting phospholipid cephalin from various tissues including dog brain. An incidental finding was the isolation of a crude fraction of hepatic tissue that inhibited coagulation. Howell named the inhibitor *heparin* to indicate its origin from animal hepatic tissue.

Heparin was first used clinically in 1935 when Clarence Crafoord of Stockholm, a surgeon with expertise in the field of venous thromboembolism (VTE), gave it intravenously to prevent thrombosis. In 1938 Gordon Murray and Charles Best from Canada reported successful treatment of a patient with deep vein thrombosis (DVT); however, it was not until a 1960 landmark open, randomized study by Barrit and Jordan (1960) demonstrating the effectiveness of heparin in treating and preventing recurrent pulmonary embolism (PE) that it became the mainstay of treatment for VTE.

12.1.1. Indications

Heparin has a variety of prophylactic and therapeutic indications including the prevention and treatment of DVT and PE, the treatment of patients with arterial embolism, unstable angina and acute myocardial infarction (MI); anticoagulation during cardiopulmonary bypass or vascular surgery; with percutaneous transluminal angioplasty (PTA), percutaneous transluminal coronary angioplasty (PTCA) or percutaneous coronary intervention (PCI); for the prevention of thrombosis in atrial fibrillation, atrial flutter and prosthetic heart valves; preventing clotting of indwelling venous or arterial devices and during dialysis; and the treatment of select patients with disseminated intravascular coagulation (DIC). It is also used for the prevention and treatment of thrombotic complications during pregnancy and is used as an in vitro anticoagulant in blood samples drawn for laboratory purposes.

12.1.2. Chemistry and Source

Heparin is a heterogeneous group of straight-chain anionic mucopolysaccharides called glycosaminoglycans. The molecular weight ranges from 5,000 to 30,000 Daltons (average 15,000). Heparin consists of unbranched chains of two repeating disaccharide units: D-glucosamine-L-iduronic acid and D-glucosamine-D-gluconic acid. Most heparin preparations contain 8–15 sequences of each disaccharide unit. Heparin is generally derived from bovine lung or porcine intestinal mucosa and is available as a sodium salt.

12.1.3. Mode of Action

The major anticoagulant effect of heparin requires binding to a plasma cofactor, originally known as heparin cofactor. Its name was later changed to antithrombin III and more recently antithrombin (AT). Antithrombin is one of the major inhibitors of the coagulation cascade (Hirsh and Levine 1992, Ross and Toth 2005).

Binding of heparin to AT has been localized to a unique pentasaccharide sequence, the third residue of which contains a 3-0 sulfated glucosamine. Approximately 30% of unfractionated heparins contain this active sequence. Heparin's anticoagulant activity results from attachment of this pentasaccharide sequence to a lysine-binding site on AT, imparting a conformational change in the molecule. This accelerates binding of AT (at its arginine reactive center) to a number of serine proteases: thrombin (IIa), IXa, Xa, XIa, XIIa although factors Xa and IIa are the most important for heparin's anticoagulant effect (Figure 12.1). Once binding of AT to thrombin takes place, the heparin molecule dissociates and binds to a new (AT) molecule. The AT–thrombin complex (TAT) is subsequently removed by the reticuloendothelial system.

For heparin to inhibit thrombin, it must contain at least 18 monosaccharide units and form a ternary complex between heparin, AT and thrombin (Figure 12.2) (Hirsh et al. 1976, Danielsson and Bjork 1981, Bjork, Olson and Shore 1989, Hirsh 1991, Hirsh and Levine 1992, Ross and Toth 2005). For the inhibition of factor Xa, direct binding of heparin is not necessary as the pentasaccharide sequence is sufficient to accelerate this reaction. Therefore, the inactivation of factor Xa can be achieved by smaller heparin chains including the LMWH preparations and the newer pentasaccharide anticoagulant, fondaparinux (Hirsh and Levine 1992, Ross and Toth 2005). The

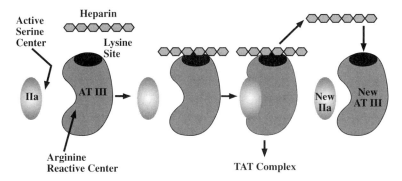

Figure 12.1 Heparin exerts its anticoagulant activity through its ability to accelerate the reaction between antithrombin (AT) and serine proteases: thrombin (IIa), IXa, Xa, XIa and XIIa. Once a thrombin–AT complex (TAT) has been formed, the heparin dissociates from the complex and binds to a new AT molecule.

anticoagulant activity of heparin is also mediated by heparin cofactor II. Unlike AT, heparin cofactor II inhibits only thrombin and can accept either heparin or dermatan sulfate as cofactors. Heparin has additional physiological effects including the release of lipoprotein lipase (lipoprotein lipase hydrolyzes triglycerides to glycerol and free fatty acids), inhibition of platelet function, inhibition of the proliferation of vascular smooth muscle cells, anti-inflammatory properties and the regulation of angiogenesis.

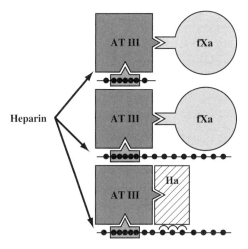

Figure 12.2 The ability of heparin to facilitate the inhibition of coagulation factors by antithrombin demonstrates a dependence on the size of the heparin chains. For heparin to inhibit thrombin (IIa), heparin must contain at least 18 monosaccharide units, with the formation of a ternary complex between antithrombin, heparin and IIa. For inhibition of factor Xa, direct binding of heparin to factor Xa is not necessary, and the pentasaccharide sequence of heparin is sufficient to accelerate the reaction. This molecular weight dependence has important implications in the laboratory monitoring of heparin and low molecular weight heparin. As low molecular weight heparin inhibits only factor Xa, it can be monitored only by factor Xa inhibition assays. The APTT and ACT are relatively unaffected by low molecular weight heparin.

12.1.4. Administration

The preferred routes of administration for heparin are continuous intravenous infusion or subcutaneous injection, although the latter method may cause erratic absorption, is uncomfortable and a less desirable route. Heparin is not administered orally because it is unstable under acidic conditions, although extensive ongoing research is working to develop this approach (Ross and Toth 2005).

Heparin is usually given subcutaneously in smaller doses for prophylactic therapy. For full dose subcutaneous injections, however, the initial dose must be sufficient to overcome the lower bioavailability of this route. Peak plasma levels occur at approximately 2–3 hours and a nomogram for full dose subcutaneous treatment of VTE has recently been published (Kearon et al. 2006). Heparin is given intravenously for the treatment of thromboembolism (venous or arterial) as well as during vascular or cardiovascular surgery and for PTA, PTCA or PCI. The anticoagulant response after intravenous injection is almost immediate.

The half-life of heparin is dose dependent (increases with the dose) ranging from 30 to 150 minutes in healthy adults (Hirsh 1991). Its half-life may be prolonged in cirrhotic individuals and in patients with severe renal disease, although reports of the influence of renal and hepatic diseases on its pharmacokinetics are not consistent (Hirsh 1991).

12.1.5. Monitoring

Heparin's anticoagulant activity can be monitored by following its effect on several coagulation assays, notably the activated partial thromboplastin time (aPTT), activated clotting time (ACT), thrombin time (TT) or heparin levels. The aPTT remains the most frequently used method except for the higher heparin doses required in PTA, PTCA, PCI or cardiopulmonary or vascular surgery where the ACT is used. An accepted therapeutic aPTT range for venous and arterial thrombosis is a ratio 1.5–2.5 times the patient's baseline value; however, the responsiveness of heparin to the different aPTT reagents (used to perform this test) can vary widely. For this reason, the College of American Pathologists, American College of Chest Physicians (ACCP) and other organizations no longer recommend using this ratio. Instead, these societies advise that all laboratories establish a heparin dose–response curve for the aPTT reagent in their facility, using concentrations that correlate to therapeutic heparin levels of 0.3–0.7 IU/mL determined by factor Xa inhibition (Hirsh and Raschke 2004a). This test is performed as a chromogenic factor Xa inhibition assay, also referred to as an anti-Xa assay. The assay measures the ability of heparin to inhibit the activity of factor Xa, which is inversely proportional to the heparin concentration. The factor Xa inhibition assay is also helpful for monitoring the anticoagulant response in patients with a "baseline"-prolonged aPTT and individuals who have an inadequate response to what is normally considered a therapeutic dose of heparin (see Sect. 12.1.6 below).

As noted above, the ACT is used when patients require higher doses of heparin for example in cardiac interventional procedures. It is also used during cardiovascular or vascular surgery to assess the adequacy of anticoagulation and to estimate reversal of heparin after the administration of protamine.

12.1.6. Heparin Resistance

Heparin binds to many different plasma proteins which reduce its anticoagulant activity and contribute to the variability of its anticoagulant response (Hirsh et al. 1976, Hirsh 1991, Hirsh and Levine 1992, Hirsh and Raschke 2004a). These include histidine-rich glycoprotein, vitronectin, platelet factor 4 (PF4), fibronectin and von Willebrand factor. This laboratory phenomenon is known as "heparin resistance", a term used when patients require abnormally large amounts of heparin to prolong their aPTT to attain a "therapeutic effect" (Young et al. 1993, Cosmi et al. 1997). Heparin resistance may be found in individuals with an underlying malignancy, elevated factor VIII or fibrinogen levels, AT deficiency, pregnancy or in patients with a lupus anticoagulant (Young et al. 1993). Drug-induced heparin resistance has also been reported in patients receiving nitroglycerin or aprotinin.

According to the seventh ACCP conference on antithrombotic therapy, heparin resistance should be suspected in individuals requiring an unusually large amount of heparin (defined as >40,000 units per 24 hours). Anti-factor Xa heparin levels should be used to measure anticoagulation if this is suspected (Hirsh and Raschke 2004a).

12.1.7. Dosing

A former commonly recommended method to heparinize patients with VTE used a loading dose of 5,000–10,000 units given slowly over 10–15 minutes, followed by a continuous infusion of 1,000 units per hour with adjustments made according to the aPTT. This approach, however, often underdosed patients and eventually led to the development of several heparin nomograms (Cruickshank et al. 1991, Raschke et al. 1993). The most commonly used nomogram (recommended by the ACCP) for the treatment of VTE is weight-based (Raschke et al. 1993). This nomogram recommends a bolus of 80 units/kg of heparin followed by an infusion rate of 18 units/kg/hr. An alternative nomogram advocates a bolus of 5,000 units followed by 1280 units per hour (Cruickshank et al. 1991). With either method, an aPTT should be obtained 6 hours after initiation and repeated at 6-hour intervals until it is within a therapeutic range. More recently fixed-dose, weight-adjusted subcutaneous heparin has been found suitable for both the inpatient and outpatient treatments of VTE. An initial dose of 333 units/kilogram is given intravenously followed by a fixed dose of 250 units/kilogram/subcutaneously every 12 hours (Kearon et al. 2006). When the subcutaneous route is used for VTE prophylaxis, the dosage is generally 5,000 units every 8–12 hours depending on the patients' risk profile. In surgical patients, it is advised that this dose be initiated 2 hours before the procedure.

The American College of Cardiology (ACC) recommends lower doses of heparin for use in patients with unstable angina or non-ST-segment elevation MI (Hirsh and Raschke 2004a). A bolus of 60–70 units/kg of heparin (maximum dose of 5,000 units) followed by an infusion of 12–15 units/kg/h (maximum of 1,000 units per hour) is advised. Larger doses are generally required for PTA, PTCA, PCI and cardiac or vascular surgery.

12.2. Low Molecular Weight Heparins (LMWHs)

The LMWHs are derived from UFH by controlled chemical or enzymatic depolymerization processes (Hirsh and Raschke 2004a). Depolymerization is achieved either by treatment with the enzyme heparinase, hydrolytic cleavage with hydrogen peroxide or by B-elimination. These processes yield products with lower molecular weights varying from 4000 to 6500 Daltons and improved pharmacokinetic properties compared to heparin (Fareed et al. 1988). The LMWHs also vary in molecular structure and function and are not clinically interchangeable, due to significant differences in the chemical and/or enzymatic procedures used for their synthesis. Due to their smaller size, LMWHs only bind their pentasaccharide sequence to AT resulting in inactivation of factor Xa, but not thrombin. Low molecular weight heparins also have a lower affinity for circulating and cellular proteins, which contributes to their higher bioavailability and more predictable anticoagulant response (Cosmi et al. 1997). They also have longer half-lives ranging from 111 to 1100 minutes and are cleared primarily by the kidneys; therefore, their half-life is increased in patients with renal failure (Hirsh and Levine 1992). Dose adjustments must be made in patients with a creatinine clearance of less than 30 ml/min and in select cases anti-factor Xa levels performed using a LMWH preparation as a reference should be used for monitoring. The available LMWH preparations in the United States include dalteparin (Fragmin, Novartis), enoxaparin (Lovenox/Clexane, Aventis) and tinzaparin (Innohep, Pharmion). In Europe they include nadroparin (Fraxiparine, GlaxoSmithKline), reviparin (Clivarine, Abbott) and parnaparin (Fluxum, Alpha-Wasserman).

12.2.1. Indications

The LMWHs are used for the prevention of VTE in patients undergoing hip and knee replacement surgery, general (e.g., abdominal, gynecologic, urologic) surgery and in acute medical conditions including cancer, prolonged bed rest, heart failure, severe lung disease and those individuals with severely restricted mobility. They are also used to reduce the risk of acute cardiac ischemic events (death and/or MI) in patients with unstable angina or non-ST-segment elevation/non-Q-wave MI (i.e., non-ST-segment elevation acute coronary syndromes). The use of a LMWH is also recommended by the ACCP as first-line or alternative therapy (instead of heparin) for prevention of VTE in selected patients undergoing intracranial neurological surgery, major trauma, acute spinal cord injury and in some patients with acute ischemic stroke (Geerts et al. 2004).Low molecular weight heparins are also used concurrently with an oral anticoagulant (warfarin or phenprocoumon) in hospitalized patients for the treatment and secondary prevention of DVT with or without PE and in selected outpatients for the treatment of acute DVT without accompanying PE. Therapy with LMWH also has been recommended for prevention or treatment of VTE occurring during pregnancy (Hirsh and Raschke 2004a). The ACCP also currently recommends "long-term" use of LMWHs following acute thrombotic events (3–6 months) in patients with cancer (Hirsh and Raschke 2004a).

12.2.2. Administration

Low molecular weight heparins are administered subcutaneously. They have no effect on the aPTT (because there is no binding to thrombin), and one of their major advantages is the lack of a need to monitor their anticoagulant effect. There are special populations where this may be necessary, however, including patients with renal insufficiency, severe obesity, during pregnancy or in the pediatric population. If required, monitoring can be performed using anti-factor Xa levels to LMWH. Levels should be checked approximately 4 hours after a subcutaneous dose and therapeutic ranges for enoxaparin (the most commonly used LMWH in the United States) are 0.5–1.0 IU/mL for the 12-hour dosing and ≥1.0 IU/mL for 24-hour dosing (Hirsh and Raschke 2004a).

12.2.3. Dosing

The LMWHs cannot be used interchangeably on a unit-for-unit (or mg-for-mg) basis. Enoxaparin has an approximate anti-factor Xa activity of 100 units/mg according to the World Health Organization (WHO) First International Low Molecular Weight Heparin Reference Standard. For the prevention of postoperative DVT in patients undergoing hip-replacement or knee-replacement surgery, several options and doses have been recommended for this particular agent: lovenox 30 mg/SC every 12 hours or 40 mg/SC daily. Enoxaparin can also be given 12 hours before surgery, 12–24 hours after surgery or 4–6 hours after surgery at half the usual prophylactic dose (Geerts et al. 2004). Prophylaxis should be given for at least 10 days following surgery and some clinicians recommend continued prophylaxis for as many as 28–35 days. For prevention of postoperative DVT in patients undergoing general surgery, including abdominal, gynecologic or urologic, the recommended dose of enoxaparin is 40 mg once daily, with an initial dose given 2 hours prior to surgery. For prevention of VTE in patients whose mobility is restricted during acute illness (cancer, heart failure, severe lung disease, confined to bed rest), 40 mg of enoxaparin is recommended daily (Geerts et al. 2004). In outpatients (and inpatients) for the treatment of VTE, the usual dose of enoxaparin is 1 mg/kg twice daily or 1.5 mg/kg/daily (Hirsh and Raschke 2004a). Dosing reductions are advised for individuals with a creatinine clearance under 30 ml/min and the LMWHs in general are not advised for patients on dialysis. For reducing the risk of ischemic complications (cardiac death or non-fatal MI) in patients with unstable angina or non-ST-segment elevation MI (non-ST-segment elevation acute coronary syndromes) who are receiving concurrent therapy with aspirin, the usual dose of enoxaparin is 1 mg/kg every 12 hours (Hirsh and Raschke 2004a).

The dose of dalteparin is also expressed in anti-factor Xa international units. Each milligram of dalteparin is equivalent to 156.25 anti-Xa units. For the prevention of postoperative VTE in patients undergoing hip-replacement surgery, therapy with dalteparin may also be initiated either before or after surgery. One method advocates a dose of 5000 units of dalteparin 10–14 hours before surgery, followed by a second dose of 5000 units 4–8 hours after surgery and 5000 units daily throughout the postoperative period. Alternatively, 2500 units may be administered within 2 hours of hip-replacement surgery, followed by 2500 units 4–8 hours after surgery and thereafter

5000 units once daily throughout the postoperative period. For the prevention of postoperative DVT in patients undergoing general (abdominal) surgery who are at high risk for DVT, 5000 units of dalteparin should be given 8–12 hours prior to surgery followed by 5000 units daily throughout the postoperative period until the risk has diminished (Geerts et al. 2004). For the treatment of acute DVT or PE, the recommended dalteparin dose is 200 units/kg daily in one or two divided doses (Hirsh and Raschke 2004a).

12.3. Adverse Effects of Heparin and Low Molecular Weight Heparins

Hemorrhage is the most commonly encountered complication of heparin and the LMWHs. Other reported complications include hypersensitivity and anaphylactoid reactions. In these conditions, patients develop minor complaints of a low-grade fever, urticaria, rhinitis or conjunctivitis (hypersensitivity reaction); however, sudden and severe hypertension, respiratory distress and chest pain have been reported with the anaphylactoid complication. Hyperkalemia, hypoaldosteronism, elevation in transaminases, osteoporosis and transient alopecia have also been described. The most devastating potential complication, HIT occurs in as many as 3–5% of all patients receiving unfractionated heparin but less than 1% of those receiving any of the LMWH preparations.

12.4. The Immune-Mediated Response to Heparin

HIT is a very prothrombotic condition due a number of contributing factors including enhanced generation of thrombin, increased platelet activation and aggregation, endothelial and monocyte activation and the release of prothrombotic microparticles. It is associated with very high morbidity and mortality.

One of the plasma proteins binding to heparin is platelet factor 4 (PF4), a basic and abundant 70-amino acid cationic glycoprotein member of the CXC subgroup of the chemokine family (Walenga et al. 2004). This is a large family of homologous proteins involved in chemotaxis, coagulation, inflammation and cell growth (Oppenheim et al. 1991, Rollins 1997, Luster 1998). Platelet factor 4 is stored in the alpha granules of platelets bound to chondroitin sulfate, forming a tetramer by sequential non-covalent association of PF4 monomers. Upon activation, the PF4–chondroitin sulfate complex is released and binds to the surface of activated platelets. Heparin (more anionic) displaces chondroitin sulfate and binds to PF4 by wrapping around the PF4 tetramer, resulting in a large linear antigenic complex that is bound to the platelet surface. The binding of heparin to PF4 causes a conformational change in the PF4 molecule, exposing neoepitopes and rendering it antigenic. This triggers an immune response that in some individuals results in the formation of antibodies (produced by B cells) that bind to this complex via their Fab terminus (Amiral et al. 1996). These antibodies are usually IgG, although IgM and IgA isotypes have been reported (Amiral et al. 1996). The Fc portion of the bound antibody then cross-links with the FcγRIIa receptor on adjacent platelets, resulting in the release of additional PF4 molecules, activation and aggregation of additional platelets and generation of procoagulant-rich microparticles (Warkentin et al. 1994). These antibodies bind and activate platelets over a narrow molar ratio of PF4 to heparin, approximating 1 mol of PF4 tetramer to 1 mol of unfractionated heparin, and are transient generally lasting no more than 80 days (Amiral et al. 2000, Warkentin and Kelton 2001).

Immune complex injury to endothelial cells lining the blood vessels may also contribute to the thrombotic process seen in HIT. Antibody binding that recognizes PF4–heparin complexes on the endothelium and the cell surface glycosaminoglycans expressed on monocytes promote prothrombotic conditions through the release of tissue factor, plasminogen activator inhibitor (PAI) and additional cytokines (Chong et al. 1989). This antibody-mediated activation of platelets, endothelial cells and monocytes results in the clinico-pathologic syndrome known as heparin-induced thrombocytopenia (HIT). It is also referred to as type II HIT or the heparin-induced thrombocytopenia and thrombosis syndrome (HITTS) (Kappers-Klunne et al. 1997, Lindhoff-Last et al. 2002, Girolami et al. 2003).

12.4.1. History of HIT

In 1958, two surgeons, Roger E. Weisman and Richard W. Tobin, became the first to report the clinical entity now known as HIT when they reported 10 cases of arterial embolism occurring during heparin therapy. All of Weisman and Tobin's patients had an appropriate indication for heparin, but between days 7 and 15 each experienced an arterial thrombosis. Six of their patients died and two required major amputations. Weisman and Tobin's (1958) report was reportedly met with skepticism because this complication had not been recognized previously. Several additional series of patients with similar complications were reported over the next 15 years, but it was not until 1972 that a group of vascular surgeons including G.R. Rhodes, R.H. Dixon and Donald Silver first suggested an immune cause for these thrombotic complications (Rhodes, Dixon and Silver 1973, 1977).

12.4.2. Incidence of HIT

HIT is now recognized as a common iatrogenic disorder that can occur in any patient population. The reported incidence of this syndrome varies but is thought to range from less than 1% for the LMWHs to as high as 5% for heparin (Lindhoff-Last et al. 2002, Mahlfeld et al. 2002, Ganzer, Gutezeit and Mayer 1999, Marx et al. 1999, Warkentin et al. 2000, Prandoni et al. 2005). Although all patients who receive these anticoagulants are at jeopardy, certain groups including orthopedic and cardiovascular surgical patients as well as individuals who have had repeated heparin exposure during diagnostic or therapeutic procedures seem to be at the highest risk (Shuster et al. 2003). HIT is uncommon in the obstetric and pediatric populations (Fausett et al. 2001, Klenner et al. 2004).

Due to their smaller size, LMWHs exhibit less non-specific binding and therefore have a lower affinity for binding to PF4 (Walenga et al. 2004). LMWH also forms a smaller complex that has been shown to cross-link fewer of the platelet $Fc\gamma RII$ receptors, thereby activating platelets less often than the larger heparin–PF4 complexes (Greinacher et al. 2006). These factors may help to explain the lower incidence of HIT with LMWH.

12.4.3. Clinical Presentation of HIT

HIT is much more likely to cause thrombosis than other hypercoagulable states including Factor V Leiden, prothrombin gene mutation, congenital protein C, S and antithrombin deficiencies or patients with the antiphospholipid syndrome (Warkentin et al. 1995). The risk of thrombosis approaches 38–76% in patients with HIT at one month if left untreated (Hirsh et al. 2004b). Thrombosis is venous, arterial or a combination of the two. Venous thromboembolism is more common (4:1 ratio compared to arterial events). Patients typically present with a lower, or less likely upper, extremity DVT or PE. Less commonly cerebral sinus thrombosis, adrenal hemorrhagic infarction or disseminated intravascular coagulation (DIC) may occur. Acute limb ischemia is the most common arterial presentation followed by stroke and MI. Cardiac intraventricular or intra-atrial thrombosis, spinal cord, bowel or renal infarction or vascular graft occlusion have also been reported.

There are several unusual presentations of HIT. These include cutaneous manifestations (heparin-induced erythematous or necrotic lesions at subcutaneous injection sites or warfarin-induced skin necrosis or WISN and warfarin-associated venous limb gangrene (VLG)), an acute systemic anaphylactoid reaction following an intravenous heparin bolus with fever, chills, tachycardia, hypertension and rarely cardiopulmonary arrest.

The site of HIT-related thrombotic events appears to be influenced by several clinical factors including localized vascular injury, placement of central venous catheters or pacemaker wires, a recent angiographic, surgical or endovascular procedure (PTA PTCA or PCI) or individuals with underlying arteriosclerosis (Levy and Hursting 2007). Approximately 9–11% of patients with HIT will require amputation and death approaches 17–30% in those untreated (Lewis et al. 2001, Lewis et al. 2003, Greinacher et al. 2000). Orthopedic patients appear to be at the highest risk of morbidity and mortality and a number of reports suggest individuals with an underlying malignancy are also at high risk (Warkentin et al. 2000, Fabris et al. 2002, Greinacher et al. 2005, Opatrny and Warner 2004).

The risk of developing HIT varies with the dose of heparin used, the preparation (bovine greater risk than porcine heparin), the duration of therapy and the patient population, although any patient receiving heparin or LMWH is at risk (Warkentin 1999). The highest incidence is reported with intravenous administration, but HIT has also been reported in patients who have only minimal exposure including through heparin-coated catheters, subcutaneous prophylactic doses or intravenous flushes to maintain arterial or central catheter line patency.

12.4.4. Definition of HIT

HIT is classically defined as a drop in a patient's platelet count to less than 100,000 mm^3 or 150,000 mm^3 while receiving heparin or LMWH. However, a 50% drop in the patients platelet count from pre-heparin treatment levels is now considered to be a more specific finding (Warkentin and Greinacher 2004). The severity of thrombocytopenia is usually moderate in most individuals, with median platelet counts of 50,000–80,000 mm^3 reported (Warkentin 2003a, Warkentin 2005a). Bleeding is rare, even when there is severe thrombocytopenia.

12.4.5. Patterns of Presentation

There are three temporal presentations of HIT (Warkentin and Kelton 2001, Warkentin 2005a). The classic presentation, sometimes referred to as "typical-onset HIT", is generally seen with a drop in the platelet count that occurs between 5 and 14 days of exposure. This time-frame represents the time it normally takes for heparin or LMWH to induce an antibody response. It is the most common presentation accounting for approximately 66% of all reported cases (Warkentin and Greinacher 2004). A less often recognized presentation (occurring roughly in 30% of all cases), referred to as rapid-onset HIT, can be seen within hours to days after heparin administration. It is the result of heparin antibodies that developed during a recent exposure to heparin or LMWH (generally within the last 30–100 days). In a series of 243 serologically proven cases of HIT, Warkentin and Kelton (2001) reported that the median time for the development of thrombocytopenia in rapid-onset HIT was 10.5 hours and most individuals had received heparin within the previous 30 days. The third presentation, delayed-onset HIT, develops anywhere from 9 to 40 days following UFH or LMWH exposure, usually after these agents have been withdrawn. This form is seen in roughly 2–3% of all HIT cases (Warkentin and Greinacher 2004). Patients are often discharged home or to a rehabilitation facility when a new thrombosis develops. Delayed-onset HIT is characterized by finding very high titers of circulating heparin antibodies. In this form, patients do not always present with thrombocytopenia (Warkentin 2003a).

Thrombocytopenia without antibody formation can also occur with heparin or LMWH therapy. This condition is referred to as type I HIT, a non-immune-mediated process. Heparin's negative charge and molecular size are thought to be responsible for binding to platelets, resulting in a transient drop in the platelet count. This generally occurs between days 1 and 4 of administration despite continuation of heparin or LMWH therapy. The platelet count rarely falls below 100,000 mm^3 and it is not associated with thromboembolic events.

12.4.6. Diagnosis

Warkentin and others have developed a practical method to calculate the pretest probability of HIT. Using their approach, one looks at the actual platelet count, the percentage decrease in the patient's platelets from pre-heparin treatment, the timing of heparin exposure, the presence of thrombosis or other related HIT complications and the potential for other causes to explain the low platelet count. Points are given depending on the variables listed above (Table 12.1). This method helps to determine the likelihood that laboratory testing will be positive or negative (Lo et al. 2006).

12.4.7. Laboratory Diagnosis

The diagnosis of HIT is based both on clinical and laboratory testing, thus the term clinicopathologic syndrome is frequently encountered. Because thrombocytopenia is a common finding in the hospital setting, other possibilities must always be considered in the differential diagnosis including pseudothrombocytopenia, DIC, thrombotic thrombocytopenia purpura (TTP), infections, alcohol, medications, bone marrow failure or dilution.

Table 12.1 Estimating the pretest probability of HIT: the 'four Ts'

	Points (0, 1 or 2 for each of 4 categories: maximum possible score = 8)		
	2	**1**	**0**
Thrombocytopenia	> 50% fall or platelet nadir 20–100 $\times 10^9$/1	30–50% fall or platelet nadir 10–19 $\times 10^9$/1	Fall < 30% or platelet nadir < 10 $\times 10$/1
Timing* of platelet count fall or other sequelae	Clear onset between d 5 and 10: or less than 1 d (if heparin exposure within past 100 d)	Consistent with immunization but not clear (e.g., missing platelet counts) or onset of thrombocytopenia after d 10	Platelet count fall too early (without recent heparin exposure)
Thrombosis or other sequelae (e.g., skin lesions)	New thrombosis: skin necrosis: post heparin bolus acute systemic reaction	Progressive or recurrent thrombosis: erythematous skin lesions: suspected thrombosis not yet proven	None
Other cause for thrombocytopenia not evident	No other cause for platelet count fall is evident	Possible other cause is evident	Definite other cause is present

Pretest probability score: 6–8 = high; 4–5 = intermediate; 0–3 = low

*First day of immunizing heparin exposure considered d 0: the day the platelet count begins to fall is considered the day of onset of thrombocytopenia (it generally takes 1–3 d more until an arbitrary threshold that defines thrombocytopenia is passed).

Source: Warkentin. T.E. & Heddle. N.M. (2003) Laboratory diagnosis of immune heparin-induced thrombocytopenia. *Current Hematology Reports.* Copyright Current Medicine, used by permission.

There is no single "gold standard" test for diagnosing HIT; however, two types of laboratory tests are readily available at most institutions. These include the functional tests which detect heparin-dependent platelet activation in the presence of the patient's sera and UFH or LMWH and the antigen assays or immunoassays which measure IgG, IgM or IgA antibodies that bind PF4 to heparin or LMWH. These tests should only be ordered when there is a clinical suspicion for HIT.

Many physicians order an antigenic assay (a solid-phase enzyme-linked immunosorbent assay, ELISA) as a screening tool, since it is more readily available, technically easier to perform and provides rapid results. The ELISA detects the presence of HIT antibodies by measuring changes in their optical density (OD). Results are reported as positive when the OD is greater than 0.4 (Sheridan, Carter and Kelton 1986).

Functional testing is generally more helpful to confirm a positive immunoassay and there are several methods available including the washed platelet assays, serotonin release assay (SRA), heparin-induced platelet aggregation assay (HIPA) and citrated plasma assay (platelet aggregation test). The washed platelet assays are recognized as more reliable than antigen assays because they have a higher sensitivity and specificity (Chong 2003, Warkentin and Heddle 2003b). Among the functional tests, the SRA is considered the gold standard. Its major disadvantage, however, is that it is technically demanding and requires the use of radioisotopes and fresh donor platelets. It is not readily available in all laboratories and most clinical laboratories prefer the less demanding platelet aggregation tests and/or immunoassays.

A rapid antigen assay (particle gel immunoassay) has also been developed (Eichler et al. 2002). It reportedly has a specificity similar to that of the functional assays with fewer false-positive results than the solid-phase immunoassays. This rapid antigen assay has the potential to fulfill a longstanding need for a quick (<30 minutes) and reliable HIT test.

Once HIT is suspected, many physicians recommend performing a combination of the two assays (washed platelet functional assay and an antigen assay) to help confirm the diagnosis. If both are negative, there is a 95% negative predictive value. If both tests are positive and the clinical picture fits, the positive predictive value is consistently 100% (Pouplard et al. 2005). Additional laboratory tests include flow cytometry and particle gel assays. These are not readily available at most hospitals and are currently used largely for research purposes.

HIT is a clinicopathologic syndrome and the diagnosis should be made by both clinical and laboratory findings. It is best to use laboratory tests only to confirm one's bedside judgment, not to make the diagnosis.

12.5. Treatment

The treatment for HIT has undergone important changes over the past decade. Until recently, clinicians had few options for treating this potentially devastating syndrome. Fortunately, with the development of several new anticoagulants, there are now a number of novel treatment options. These include the heparinoid danaparoid (organ®) and the direct thrombin inhibitors (DTIs); recombinant hirudin (r-hirudin) (e.g., lepirudin®); the small molecule argatroban; and bivalirudin (Angiomax®). The synthetic pentasaccharide (fondaparinux or Arixtra®), an indirect factor Xa inhibitor, has also been used "off-label" to treat HIT (Spinler 2006). The oral anticoagulants of the coumarin class, either warfarin or phenprocoumon, are used for long-term treatment. These agents should only be initiated when the patients' clinical condition and platelet counts have sufficiently recovered from their acute HIT event.

Once the diagnosis is suspected, all heparin or LMWH products should be stopped, and a fast-acting non-heparin alternative anticoagulant started immediately, even if there is no evidence for thrombosis (Warkentin 1999). Treatment should not be delayed while awaiting laboratory results as this only increases the risk for new thrombosis (Warkentin 1999). Cessation of heparin alone is not sufficient as studies have consistently shown a cumulative risk for new thrombosis rates approaching 53% if this approach is taken (Hirsh, Heddle and Kelton 2004b, Wallis et al. 1999, Warkentin and Kelton 1996).

Direct thrombin inhibitors have proven useful because of their ability to inhibit the generation of thrombin, reduce the incidence of new thrombosis and continue treatment for the initial heparin or LMWH indication. These anticoagulants inhibit thrombin without the need for the cofactor AT and do not generate or interact with heparin–PF4 antibodies. In previous studies, Argatroban and Lepirudin have been shown to significantly improve outcomes in patients with HIT (decreasing rates of new thrombosis) when compared to historical controls (Hirsh, Heddle and Kelton 2004b, Lewis et al. 2001, Lewis et al. 2003, Greinacher et al. 2000, Warkentin and Kelton 1996). Both are Federal Drug Administration (FDA) approved in the United States, while the DTI bivalirudin is FDA approved only in patients with HIT who require PCI.

12.5.1. Lepirudin

Lepirudin (*Refludan, Refludin, Aventis, Berlex, Hoechst, Pharmion, Pharma, Schering*) is a hirudin derived from the salivary glands of the medicinal leech, *Hirudo medicinalis*. It is produced by recombinant biotechnology from the yeast *Saccharomyces cerevisiae*, yielding recombinant hirudin (r-hirudin). Lepirudin differs from the natural hirudins by substitution of a leucine for isoleucine at the NH_2-terminal end of the molecule and by the absence of a sulfate group at tyrosine (position 63). Its molecular weight is approximately 7000 Daltons. Lepirudin was the first DTI approved for use in the United States by the FDA for anticoagulation in patients with HIT, based largely on the studies by Dr Andreas Greinacher and colleagues (Greinacher et al. 2000, Lubenow et al. 2005).

Lepirudin is a bivalent inhibitor of thrombin that inhibits all of its biological activities. It is a polypeptide composed of 65 amino acids that has two binding sites: an active site which catalyzes most of the functions of the thrombin molecule and a fibrinogen-binding site which mediates the binding of thrombin to fibrinogen. This binding is very specific and irreversible and inactivates both free (soluble) and clot-bound (fibrin-bound) thrombin.

Lepirudin is given intravenously, although there are numerous case reports of subcutaneous administration. It has a relatively short half-life of approximately 1.7 hours. Therapeutic levels are usually reached within 30–60 minutes following intravenous infusion and its lack of plasma protein binding leads to a more predictable bioavailability and therapeutic effect. Lepirudin is cleared by the kidneys and therefore significant dose adjustments are required in patients with renal insufficiency.

Lepirudin is monitored by the aPTT for most indications; however, the ACT is used in patients undergoing PTA, PTCA, PCI or other interventional procedures. The target aPTT is 1.5–2.5 times the baseline level and should be measured 4–6 hours after initiation and following any dose adjustments. Lepirudin can also prolong the prothrombin time (PT), although it causes less of an effect when compared to other DTIs including argatroban or bivalirudin.

The recommended dosage for lepirudin in patients with HIT is shown in Table 12.2. The maximum dose (recommended by the manufacturer) should not exceed a dose based on a maximum weight of 110 kg. In patients with a creatinine clearance below 60 ml/min, the dose should be reduced. Lepirudin is not recommended for use in patients with a creatinine clearance below 15 ml/min or in individuals on dialysis.

Lepirudin is a foreign protein; therefore, antibodies (IgG, but not IgE) develop in as many as 44–75% of patients after initial or re-exposure (Lubenow et al. 2005). This generally occurs after 5 days or more of therapy (more rapidly if repeat exposure) and is the amount of time required for an immune response to develop. These antibodies do not neutralize lepirudin, but cause decreased renal elimination leading to an enhanced anticoagulant effect by extending lepirudin's half-life. In this condition close monitoring and appropriate dose reductions are necessary (Lubenow et al. 2005, Greinacher, Lubenow and Eichler 2003b, Eichler et al. 2000). There have been several reports of anaphylaxis associated with lepirudin including four deaths. These severe adverse reactions generally occur within minutes of an intravenous bolus and are more likely to occur upon re-exposure (Greinacher et al. 2003a). Anaphylaxis is believed to be reduced by omitting the bolus dose (Greinacher, Lubenow and Eichler 2003b, Eichler et al. 2000, Greinacher et al. 2003a). Other authors, however, have not identified allergic reactions or anaphylaxis related to initial or re-exposure to lepirudin; nevertheless, caution is urged, especially if the patient has previous lepirudin exposure (Cardenas and Deitcher 2005). There is no cross-reactivity with PF4, therefore no risk of thrombosis is associated with these antibodies.

There are additional side-effects of lepirudin including eczema, pruritus, hot flashes, fever, chills, urticaria, bronchospasm, cough, angioedema and injection-site reactions when given subcutaneously. The main adverse effect of lepirudin is bleeding; unfortunately, there is no antidote, although in most cases, stopping the drug is sufficient. In severe bleeding cases, desmopressin, prothrombin complex and hemofiltration have been tried (Amin et al. 1997, Ibbotson et al. 1991, Irani, White and Sexon 1995, Mon et al. 2006).

12.5.2. Bivalirudin

Bivalirudin (*Angiomax or Angiox, Oryx, The Medicines Company, Angiox, Nycomed, CSL*) is a synthetic hirudin analog initially approved for use as an alternative to heparin for PCI in the United States. Bivalirudin is also approved in the United States, Canada, New Zealand, Israel, Argentina and the 25 members of the EU for use as an anticoagulant in patients undergoing

Table 12.2 Currently Available Anticoagulants

	Heparin (UFH)	Low Molecular Weight Heparin (LMWH)	Lepirudin	Bivalirudin	Argatroban	Fondaparinux	Danaparoid	Coumarins
Administration	IV, SC	SC	IV (some reports of SC)	IV	IV	SC	IV, SC	Oral, IV
Indication Dosage	VTE: 80 U/kg bolus IV followed by infusion of 18 units/kg/hr IV or 5000 units IV followed by 1280 units/hr IV or 333 units/kg SC followed by 250 units/kg SC Q12°

Unstable angina or NSTEMI: 60–70 units/kg/hr (max 5,000 units) IV followed by 12–15 units/kg/hr

— | VTE: Enoxaparin 1 mg/kg SC Q12° Dalteparin 200 units/kg SC qd or divided into 2 doses

Unstable angina or NSTEMI: Enoxaparin 1 mg/kg Q12° SC

VTE prophylaxis Enoxaparin 40 mg QD SC or | HIT: Bolus 0.4 mg/kg followed by 0.15 mg/kg/h infusion (max dose based on a weight of 110 kg) now advised by the manufacturer to eliminate the bolus and begin with a dose of 0.05 to 0.10 mg/kg/hr | NOT FDA approved for HIT except in PCI: doses reported for the treatment of "off label" VTE in HIT range from 0.10 to 0.2 mg/kg/hr

—

PCI: bolus: 0.75 mg/kg, followed by continuous infusion: 1.75 mg/kg/hour for the duration of procedure and up to 4 hours | HIT: 2 µg/kg/min not to exceed 10 µg/kg/min

PCI: 350 µg/kg/min bolus followed by an infusion of 25 µg/kg/min

— | VTE: "off label" used for HIT <50 kg5 mg SC QD 50–100 kg 7.5 mg SC QD >100 kg 10 mg SC QD

VTE prophylaxis: 2.5 mg SC QD | HIT: 2500 bolus of anti-Xa units followed by a step-down infusion of 400 anti-Xa units for 4 hours, then 300 anti-Xa units for 4 hours, followed by a maintenance infusion of 150–200 anti-Xa units

—

VTE prophylaxis: 750 anti-Xa units SC BID or TID | VTE: 2–10 mg once daily not to be used in HIT unless the platelet countless recovered to >100,000 mm^3 and preferably >150,000 mm^3

— |

VTE prophylaxis	VTE prophylaxis 5000 units SC Q8° or 12°	30 mg Q12° SC Dalteparin 5000 units QD SC						
Dosage adjustments	N/A	CrCl <30ml/min Treatment of VTE: 1 mg/kg SC/d VTE prophylaxis dose: 30 mg SC/d	Dosage adjustment required for renal failure: Defined as a CrCl <60: not recommended for patients on dialysis	Dosage adjustment required for patients with moderate or severe renal impairment	0.5 μg/kg/min with hepatic dysfunction 0.2 μg/kg/min with multiple organ dysfunction	Contraindicated in renal failure or CrCl <30 ml/min	Dose reduction recommended in patients with CrCl <30 ml/min	Begin with lower doses in geriatric patients and HIT
Monitoring	aPTT 1.5–2.5X baseline or Anti-XA assay 0.3–0.7 IU/mL in patients with a baseline prolonged aPTT or heparin resistance Check 6 hours after initiation and dosage adjustments	No need to monitor but there are exceptions: for pregnancy, pediatric, obese and renal failure patients Target is an anti-Xa assay to LMWH with levels of 0.5–1.0 IU/mL for Q12-hour dosing or 1.0–2.0 IU/mL for Q24-hour dosing	aPTT 1.5–2.5X baseline Check 4–6 hours after initiation and dosage adjustments Use ACT during interventional procedures	aPTT 1.5–2.5X baseline Use ACT during interventional procedures	aPTT 1.5–3X baseline Check 2 hours after initiation and any dosage adjustments Use ACT during interventional procedures	No monitoring necessary	Use anti-Xa 0.5–0.8 IU/mL using danaparoid as the standard	INR with goal of 2–3

(Continued)

Table 12.2 (*Continued*)

	Heparin (UFH)	Low Molecular Weight Heparin (LMWH)	Lepirudin	Bivalirudin	Argatroban	Fondaparinux	Danaparoid	Coumarins
Administration	IV, SC	SC	IV (some reports of SC)	IV	IV	SC	IV, SC	Oral, IV
	Use the ACT during interventional procedures or cardiac or vascular surgery	Check anti-factor Xa to LMWH 4 hours after 12-hour and 6 hours dosing						
Mechanism of action	Binds to antithrombin, accelerating its inactivation of thrombin and factor Xa	Binds to a specific pentasaccharide sequence to antithrombin resulting in the inactivation of Xa	Irreversible binding to thrombin inhibits both free and clot bound thrombin	Reversible non-competitive bivalent inhibitor of free and clot bound thrombin	Competitively inhibits free and clot-bound thrombin	Synthetic pentasaccharide selectively inhibiting factor Xa by binding to antithrombin	Inhibition of factor Xa	Interferes with the hepatic synthesis of vitamin K-dependent clotting factors and natural anticoagulants protein C and S
Peak onset	2–3 hours	1–5 hours	30–60 minutes	5 minutes	1–3 hours	3 hours	2–5 hours	72–96 hours

Half-life	Dose dependent, ranging from 30 to 150 minutes	111–1100 minutes (agent dependent)	1.3 hours	25 minutes	39–51 minutes	17–21 hours	24 hours	1 week
Route of elimination	Cellular mechanism at lower doses and renal clearance at higher doses	Renal	Renal	Mainly proteolytic, some renal (reportedly 20%)	Hepatic	Renal	Renal	Hepatic
Notes			Can prolong PT/INR (least of the DTIS)	Minimal effect on PT/INR	Prolongs INR; a target INR of 4 should be used if on Coumadin before argatroban is discontinued			

PTCA. In the EU it is marketed under the trade name Angiox™. More recently, bivalirudin has been approved in the United States for use in patients requiring PCI with HIT.

Bivalirudin is a small synthetic 20-amino acid peptide that shares an 11-amino acid sequence with hirudin. It has a molecular mass of 2180 Daltons and is a specific and reversible non-competitive inhibitor of thrombin, rendering it inactive. Like other bivalent DTIs, it also binds to both free and clot-bound thrombin. Bivalirudin binds two distinct regions on thrombin at the same time: it binds its amino-terminal segment, the active (catalytic) site of thrombin, and its carboxy-terminal segment to the fibrinogen-binding site of thrombin. Once inhibition occurs, circulating proteases cleave bivalirudin, releasing the amino-terminal segment from the active site region of thrombin (Reed and Bell 2002, Sciulli and Mauro 2002). This allows thrombin to resume catalytic function and differentiates it from lepirudin, whose binding is irreversible. Bivalirudin is not inactivated by PF4 nor does it require any cofactor for its activity. It does not bind to proteins other than thrombin.

Bivalirudin has predictable pharmacokinetics and exhibits a linear dose–response relationship when given intravenously, producing an immediate effect after this mode of administration. It has the shortest half-life of the currently available DTIs (approximately 25 minutes) and is metabolized by both proteolytic and renal mechanisms, the majority being proteolytic (Reed and Bell 2002, Sciulli and Mauro 2002, Robson 2000, Robson et al. 2002). Patients with renal insufficiency may need dose adjustments according to their degree of impairment; however, given the minor renal excretion there is much less risk of overdosing in renal failure compared to lepirudin and a lower risk of bleeding (Robson 2000, Robson et al. 2002). Because bivalirudin is only approved for patients with HIT undergoing PCI, there are no well-established dosing regimens in other patient populations (Bartholomew, Begelman and Almahameed 2005a). Studies that have used bivalirudin in these clinical situations (individuals with both clinically suspected and confirmed HIT) have found that doses between 0.05 and 0.2 mg/kg/hr are effective, with dose reduction in patients with moderate to severe renal impairment (see Table 12.2) (Bufton et al. 2002, Berilgen et al. 2003, Ramirez et al. 2005).

The PT, aPTT, ACT and thrombin time (TT) all rise linearly with increased doses of bivalirudin. The aPTT is generally used in patients treated for HIT with a goal of 1.5–2.5 times the patient's baseline. There is a minimal effect on the INR, which simplifies transition to oral anticoagulation. Although it is not approved for all patients with HIT (except PCI), it has demonstrated favorable outcomes in these patients (Campbell et al. 2000, Mahaffey et al. 2003).

Bivalirudin has also been used with favorable results in both "on-pump" and "off-pump" cardiac surgery cases in HIT. A clinical trial completed by Merry and colleagues compared bivalirudin with UFH (with protamine reversal) in non-HIT patients requiring off-pump coronary artery bypass (OPCAB) surgery (Merry et al. 2004). Favorable results, including improved graft patency and comparable hemorrhage and transfusion requirements, led to two subsequent multicenter trials. The *CABG HIT/TS On* and *OFF*-Pump *Safety* and *Efficacy* (CHOOSE-ON and CHOOSE-OFF) studies for patients with HIT and the *EValuation* of patients during coronary artery bypass graft *Operations: Linking UTilization* of bivalirudin to *Improved Outcomes* and

*N*ew anticoagulation strategies (EVOLUTION-OFF and EVOLUTION-ON) trials were conducted to evaluate the safety and efficacy of bivalirudin as an alternative to UFH (and protamine reversal) in the HIT and non-HIT settings, respectively. To date, results of these studies have revealed comparable safety and efficacy endpoints (Dyke et al. 2005, Dyke et al. 2006, Smedira et al. 2006, Koster et al. 2007).

Adverse effects include headache, diarrhea, nausea and abdominal cramps. Bleeding is the major adverse effect and occurs more commonly in patients with renal impairment. There is no specific antidote to bivalirudin; however, the use of recombinant factor VIIa, desmopressin, dialysis, hemofiltration and plasmapheresis have all been suggested (Irvin et al. 1999). If bleeding does occur, the anticoagulant should be discontinued immediately. The anticoagulant effect clears within a few hours after discontinuing the infusion.

Bivalirudin lacks significant antigenicity. A review of bivalirudin-treated patients from nine different studies involving 494 patients reported 11 patients with antibivalirudin antibodies; 9 of them were false positives (Berkowitz 1999). None of the patients experienced anaphylactic reactions.

Since bivalirudin shares an 11-amino acid sequence with hirudin, it is at least theoretically possible that patients with antilepirudin antibodies resulting from treatment with lepirudin could cross-react with bivalirudin. Eichler and colleagues found that 22 of 43 sera containing antilepirudin antibodies showed reactivity in vitro against bivalirudin (Eichler et al. 2004). This suggests that if bivalirudin is used in patients previously treated with lepirudin, extra caution should be used, e.g., careful anticoagulant monitoring, as antilepirudin antibodies sometimes influence pharmacokinetics.

12.5.3. Argatroban

Argatroban *(Argatroban, Novastan®, GlaxoSmithKline)* was originally known as MD-805. It was later given the trademark Novastan®, but in 2000 the US FDA required a name change because of other similar named drugs. It is now known as Argatroban in the United States, but still bears the name Novastan in other countries. Argatroban is a small synthetic (molecular weight of 526.66 Daltons) DTI derived from L-arginine. It is approved in the United States and Canada for the treatment and prevention of thrombosis in patients with HIT and for use in patients with HIT who require PCI. Argatroban has also been approved in a number of European countries for this indication as well.

Historically, argatroban was first found useful in conjunction with thrombolysis for treatment of arterial thrombosis in animals. Later its role as adjunctive treatment of thrombolysis in combination with glycoprotein IIb/IIIa inhibition in canine models with coronary thrombosis led to further studies in humans. Argatroban has been used in clinical trials in patients with non-ST-segment elevation acute coronary syndrome, acute ST-segment elevation MI (ARGAMI and ARGAMI-2), cardiac surgery, ischemic stroke and hemodialysis (Yeh and Jang 2006).

Argatroban is a univalent active-site thrombin inhibitor that competitively blocks the catalytic action of thrombin by way of multiple binding mechanisms. Argatroban effectively inhibits free and clot-bound thrombin. It is more potent than r-hirudin in its ability to inhibit clot-bound versus free thrombin (Berry et al. 1994).

Approximately fifty percent of argatroban binds to human proteins in the circulation, particularly albumin and glycoprotein (Yeh and Jang 2006, Linkins and Weitz 2005). It has a fast onset of action and is rapidly eliminated. Argatroban has a short half-life of 39–51 minutes and in healthy volunteers, aPTT and ACT times return to normal in 1–2 hours after stopping the infusion. Argatroban undergoes no significant renal clearance. It is hepatically metabolized via hydroxylation and aromatization of the 3-methyltetrahydroquinoline ring in the liver and its metabolites are excreted primarily in the feces by biliary excretion. Dose adjustments are recommended in patients with moderate to severe liver disease and the critically ill patient (Beiderlinden et al. 2007). There is no cross-reactivity with UFH.

The recommended dose for treating HIT is 2 µg/kg/minute in patients with normal liver function and 0.5 µg/kg/minute in those with hepatic impairment. No bolus is needed and the manufacturer recommends that the infusion rate not exceed 10 µg/kg/minute. Lower doses have been recommended (Beiderlinden et al. 2007) in critically ill patients with multiple organ dysfunction (see Table 12.2).

Argatroban can be monitored via the aPTT and ACT and these tests are increased in a dose-dependent manner. Steady-state levels are achieved within 1–3 hours after starting the infusion (Yeh and Jang 2006). The targeted aPTT is generally 1.5–3.0 times the baseline level and this should be checked two hours after initiation or with any dose adjustments. Argatroban prolongs the INR without bleeding complications; therefore, assessing the anticoagulant effects of warfarin can be challenging. The manufacturer recommends that a target INR of 4.0 be used during cotherapy before argatroban is discontinued (after a minimum of 5 days of combined therapy), and that the INR be checked 4–6 hours after discontinuation to ensure that it remains in a therapeutic range. The aPTT should also be monitored at this time because if it remains elevated it may also have an effect on the INR (Bartholomew and Hursting 2005b). Although an INR ≥4 while on warfarin is historically associated with a significantly increased risk of bleeding, values ≥7 while on argatroban and warfarin cotherapy have been reported to occur without bleeding in both healthy subjects and HIT patients (Sheth et al. 2001). No antibody formation has been demonstrated to date with argatroban.

The benefits of using argatroban were clearly demonstrated in two studies (including ARG-911 and ARG-915) which enrolled a total of 722 patients. Reductions in the risk for new thrombosis and thromboembolic complications compared with historical controls were reported (Hirsh, Heddle and Kelton 2004b, Lewis et al. 2001, Lewis et al. 2003).

There is no antidote available to reverse argatroban; however, if bleeding occurs the drug should be discontinued immediately. Reportedly, argatroban can be cleared using high-flux dialysis membranes, and recombinant activated factor VII has been used in this setting.

The choice of an anticoagulant for the treatment or prevention of HIT should be based on the availability of the agent, the patient's hepatic and renal function and the physician's familiarity with the anticoagulant. Although there have been no comparative studies evaluating the clinical efficacies of the DTIs due in part to the different patient baseline characteristics and the lack of significant numbers of patients at most institutions, one recent study did compare the efficacy and safety outcomes of lepirudin and argatroban over a two-year period (Smythe et al. 2005). Results demonstrated comparable efficacy and safety for these two DTIs.

Monitoring DTIs may not be reliable if the patient has a lupus anticoagulant, hypofibrinogenemia or elevated fibrinogen–fibrin degradation products. If present these conditions lead to difficulties in judging appropriate drug levels (Kaplan and Francis 2002).

12.5.4. Other Agents

12.5.4.1. Fondaparinux

Fondaparinux, *Arixtra® (Sanofi-Synthelabo, Toulouse, France)*, is a synthetic pentasaccharide that was formerly named Org31540/SR90107A. It has a molecular weight of 1728 Daltons and is generated by total chemical synthesis (Herbert, Petitou and Lormeau 1997, Savi et al. 2005). Fondaparinux is a selective indirect factor Xa inhibitor that binds specifically to the arginine-rich domain of AT. Fondaparinux does not inactivate thrombin and has no known effect on platelet function. At the recommended dose, fondaparinux does not affect fibrinolytic activity or bleeding time.

Fondaparinux is given subcutaneously, has 100% bioavailability and a half-life of 17–21 hours. It is excreted by the kidneys and therefore elimination is prolonged in patients with renal impairment. The pharmacokinetic properties of fondaparinux have not been studied in patients with hepatic impairment.

Fondaparinux has a minimal effect on the aPTT and PT/INR. There is generally no need for laboratory monitoring, although it may be useful for assessing its anticoagulation effect in patients with low body weight, the elderly or renally impaired.

Fondaparinux is approved in the United States for prevention of VTE in orthopedic patients (total knee and hip replacement and hip fracture), abdominal surgery and for the treatment of VTE in hospitalized individuals; the latter is based on the MATISSE DVT and PE trials (Herbert, Petitou and Lormeau 1997, Savi et al. 2005, Bauer et al. 2001, Turpie et al. 2002, Buller et al. 2003, Buller et al. 2004). More recently it has been used for patients with acute coronary syndrome (ACS) including unstable angina, non-ST-segment elevation MI and ST elevation MI (Yusuf et al. 2006a,b).

The recommended prophylaxis dose for fondaparinux is 2.5 mg subcutaneously given daily. For the treatment of VTE the recommended dose for patients weighing less than 50 kg is 5 mg subcutaneously daily, for 50–100 kg it is 7.5 mg subcutaneously daily, and 10 mg for individuals greater than 100 kg (see Table 12.2).

Fondaparinux has been used "off-label" in a number of patients with HIT and until recently no episodes of HIT have been reported in clinical trials (Efird and Kockler 2006). In studies involving 2726 patients, Warkentin et al. (2005b) reported similar immunogenicity between fondaparinux and low molecular weight heparin; however, PF4/fondaparinux was recognized poorly by the antibodies generated suggesting that the risk of HIT was very low. To date, Warkentin and colleagues have reported the only known case of HIT associated with fondaparinux (Warkentin, Maurer and Aster 2007).

12.5.4.2. Danaparoid

Danaparoid *(danaparoid sodium, Organ® Oss, the Netherlands)* is a non-heparin low molecular weight (approximately 5,500 Daltons) polysulfated glycosaminoglycan derived from porcine intestinal mucosa. It is a heparinoid whose active components are heparan sulfate, dermatan sulfate and chondroitan sulfate. Compared with LMWH and UFH, it has a lower degree of sulfation and a lower charge density making it less likely to bind to plasma proteins or platelets (Chong et al. 2001).

Danaparoid is approved for the treatment and prevention of HIT-associated thrombosis in Canada, continental Europe, Australia, New Zealand and Japan (Chong et al. 2001, Farner et al. 2001, Newman, Swanson and Chong 1998, Magnani and Gallus 2006). It is also used for the prophylaxis of DVT. It is no longer available in the United States.

Danaparoid exerts its activity by the highly selective antithrombin-mediated inhibition of factor Xa. It has minimal activity on thrombin; therefore, it does not prolong the aPTT and does not interfere with conversion to warfarin or phenprocoumon as is seen with the DTIs.

Danaparoid can be administered either intravenously or subcutaneously with a bioavailability approaching 100%. It has a predictable anticoagulant response, a half-life of approximately 24 hours and is mainly eliminated by the kidneys. In patients requiring prophylaxis for elective hip-replacement surgery, the recommended dose is 750 anti-Xa units given two to three times per day subcutaneously. For full dose intravenous treatment of HIT, a bolus is given followed by step-down infusions and a maintenance dose (Table 12.2). Dose reductions are recommended (similar to those advised for the LMWHs) if the creatinine clearance is less than 30 ml/min. Monitoring of anti-factor Xa (using danaparoid as the standard) may be indicated in the pediatric population, individuals with low or high body weight (<45 or >90 kilograms) and in patients with renal insufficiency, especially those with end-stage renal disease. It is also advised that patients be monitored every 1–2 months if they are receiving chronic therapy (Magnani and Gallus 2006). Therapeutic levels are 0.5–0.8 IU/ml.

There is no antidote to danaparoid and if bleeding complications occur, the agent should be stopped immediately. Protamine sulfate will only partially antagonize the anti-Xa activity, and blood products should therefore be administered as necessary.

Danaparoid has been used effectively in patients with HIT (Chong 2003, Chong et al. 2001, Farner et al. 2001, Newman, Swanson and Chong 1998, Magnani and Gallus 2006). It interferes with the binding of HIT antibodies to platelets, reduces the adverse effects of heparin remaining in the circulation after it has been discontinued and may decrease endothelial damage (Magnani and Gallus 2006). In a report of 1,478 patients treated with danaparoid over a 22-year period, Magnani and Gallus (2006) found clinical outcomes comparable to accounts using the other commercially available DTIs (argatroban and lepirudin). Danaparoid has also been compared favorably to lepirudin and dextran with findings of similar efficacies (Chong et al. 2001, Farner et al. 2001). Because it is a mixture of glycosaminoglycans, a small percentage of patients with HIT antibodies have cross-reactivity to danaparoid (as high as 20%), although they are generally weak and do not appear to be clinically significant (Warkentin and Greinacher 2004). Nevertheless, some authors including Magnani and Gallus (2006) recommend testing patients for danaparoid cross-reactivity prior to treatment.

12.5.4.3. Coumarins

Members of the coumarin class, either warfarin or phenprocoumon are the main choice of therapy for the long-term management of HIT. Of note, however, initiation of warfarin therapy prior to the patient's and platelet recovery, or without bridging using a non-heparin-based anticoagulant, can result in an accelerated prothrombotic state (Warkentin and Greinacher 2004). This condition, now well described in the literature, can lead to WISN or VLG and is more likely to be seen in patients with a supratherapeutic INR or when the alternative anticoagulant (DTI or danaparoid) is stopped too soon (not adequate overlap with a non-heparin anticoagulant) or before the platelet count has recovered from the acute event (Warkentin and Greinacher 2004, Srinivasan et al. 2004). It is believed to result from a rapid decline in the levels of protein C in addition to the prothrombotic affects of HIT. Current practice guidelines recommend initiating the coumarin class anticoagulants only after the patient has improved clinically, is adequately anticoagulated with a DTI or other non-heparin anticoagulant, platelet counts have recovered to at least 100,000 mm^3 and preferably 150,000 mm^3 and low doses of the oral anticoagulant are initiated (Warkentin and Greinacher 2004, Srinivasan et al. 2004). Warfarin or phenprocoumon should be overlapped with a DTI for a minimum of 5 days, and the INR should be in the accepted therapeutic range for at least 2 consecutive days before discontinuing the DTI or alternative anticoagulant (Srinivasan et al. 2004).

The DTIs can produce a misleading elevation in the PT/INR making transitioning to warfarin or phenprocoumon challenging at times. This is largely attributed to the differences in the required molar concentrations among the DTIs to achieve the desired inhibition of thrombin (Warkentin et al. 2005c). The increased INR is most pronounced with argatroban and the least pronounced with lepirudin (Gosselin et al. 2004). It should also be recognized that warfarin can independently elevate the aPTT (Kearon et al. 1998).

In order to help with transition, the INR and aPTT should be checked after the DTI is held for approximately 4–6 hours once the desired overlap target INR is reached. If at this point the INR is within the targeted range (generally 2–3) and the aPTT is close to baseline, the DTI can be safely discontinued (Kearon et al. 1998). Another management strategy that may prove helpful is to measure a chromogenic factor Xa or factor IIa level to determine if an adequate response to the oral anticoagulant has been attained (Arpino, Demirjian and Van Cott 2005, Trask et al. 2004). The length of therapy following an episode of acute HIT is not well known, but given the higher risk of thrombosis within the first 30 days, most physicians recommend at least 3 months of anticoagulation.

12.5.5. Re-exposure to Heparin

Heparin or the LMWHs should normally be avoided after an acute episode of HIT, at least as long as heparin antibodies are detectable. Previous studies have demonstrated that these antibodies are transient and are generally not detectable by antigen assays after 80 days (Warkentin and Kelton 2001). Warkentin and Kelton (2001) reported that 10 patients, who were accidentally (or deliberately) readministered heparin, had no adverse effects. Others have reported different outcomes including Magnani's and Gallus' (2006) review of the clinical complications involving 18 patients unintentionally re-exposed to LMWH during or after danaparoid use. The authors found a delay in platelet recovery and/or platelet count reductions in 14 patients, 8 deaths (3 thrombotic) and 1 reversible cardiac arrest (patient died one month later due to cardio-respiratory failure) and 2 non-fatal thrombotic events (Magnani and Gallus 2006).

Once the antibodies have cleared by any of the available sensitive laboratory assays, patients may tolerate brief exposures to heparin (during cardiac or vascular surgery or interventional procedures) where it may be considered less risky to use heparin (where an antidote is available) than an alternative anticoagulant that cannot be rapidly reversed. This strategy has been used in a limited number of patients without major complications (Olinger et al. 1984, Makhoul et al. 1987, Selleng et al. 2001, Potzsch, Klovekorn and Madlener 2000, Lubenow et al. 2002). Regardless, full re-exposure (over a period of several days) is generally not recommended.

12.5.6. Other Modes of Treatment

Platelet transfusions are not recommended even when there is profound thrombocytopenia, unless there is active bleeding. Transfused platelets are believed to be activated by the same immune mechanisms responsible for acute HIT and have been linked to thrombotic events in previous reports (Warkentin and Greinacher 2004, Cimo et al. 1979).

A number of adjunctive therapies have been tried, including antiplatelet agents (dextran, acetylsalicylic acid, dipyridamole), the glycoprotein IIb/IIIa inhibitors, ancrod, plasmapheresis and intravenous gammaglobulin. Two of the more promising appear to be plasmapheresis and intravenous gammaglobulin. Plasmapheresis, a process in which the patient's plasma is removed and replaced with normal plasma, has been used successfully in a number of uncontrolled studies (Antonijevic et al. 2006, Robinson and Lewis 1999, Greinacher and Warkentin 2004). This approach has been taken in part because not all currently available treatment methods are successful (Antonijevic et al. 2006). Plasmapheresis has been shown to result in the normalization of both the platelet count and aggregation studies (Robinson and Lewis 1999, Greinacher and Warkentin 2004). Although the mechanism is unknown it may result from removing the HIT antibody or by the correction of an anticoagulant deficiency by the addition of normal plasma replacement (Robinson and Lewis 1999). J.A. Robinson and Bruce Lewis reported the benefits of plasmapheresis in the management of 21 patients with HIT. If plasmapheresis was initiated early in the management (within four days of thrombocytopenia developing), there was a reduction in mortality; however, if started later mortality increased (Robinson and Lewis 1999). Antonijevic et al. (2006) found a mortality benefit when plasmapheresis was added to a DTI speculating that the combination of therapy may be of benefit in patients resistant to treatment.

The use of intravenous gammaglobulin has also been reported in several small series (Greinacher and Warkentin 2004, Winder et al. 1998, Frame et al. 1989). Patients generally had severe thrombocytopenia but had an increase in their platelet count with treatment. Intravenous gammaglobulin is believed to interrupt platelet activation by the HIT antibodies (Frame et al. 1989).

12.6. Conclusion

Heparin-induced thrombocytopenia is a serious complication of unfractionated heparin or LMWH preparations that affects both the venous and arterial circulation. It is an immune-mediated process (commonly referred to as a clinicopathologic syndrome) that requires both clinical and laboratory findings to confirm the diagnosis. Thrombocytopenia is no longer essential for the diagnosis since a 50% drop in the platelet count from pre-heparin treatment levels may be a more specific indicator. Once HIT is clinically suspected, all forms of heparin (or LMWH) should be discontinued immediately and an alternative non-heparin anticoagulant initiated.

References

Amin, D. M., Mant, T. G., Walker, S. M., Kerry, R., Lloyd, P., Lefevre, G., and Close, P. 1997. Effect of a 15-minute infusion of DDAVP on the pharmacokinetics and pharmacodynamics of REVASC during a four-hour intravenous infusion in healthy male volunteers. J. Thromb. Haemost. 77:127–132.

Amiral, J., Wolf, M., Fischer, A., Boyer-Neumann, C., Vissac, A., and Meyer, D. 1996. Pathogenicity of IgA and/or IgM antibodies to heparin-PF4 complexes in patients with heparin-induced thrombocytopenia. Br. J. Haematol. 92:954–959.

Amiral, J., Pouplard, C., Vissac, A. M., Walenga, J. M., Jeske, W., and Gruel, Y. 2000. Affinity purification of heparin-dependent antibodies to platelet factor 4 developed in heparin-induced thrombocytopenia: biological characteristics and effects on platelet activation. Br. J. Haematol. 109:336–341.

Ancalmo, N., and Ochsner, J. 1990. Heparin, the miracle drug: a brief history of its discovery. J. La. State Med. Soc. 142:22–24.

Antonijevic, N. M., Savic, N. B., Perunicic, J., Kovac, M., Mikovic, D., Stanojevic, M., Calija, B., Milosevic, R. A., Obradovic, S. D., and Vasiljevic, Z. 2006. Salvage late plasmapheresis in a patient with pulmonary embolism caused by heparin-induced thrombocytopenia primarily resistant to danaparoid sodium and lepirudin. J. Clin. Apher. 21:252–255.

Arpino, P. A., Demirjian, Z., and Van Cott, E. M. 2005. Use of the chromogenic factor X assay to predict the international normalized ratio in patients transitioning from argatroban to warfarin. Pharmacotherapy 25:157–164.

Barrit, D. W., and Jordan, S. C. 1960. Anticoagulant drugs in the treatment of pulmonary embolism. A controlled trial. Lancet 1:1309–1312.

Bartholomew, J. R., Begelman, S. M., and Almahameed, A. 2005a. Heparin-induced thrombocytopenia: principles for early recognition and management. Cleve. Clin. J. Med. 72 (Suppl 1):S31–36.

Bartholomew, J. R., and Hursting, M. J. 2005b. Transitioning from argatroban to warfarin in heparin-induced thrombocytopenia: an analysis of outcomes in patients with elevated international normalized ratio (INR). J. Thromb. Thrombolysis 19:183–188.

Bauer, K. A., Eriksson, B. I., Lassen, M. R., and Turpie, A. G. 2001. Steering Committee of the Pentasaccharide in Major Knee Surgery Study. Fondaparinux compared with enoxaparin for the prevention of venous thromboembolism after elective major knee surgery. N. Engl. J. Med. 345:1305–1310.

Beiderlinden, M., Treschan, T. A., Gorlinger, K., and Peters, J. 2007. Argatroban anticoagulation in critically ill patients. Ann. Pharmacother. 41:749–754.

Berilgen, J. E., Nguyen, P. H., Baker, K. R., and Rice, L. 2003. Bivalirudin treatment of heparin-induced thrombocytopenia [abstr]. Blood 102:537a.

Berkowitz, S.D. 1999. Antigenic potential of bivalirudin [abstr]. Blood 94 (suppl 1):102.

Berry, C. N., Girardot, C., Lecoffre, C., and Lunven, C. 1994. Effects of the synthetic thrombin inhibitor argatroban on fibrin- or clot-incorporated thrombin: comparison with heparin and recombinant Hirudin. Thromb. Haemost. 72:381–386.

Bjork, I., Olson, S. T., and Shore, J. D. 1989. Molecular mechanisms of the accelerating effect of heparin on the reactions. between antithrombin and clottingproteinases. In Lane, D. A., and Lindhal, U. (eds.), Heparin. Clinical and biological properties clinical application, Boca Raton, Fla, CRC Press.

Bufton, M. G., et al. 2002. Bivalirudin effect on the INR and experience with prolonged inpatient and outpatient anticoagulation with bivalirudin for treatment of leg ischemia and arterial thrombosis due to HIT-TS (abstr). Blood 100:124b.

Buller, H. R., Davidson, B. L., Decousus, H., Gallus, A., Gent, M., Piovella, F., Prins, M. H., Raskob, G., Segers, A. E. M., Cariou, R., Leeuwenkamp, O., and Lensing, A. W. A. 2004. Fondaparinux or enoxaparin for the initial treatment of symptomatic deep venous thrombosis: a randomized trial. Ann. Intern. Med. 140:867–873.

Buller, H. R., Davidson, B. L., Decousus, H., Gallus, A., Gent, M., Piovella, F., Prins, M. H., Raskob, G., van den Berg-Segers, A. E. M., Cariou, R., Leeuwenkamp, O., and Lensing, A. W. A. 2003. Subcutaneous fondaparinux versus intravenous unfractionated heparin in the initial treatment of pulmonary embolism. N. Engl. J. Med. 349:1695–1702.

Campbell, K. R., Mahaffey, K. W., Lewis, B. E., Weitz, J. I., Berkowitz, S. D., Ohman, E. M., and Califf, M. 2000. Bivalirudin in patients with heparin-induced thrombocytopenia undergoing percutaneous coronary intervention. J. Invasive Cardiol. 12 (Suppl F):14F–19F.

Cardenas, G. A., and Deitcher, S. R. 2005. Risk of anaphylaxis after reexposure to intravenous lepirudin in patients with current or past heparin-induced thrombocytopenia. Mayo Clin. Proc. 80:491–493.

Chong, B. H., Fawaz, I., Chesterman, C. N., and Berndt, M. C. 1989. Heparin-induced thrombocytopenia: mechanism of interaction of the heparin-dependent antibody with platelets. Br. J. Haematol. 73:235–240.

Chong, B. H. 2003. Heparin-induced thrombocytopenia. J. Thromb. Haemost. 1: 1471–1478.

Chong, B. H., Gallus, A. S., Cade, J. F., Magnani, H., Manoharan, A., Oldmeadow, M., Arthur, C., Richard, K., Gallo, J, Lloyd, J., Seshadri, P., and Chesterman, N. 2001 Prospective randomised open-label comparison of danaparoid with dextran 70 in the treatment of heparin-induced thrombocytopaenia with thrombosis: a clinical outcome study. J. Thromb. Haemost. 86:1170–1175.

Cimo, P. L., Moake, J. L., Weinger, R. S., Ben-Menachem, Y. B., and Khalil, K. G. 1979. Heparin-induced thrombocytopenia: association with a platelet aggregating factor and arterial thromboses. Am. J. Hematol. 6:125–133.

Cosmi, B., Fredenburgh, J. C., Rischke, J., Hirsh, J., Young, E., and Weitz, J. I. 1997. Effect of nonspecific binding to plasma proteins on the antithrombin activities of unfractionated heparin, low-molecular-weight heparin, and dermatan sulfate. Circulation 95:118–124.

Cruickshank, M. K., Levine, M. N., Hirsh, J., Roberts, R., and Siguenza, M. 1991. A standard heparin nomogram for the management of heparin therapy. Arch. Intern. Med. 151:333–337.

Danielsson, A., and Bjork, I. 1981. Binding to antithrombin of heparin fractions with different molecular weights. Biochem. J. 193:427–433.

Dyke, C. M., Koster, A., Veale, J. J., Maier, G. W., McNiff, T., and Levy, J. H. 2005. Preemptive use of bivalirudin for urgent on-pump coronary artery bypass grafting in patients with potential heparin-induced thrombocytopenia. Ann. Thorac. Surg. 80:299–303.

Dyke, C. M., Smedira, N. G., Koster, A., Aronson, S., McCarthy, H. L., Kirshner, R., Lincoff, A. M., and Spiess, B. D. 2006. A comparison of bivalirudin to heparin with protamine reversal in patients undergoing cardiac surgery with cardiopulmonary bypass: The EVOLUTION-ON study. J. Thorac. Cardiovasc. Surg. 131:533–539.

Efird, L. E., and Kockler, D. R. 2006. Fondaparinux for thromboembolic treatment and prophylaxis of heparin-induced thrombocytopenia. Ann. Pharmacother. 40: 1383–1387.

Eichler, P., Raschke, R., Lubenow, N., Meyer, O., Schwind, P., and Greinacher, A. 2002. The new ID-heparin/PF4 antibody test for rapid detection of heparin-induced antibodies in comparison with functional and antigenic assays. Br. J. Haematol. 116:887–891.

Eichler, P., Lubenow, N., Strobel, U., and Greinacher, A. 2004. Antibodies against lepirudin are polyspecific and recognize epitopes on bivalirudin. Blood 103: 613–616.

Eichler, P., Friesen, H. J., Lubenow, N., Jaeger, B., and Greinacher, A. 2000. Antihirudin antibodies in patients with heparin-induced thrombocytopenia treated with lepirudin: Incidence, effects on aPTT, and clinical relevance. Blood 96: 2373–2378.

Fabris, F., Luzzatto, G., Soini, B., Ramon, R., Scandellari, R., Randi, M. L., and Girolami, A. 2002. Risk factors for thrombosis in patients with immune mediated heparin-induced thrombocytopenia. J. Intern. Med. 252:149–154.

Fareed, J., Walenga, J. M., Hoppensteadt, D., Huan, X., and Racanelli, A. 1988. Comparative study on the in vitro and in vivo activities of seven low-molecular-weight heparins. Haemostasis 18 (Suppl 3):3–15.

Farner, B., Eichler, P., Kroll, H., and Greinacher, A. 2001. A comparison of danaparoid and lepirudin in heparin-induced thrombocytopenia. J. Thromb. Haemost. 85: 950–957.

Fausett, M. B., Vogtlander, M., Lee, R. M., Esplin, M. S., Branch, D. W., Rodgers, G. M., and Silver, R. M. 2001. Heparin-induced thrombocytopenia is rare in pregnancy. Am. J. Obstet. Gynecol. 185:148–152.

Frame, J. N., Mulvey, K. P., Phares, J. C., and Anderson, M. J. 1989. Correction of severe heparin-associated thrombocytopenia with intravenous immunoglobulin. Ann. Intern. Med. 111:946–947.

Ganzer, D., Gutezeit, A., and Mayer, G. 1999. Potentials risks in drug prevention of thrombosis—low-molecular-weight heparin versus standard heparin. Z. Orthop. Ihre. Grenzgeb. 137:457–461.

Geerts, W. H., Pineo, G. F., Heit, J. A., Bergqvist, D., Lassen, M. R., Colwell, C. W., and Ray, J. G. 2004. Prevention of venous thromboembolism: the Seventh ACCP Conference on Antithrombotic and Thrombolytic Therapy. Chest 126 (Suppl 3):338S–400S.

Girolami, B., Prandoni, P., Stefani, P. M., Tanduo, C., Sabbion, P., Eichler, P., Ramon, R., Baggio, G., Fabris, F., and Girolami, A. 2003. The incidence of heparin-induced thrombocytopenia in hospitalized medical patients treated with subcutaneous unfractionated heparin: a prospective cohort study. Blood 101: 2955–2959.

Gosselin, R. C., Dager, W. E., King, J. H., Janatpour, K., Mahackian, K., Larkin, E. C., and Owings, E. T. 2004. Effect of direct thrombin inhibitors, bivalirudin, lepirudin, and argatroban, on prothrombin time and INR values. Am. J. Clin. Pathol. 121: 593–599.

Greinacher, A., Gopinadhan, M., Gunther, J. U., Omer-Adam, M. A., Strobel, U., Warkentin, T. E., Papastravou, G. Weitschies, W., and Helm, C. A. 2006. Close approximation of two platelet factor 4 tetramers by charge neutralization forms the antigens recognized by HIT antibodies. Arterioscler. Thromb. Vasc. Biol. 26: 2386–2393.

Greinacher, A., Eichler, P., Lubenow, N., Kwasny, H., and Luz, M. 2000. Heparin-induced thrombocytopenia with thromboembolic complications: meta-analysis of 2 prospective trials to assess the value of parenteral treatment with lepirudin and its therapeutic aPTT range. Blood 96:846–851.

Greinacher, A., Farner, B., Kroll, H., Kohlmann, T., Warkentin, T. E., and Eichler, P. 2005. Clinical features of heparin-induced thrombocytopenia including risk factors for thrombosis. A retrospective analysis of 408 patients. J. Thromb. Haemost. 94:132–135.

Greinacher, A., Eichler, P., Albrecht, D., Strobel, U., Potzsch, B., and Eriksson, B. I. 2003a. Antihirudin antibodies following low-dose subcutaneous treatment with desirudin for thrombosis prophylaxis after hip-replacement surgery: incidence and clinical relevance. Blood 101:2617–2619.

Greinacher, A., Lubenow, N., and Eichler, P. 2003b. Anaphylactic and anaphylactoid reactions associated with lepirudin in patients with heparin-induced thrombocytopenia. Circulation 108:2062–2065.

Greinacher, A., and Warkentin, T. E. 2004. Treatment of heparin-induced thrombocytopenia: an overview. In Heparin-induced thrombocytopenia, 3rd edition. Marcel Dekker Inc, Basel, pp. 355–370.

Herbert, J.-M., Petitou, M., and Lormeau, J.-C. 1997. SR90107A/Org31540, a novel anti-factor Xa antithrombotic agent. Cardiovasc. Drug Ref. 15:1–26.

Hirsh, J., and Levine, M. N. 1992. Low molecular weight heparin. Blood 79:1–17.

Hirsh, J., van Aken, W. G., Gallus, A. S., Dollery, C. T., Cade, J. F., and Yung, W. L. 1976. Heparin kinetics in venous thrombosis and pulmonary embolism. Circulation 53:691–695.

Hirsh, J. 1991. Heparin. N. Engl. J. Med. 324:1565–1574.

Hirsh, J., and Raschke, R. 2004a. Heparin and low-molecular-weight heparin: the Seventh ACCP Conference on Antithrombotic and Thrombolytic Therapy. Chest 126(Suppl 3):188S–203S.

Hirsh, J., Heddle, N., and Kelton, J. G. 2004b. Treatment of heparin-induced thrombocytopenia: a critical review. Arch. Intern. Med. 164:361–369.

Ibbotson, S. H., Grant, P. J., Kerry, R., Findlay, V. S., and Prentice, C. R. 1991. The influence of infusions of 1-desamino-8-D-arginine vasopressin (DDAVP) in vivo on the anticoagulant effect of recombinant hirudin (CGP39393) in vitro. J. Thromb. Haemost. 65:64–66.

Irani, M. S., White, H. J. Jr., Sexon, R. G. 1995. Reversal of hirudin-induced bleeding diathesis by prothrombin complex concentrate. Am. J. Cardiol. 75(5):422–423.

Irvin, W., Sica, D., Gehr, T., McAllister, A., Rogge, M., Charenkavanich, S., and Adelman, B. 1999. Pharmacodynamics (PD) and kinetics (PK) of bivalirudin (BIV) in renal failure (RF) and hemodialysis (HD) [abstr]. Clin. Pharmacol. Ther. 65:202.

Kaplan, K. L., and Francis, C. W. 2002. Direct thrombin inhibitors. Semin. Hematol. 39:187–196.

Kappers-Klunne, M. C., Boon, D. M., Hop, W. C., Michiels, J. J., Stibbe, J., van der Zwaan, C., Koudstaal, P. J., and van Vliet, H. H. D. M. 1997. Heparin-induced thrombocytopenia and thrombosis: a prospective analysis of the incidence in patients with heart and cerebrovascular diseases. Br. J. Haematol. 96:442–446.

Kearon, C., Ginsberg, J. S., Julian, J. A., Douketis, J., Solymoss, S., Ockelford, P., Jackson, S., Turpie, A. G., MacKinnon, B., Hirsh, J., and Gent, M. 2006. Comparison of fixed-dose weight-adjusted unfractionated heparin and low-molecular-weight heparin for acute treatment of venous thromboembolism. JAMA 296:935–942.

Kearon, C., Johnston, M., Moffat, K., McGinnis, J., and Ginsberg, J. S. 1998. Effect of warfarin on activated partial thromboplastin time in patients receiving heparin. Arch. Intern. Med. 158:1140–1143.

Klenner, A. F., Lubenow, N., Raschke, R., and Greinacher, A. 2004. Heparin-induced thrombocytopenia in children: 12 new cases and review of the literature. J. Thromb. Haemost. 91:719–724.

Koster, A., Dyke, C. M., Aldea, G., Smedira, N. G., McCarthy, H. L., Aronson, S., Hetzer, R., Avery, E., Spiess, B., and Lincoff, A. M. 2007. Bivalirudin during cardiopulmonary bypass in patients with previous or acute heparin-induced thrombocytopenia and heparin antibodies: results of the CHOOSE-ON trial. Ann. Thorac. Surg. 83:572–577.

Levy, J. H., and Hursting, M. J. 2007. Heparin-induced thrombocytopenia, a prothrombotic disease. Hematol. Oncol. Clin. North Am. 21:65–88.

Lewis, B. E., Wallis, D. E., Berkowitz, S. D., Matthai, W. H., Fareed, J., Walenga, J. M., and Bartholomew, J. 2001. Argatroban anticoagulant therapy in patients with heparin-induced thrombocytopenia. Circulation 103:1838–1843.

Lewis, B. E., Wallis, D. E., Leya, F., Hursting, M. J., and Kelton, J. G. 2003. Argatroban-915 Investigators. Argatroban anticoagulation in patients with heparin-induced thrombocytopenia. Arch. Intern. Med. 163:1849–1856.

Lindhoff-Last, E., Nakov, R., Misselwitz, F., Breddin, H. K., and Bauersachs, R. 2002. Incidence and clinical relevance of heparin-induced antibodies in patients with deep vein thrombosis treated with unfractionated or low-molecular-weight heparin. Br. J. Haematol. 118:1137–1142.

Linkins, L. A., and Weitz, J. I. 2005. Pharmacology and clinical potential of direct thrombin inhibitors. Curr. Pharm. Des. 11:3877–3884.

Lo, G. K., Juhl, D., Warkentin, T. E., Sigouin, C. S., Eichler, P., and Greinacher, A. 2006. Evaluation of pretest clinical score (4 T's) for the diagnosis of heparin-induced thrombocytopenia in two clinical settings. J. Thromb. Haemost. 4: 759–765.

Lubenow, N., Kempf, R., Eichner, A., Eichler, P., Carlsson, L. E., and Greinacher, A. 2002. Heparin-induced thrombocytopenia: temporal pattern of thrombocytopenia in relation to initial use or reexposure to heparin. Chest 122:37–42.

Lubenow, N., Eichler, P., Lietz, T., and Greinacher, A, Hit Investigators Group. 2005. Lepirudin in patients with heparin-induced thrombocytopenia – results of the third prospective study (HAT-3) and a combined analysis of HAT-1, HAT-2, and HAT-3. J. Thromb. Haemost. 3:2428–2436.

Luster, A. D. 1998. Chemokines—chemotactic cytokines that mediate inflammation. N. Engl. J. Med. 338:436–445.

Magnani, H. N., and Gallus, A. 2006. Heparin-induced thrombocytopenia (HIT). A report of 1,478 clinical outcomes of patients treated with danaparoid (Orgaran) from 1982 to mid-2004. J. Thromb. Haemost. 95:967–981.

Mahaffey, K. W., Lewis, B. E., Wildermann, N. M., Berkowitz, S. D., Oliverio, R. M., Turco, M. A., Shalev, Y., Ver Lee, P., Traverse, J. H., Rodriguez, A. R., Ohman, E. M., Harrington, R. A., and Califf, R. M. 2003. The anticoagulant therapy with bivalirudin to assist in the performance of percutaneous coronary intervention in patients with heparin-induced thrombocytopenia (ATBAT) study: main results. J. Invasive Cardiol. 15:611–616.

Mahlfeld, K., Franke, J., Schaeper, O., Kayser, R., and Grasshoff, H. 2002. Heparin-induced thrombocytopenia as a complication of postoperative prevention of thromboembolism with unfractionated heparin/low molecular weight heparin after hip and knee prosthesis implantation. Unfallchirurg 105:327–331.

Makhoul, R. G., McCann, R. L., Austin, E. H., Greenberg, C. S., and Lowe, J. E. 1987. Management of patients with heparin-associated thrombocytopenia and thrombosis requiring cardiac surgery. Ann. Thorac. Surg. 43:617–621.

Marx, A., Huhle, G., Hoffmann, U., Wang, L. C., Schule, B., Jani, L., and Harenberg, J. 1999. Heparin-induced thrombocytopenia after elective hip joint replacement with postoperative prevention of thromboembolism with low-molecular-weight heparin. Z. Orthop. Ihre. Grenzgeb. 137:536–539.

Merry, A. F., Raudkivi, P. J., Middleton, N. G., McDougall, J. M., Nand, P., Mills, B. P., Webber, B. J., Frampton, C. M., and White, H. D. 2004. Bivalirudin versus heparin and protamine in off-pump coronary artery bypass surgery. Ann. Thorac. Surg. 77:925–931; discussion 931.

Mon, C., Moreno, G., Ortiz, M., Diaz, R., Herrero, J. C., Oliet, A., Rodriguez, I., Ortega, O., Gallar, P., and Vigil, A. 2006. Treatment of hirudin overdosage in a dialysis patient with heparin-induced thrombocytopenia with mixed hemodialysis and hemofiltration treatment. Clin. Nephrol. 66:302–305.

Newman, P. M., Swanson, R. L., and Chong, B. H. 1998. Heparin-induced thrombocytopenia: IgG binding to PF4-heparin complexes in the fluid phase and cross-reactivity with low molecular weight heparin and heparinoid. J. Thromb. Haemost. 80:292–297.

Olinger, G. N., Hussey, C. V., Olive, J. A., and Malik, M. I. 1984. Cardiopulmonary bypass for patients with previously documented heparin-induced platelet aggregation. J. Thorac. Cardiovasc. Surg. 87:673–677.

Opatrny, L., and Warner, M. N. 2004. Risk of thrombosis in patients with malignancy and heparin-induced thrombocytopenia. Am. J. Hematol. 76:240–244.

Oppenheim, J. J., Zachariae, C. O., Mukaida, N., and Matsushima, K. 1991. Properties of the novel proinflammatory supergene "intercrine" cytokine family. Annu. Rev. Immunol. 9:617–648.

Potzsch, B., Klovekorn, W. P., and Madlener, K. 2000. Use of heparin during cardiopulmonary bypass in patients with a history of heparin-induced thrombocytopenia. N. Engl. J. Med. 343:515.

Pouplard, C., May, M. A., Regina, S., Marchand, M., Fusciardi, J., and Gruel, Y. 2005. Changes in platelet count after cardiac surgery can effectively predict the development of pathogenic heparin-dependent antibodies. Br. J. Haematol. 128: 837–841.

Prandoni, P., Siragusa, S., Girolami, B., and Fabris, F., BELZONI Investigators Group. 2005. The incidence of heparin-induced thrombocytopenia in medical patients treated with low-molecular-weight heparin: a prospective cohort study. Blood 106:3049–3054.

Ramirez, L. M., Carman, T. L., Begelman, S. M., AlMahameed, A., Joseph, D., Kashyap, V., White, D. A., Andersen-Harris, K., and Bartholomew, J. R. 2005. Bivalirudin in patients with clinically suspected HIT or history of HIT [abstr]. Blood 106:269a.

Raschke, R. A., Reilly, B. M., Guidry, J. R., Fontana, J. R., and Srinivas, S. 1993. The weight-based heparin dosing nomogram compared with a "standard care" nomogram. A randomized controlled trial. Ann. Intern. Med. 119:874–881.

Reed, M. D. and Bell, D. 2002. Clinical pharmacology of bivalirudin. Pharmacotherapy 22(6 Pt 2):105S–111S.

Rhodes, G. R., Dixon, R. H., and Silver, D. 1973. Heparin induced thrombocytopenia with thrombotic and hemorrhagic manifestations. Surg. Gynecol. Obstet. 136: 409–416.

Rhodes, G. R., Dixon, R. H., and Silver, D. 1977. Heparin induced thrombocytopenia: eight cases with thrombotic-hemorrhagic complications. Ann. Surg. 186:752–758.

Robinson, J. A., and Lewis, B. E. 1999. Plasmapheresis in the management of heparin-induced thrombocytopenia. Semin. Hematol. 36(Suppl 1):29–32.

Robson, R. 2000. The use of bivalirudin in patients with renal impairment. J. Invasive Cardiol. 12 (Suppl F):33F–36F.

Robson, R., White, H., Aylward, P., and Frampton, C. 2002. Bivalirudin pharmacokinetics and pharmacodynamics: effect of renal function, dose, and gender. Clin. Pharmacol. Ther. 71:433–439.

Rollins, B. J. 1997. Chemokines. Blood 90:909–928.

Ross, B. P., and Toth, I. 2005 Gastrointestinal absorption of heparin by lipidization or coadministration with penetration enhancers. Current Drug Delivery. 2:277–287.

Savi, P., Chong, B. H., Greinacher, A., Gruel, Y., Kelton, J. G., Warkentin, T. E., Eichler, P., Meuleman, D., Petitou, M., Herault, J.-P., Cariou, R., and Herbert, J.-M. 2005. Effect of fondaparinux on platelet activation in the presence of heparin-dependent antibodies: a blinded comparative multicenter study with unfractionated heparin. Blood 105:139–144.

Sciulli, T. M. and Mauro, V. F. 2002. Pharmacology and clinical use of bivalirudin. Ann. Pharmacother. 36:1028–1041.

Selleng, S., Lubenow, N., Wollert, H. G., Mullejans, B., and Greinacher, A. 2001. Emergency cardiopulmonary bypass in a bilaterally nephrectomized patient with a history of heparin-induced thrombocytopenia: successful reexposure to heparin. Ann. Thorac. Surg. 71:1041–1042.

Sheridan, D., Carter, C., and Kelton, J. G. 1986. A diagnostic test for heparin-induced thrombocytopenia. Blood 67:27–30.

Sheth, S. B., DiCicco, R. A., Hursting, M. J., Montague, T., and Jorkasky, D. K. 2001. Interpreting the International Normalized Ratio (INR) in individuals receiving argatroban and warfarin. J. Thromb. Haemost. 85:435–440.

Shuster, T. A., Silliman, W. R., Coats, R. D., Mureebe, L., and Silver, D. 2003. Heparin-induced thrombocytopenia: twenty-nine years later. J. Vasc. Surg. 38:1316–1322.

Smedira, N. G., Dyke, C. M., Koster, A., Jurmann, M., Bhatia, D. S., Hu, T., McCarthy, H. L., Lincoff, A. M., Spiess, B. D., and Aronson, S. 2006. Anticoagulation with bivalirudin for off-pump coronary artery bypass grafting: the results of the EVOLUTION-OFF study. J. Thorac. Cardiovasc. Surg. 131:686–692.

Smythe, M. A., Stephens, J. L., Koerber, J. M., and Mattson, J. C. 2005. A comparison of lepirudin and argatroban outcomes. Clin. Appl. Thromb. Hemost. 11:371–374.

Spinler, S. A. 2006. New concepts in heparin-induced thrombocytopenia: diagnosis and management. J. Thromb. Thrombolysis 21:17–21.

Srinivasan, A. F., Rice, L., Bartholomew, J. R., Rangaswamy, C., La Perna, L., Thompson, J. E., Murphy, S., and Baker, K. R. 2004. Warfarin-induced skin necrosis and venous limb gangrene in the setting of heparin-induced thrombocytopenia. Arch. Intern. Med. 164:66–70.

Trask, A. S., Gosselin, R. C., Diaz, J. A., and Dager, W. E. 2004. Warfarin initiation and monitoring with clotting factors II, VII, and X. Ann. Pharmacother. 38:251–256.

Turpie, A. G., Bauer, K. A., Eriksson, B. I., and Lassen, M. R., PENTATHALON 2000 Study Steering Committee. 2002. Postoperative fondaparinux versus postoperative enoxaparin for prevention of venous thromboembolism after elective hip-replacement surgery: a randomised double-blind trial. Lancet 359:1721–1726.

Walenga, J. M., Jeske, W. P., Prechel, M. M., Bacher, P., and Bakhos, M. 2004. Decreased prevalence of heparin-induced thrombocytopenia with low-molecular-weight heparin and related drugs. Semin. Thromb. Hemost. 30 (Suppl 1):69–80.

Wallis, D. E., Workman, D. L., Lewis, B. E., Steen, L., Pifarre, R., and Moran, J. F. 1999 Failure of early heparin cessation as treatment for heparin-induced thrombocytopenia. Am. J. Med. 106:629–635.

Warkentin, T. E., Hayward, C. P., Boshkov, L. K., Santos, A. V., Sheppard, J. A., Bode, A. P., and Kelton J. G. 1994. Sera from patients with heparin-induced thrombocytopenia generate platelet-derived microparticles with procoagulant activity: an explanation for the thrombotic complications of heparin-induced thrombocytopenia. Blood 84:3691–3699.

Warkentin, T. E. and Kelton, J. G. 2001. Temporal aspects of heparin-induced thrombocytopenia. N. Engl. J. Med. 344:1286–1292.

Warkentin, T. E. and Greinacher, A. 2004. Heparin-induced thrombocytopenia: recognition, treatment, and prevention: the Seventh ACCP Conference on Antithrombotic and Thrombolytic Therapy. Chest 126(Suppl 3):311S–337S.

Warkentin, T. E., Sheppard, J. A., Horsewood, P., Simpson, P. J., Moore, J. C., and Kelton, J. G. 2000. Impact of the patient population on the risk for heparin-induced thrombocytopenia. Blood 96:1703–1708.

Warkentin, T. E., Levine, M. N., Hirsh, J., Horsewood, P., Roberts, R. S., Gent, M., and Kelton, J. G. 1995. Heparin-induced thrombocytopenia in patients treated with low-molecular-weight heparin or unfractionated heparin. N. Engl. J. Med. 332:1330–1335.

Warkentin, T. E. and Kelton, J. G. 1996. A 14-year study of heparin-induced thrombocytopenia. Am. J. Med. 101:502–507.

Warkentin, T. E. 1999. Heparin-induced thrombocytopenia: a clinicopathologic syndrome. J. Thromb. Haemost. 82:439–447.

Warkentin, T. E. 2003a. Heparin-induced thrombocytopenia: pathogenesis and management. Br. J. Haematol. 121:535–555.

Warkentin, T. E. and Heddle, N. M. 2003b. Laboratory diagnosis of immune heparin-induced thrombocytopenia. Curr. Hematol. Rep. 2:148–157.

Warkentin, T. E. 2005a. New approaches to the diagnosis of heparin-induced thrombocytopenia. Chest 127(Suppl 2):35S–45S.

Warkentin, T. E., Cook, R. J., Marder, V. J., Sheppard, J. A., Moore, J. C., Eriksson, B. I., Greinacher, A., and Kelton, J. G. 2005b. Anti-platelet factor 4/heparin antibodies in orthopedic surgery patients receiving antithrombotic prophylaxis with fondaparinux or enoxaparin. Blood 106:3791–3796.

Warkentin, T. E., Greinacher, A., Craven, S., Dewar, L., Sheppard, J. A., and Ofosu, F. A. 2005c. Differences in the clinically effective molar concentrations of four direct thrombin inhibitors explain their variable prothrombin time prolongation. J. Thromb. Haemost. 94:958–964.

Warkentin, T. E., Maurer, B. T., and Aster, R. H. 2007. Heparin-induced thrombocytopenia associated with fondaparinux. N. Engl. J. Med. 356:2653–2655.

Weisman, R. E. and Tobin, R. W. 1958. Arterial embolism occurring during systemic heparin therapy. Arch. Surg. 76:219–225; discussion 225–227.

Winder, A., Shoenfeld, Y., Hochman, R., Keren, G., Levy, Y., and Eldor, A. 1998. High-dose intravenous gamma-globulins for heparin-induced thrombocytopenia: a prompt response. J. Clin. Immunol. 18:330–334.

Yeh, R. W. and Jang, I. K. 2006. Argatroban: update. Am. Heart J. 151:1131–1138.

Young, E., Cosmi, B., Weitz, J., and Hirsh, J. 1993. Comparison of the non-specific binding of unfractionated heparin and low molecular weight heparin (Enoxaparin) to plasma proteins. J. Thromb. Haemost. 70:625–630.

Yusuf, S., Mehta, S. R., Chrolavicius, S., Afzal, R., Pogue, J., Granger, C. B., Budaj, A, Peters, R. J., Bassand, J. P., Wallentin, L., Joyner, C., and Fox, K. A. 2006a. Effects of fondaparinux on mortality and reinfarction in patients with acute ST-segment elevation myocardial infarction: the OASIS-6 randomized trial. JAMA 295: 1519–1530.

Yusuf, S., Mehta, S. R., Chrolavicius, S., Afzal, R., Pogue, J., Granger, C. B., Budaj, A, Peters, R. J., Bassand, J. P., Wallentin, L., Joyner, C., and Fox, K. A. 2006b. Fifth Organization to Assess Strategies in Acute Ischemic Syndromes Investigators, Comparison of fondaparinux and enoxaparin in acute coronary syndromes. N. Engl. J. Med. 354:1464–1476.

13

Presenting an Immunogenicity Risk Assessment to Regulatory Agencies

Paul Chamberlain

13.1. Purpose

The purpose of this chapter is to provide a working method for constructing a risk management plan for undesirable immunogenicity of biopharmaceutical products. The approach is based on an accumulation of experience of diverse product types, including biosimilar medicinal products, unconjugated and conjugated recombinant therapeutic proteins, plant-derived monoclonal antibodies, biologic-device combinations and diagnostic imaging agents. In all cases, it has been useful to apply a common framework of questions to the specific risk scenario, in order to present a balanced assessment of risk for discussion with regulatory agencies. This chapter has been formatted around these questions to illustrate the weighting that might be attributed to different factors.

Typically, this process is initiated during the preparation of an IND or Clinical Trial Application, in order to interpret signals observed in non-clinical studies, and/or to demonstrate the suitability of bioanalytical methods to detect signals should these occur. This will underpin the proposed benefit-to-risk ratio to support initiation of the clinical programme. The risk management exercise then becomes an iterative process that must consider the changing risk status associated with wider exposure in the human population, as well as more stringent regulatory requirements in the approach to marketing authorisation. The process continues as an obligatory feature of the post-marketing pharmacovigilance plan for most biopharmaceutical products, to enable an ongoing re-evaluation of the probability of a host immune response to the product and its possible associated effects.

It may even be important to incorporate an assessment of relative risk to support the selection of a lead candidate for progression into the development cycle. Thus, a sponsor might apply such a structured analysis at the discovery stage to eliminate product candidates that present a high level of risk of provoking an anti-product immune response, in cases where such a response could be associated with serious consequences for the target population.

13.2. Regulatory Guidance

Although US and European regulatory agencies have been diligent in providing guidance on the need for a scientifically rigorous evaluation of immunogenicity during the development of biopharmaceutical products (an excellent review is provided in Shankar et al. 2006), the case-specific nature of the risk can make it difficult to interpret the level of risk associated with any signals observed (Koren et al. 2002).

This is why the FDA-led approach to risk assessment, which advocated a need to balance probability versus consequences of an undesirable anti-product immune response, provided an important advance in the regulatory process (Rosenberg and Worobec 2004a, Rosenberg and Worobec 2004b, Rosenberg and Worobec 2005). European regulatory agencies have recently drafted additional guidance (EMEA 2007) that represents a valuable summary of the various factors that should be taken into account in the evaluation of immunogenic potential of biopharmaceutical products.

Immunogenicity risk assessment is highly relevant to the demonstration of product comparability following manufacturing changes (ICH 2005) and to the development of biosimilar medicinal products (EMEA 2006a). The FDA has provided helpful guidance on the evaluation of immunogenicity of monoclonal antibody products in relation to potential clinical sequelae (FDA 1997).

In the post-marketing setting, an ongoing assessment of risk, including that associated with immune-mediated adverse drug reactions, will be required. For certain products, e.g. biosimilar medicinal products, immunogenicity monitoring will represent a major component of the post-authorisation risk management programme.

13.3. Risk Assessment

A risk assessment should involve three main elements:

1. Identification of risk factors
2. Evaluation of risk in terms of rate of occurrence (probability vector) and impact (consequences vector)
3. Strategy for managing the risk.

These elements are discussed in more detail below.

13.3.1. Identification of Risk Factors

As immunogenicity of biopharmaceutical products is a multifactorial phenomenon, it will be necessary to consider different sources of risk:

- Intrinsic immunogenicity of the product (see earlier chapters of this book)
- Abundance and uniqueness/redundancy of function of endogenous counterparts of the drug product
- Manufacturing process and rigour of product quality control
- Formulation and drug product stability
- Characteristics of the target population, including immune competence, prior exposure to the drug product or to related products, and genetic factors that may influence immune recognition
- Clinical dosing regimen, including route of administration, level and frequency of dosing.

13.3.2. Evaluation of Risk: Probability Versus Consequences

The evaluation of risk should be data-driven, and is most likely to emphasise the following:

- Validation of specificity and sensitivity of bioanalytical methods to detect immune responses to the product
- Observations from non-clinical studies on the effect of host anti-product antibody on pharmacokinetic and/or pharmacodynamic parameters (although relevance is highly dependent on the extent of sequence conservation between species, as discussed below)
- Controlled clinical studies that feature real-time monitoring of anti-product antibody responses using appropriately validated methods.

13.3.3. Management of Risk

Having evaluated the risk in terms of probability relative to consequences of an undesirable host immune response to the biopharmaceutical product, it will be necessary to propose a strategy for managing the risk. This could involve the following:

- Avoidance, e.g. terminate development or attempt to de-immunise the protein via deletion of immunogenic motifs
- Reduction, e.g. restrict use to intravenous administration or apply a tolerising dose regimen
- Retention, e.g. introduce appropriate precautions for use in product labelling
- Transfer, e.g. develop an effective post-marketing pharmacovigilance plan so that risk may be re-evaluated from a larger clinical database.

13.4. Key Questions for Risk Assessment

The pertinent information for a written risk assessment may be compiled through consideration of a set of questions that could be relevant for all biopharmaceutical products. The sequence of questions seeks to progress logically from a review of intrinsic and extrinsic causal factors, through an assessment of the suitability of bioanalytical methods and the results obtained from non-clinical and clinical studies, to a balancing of probability and consequences.

Question 1: What is the structural relationship of the therapeutic protein to endogenous counterparts?

The intrinsic immunogenicity of a biopharmaceutical product will depend on the presence of self and foreign structural motifs that are recognised by the host immune system (Koren et al. 2002, Schellekens 2002a, Chirino, Ary, and Marshall 2004, Rosenberg 2006, Strand, Kimberly, and Isaacs 2007).

Products that contain both foreign and self antigens are likely to be associated with the highest level of risk, since the presence of xenodeterminants will strongly increase the likelihood of breaking of immune tolerance to co-presenting self antigens. The administration of completely foreign proteins is associated with the highest risk of hypersensitivity reactions.

Because T-cell help is required for the development of a mature, high-affinity, antibody response, therapeutic proteins that contain T_H epitopes that bind common MHC Class II haplotypes would represent a potential risk. Equally, since B-cell receptors – as well as the antibodies produced by these B-cells – are able to recognise conformational epitopes (comprising amino acid residues that may be remote in the primary sequence), there is also merit in identifying B cell-binding motifs. Accordingly, in silico and ex vivo methods (Chapter 4) have been applied to identify immunogenic potential based on the presence of T- and B-cell binding motifs (Roggen 2006, Jaber and Baker 2007, Van Walle et al. 2007).

It is important to remember that identification of a T_H epitope using an in silico method, or even ex vivo T-cell stimulation, does not necessarily imply the generation of high-affinity anti-product antibodies in vivo, since the development of the mature response depends on the efficiency of antigen processing and presentation in the context of highly polymorphic MHC Class II proteins, co-stimulation of B- and T-cells, as well as central and peripheral tolerance mechanisms. The latter are able to delete antigen-specific T-cells or to suppress their activity via $CD4^+CD25^+T_{Reg}$ cell subset. Thus, although some proteins contain degenerate immunodominant T_H-epitopes (Tangri et al. 2005), anti-product antibodies may be generated in very rare circumstances – this appears to be the case for rhEPO. Nevertheless, the potential to form antibodies that could cross-react with self-antigens requires a critical (and conservative) appraisal of the probability of developing an anti-product antibody response, and the development of bioanalytical methods of appropriate specificity and sensitivity to detect such responses should they occur.

The experience gained with 'humanised' or even 'fully human' monoclonal antibody products clearly indicates that host responses may be directed to unique motifs presented in the idiotype, as well as to allotypic variants in the constant regions that reflect polymorphism of immunoglobulins across the human population (Strand, Kimberly, and Isaacs 2007). This requires evaluation of the specificity of the host anti-product antibodies, since these may be associated with different consequences for the performance of the product.

If there is high sequence conservation between species, non-clinical studies might provide useful data about the consequences of neutralisation of an endogenous factor (EMEA 2007). Therefore, the justification for non-clinical safety testing strategy should reflect the structural relationship of the therapeutic protein to endogenous counterparts in the selected animal species.

Question 2: What is the target of the drug product and how unique is its function?

The probability of inducing a host immune response to a product may be related to the physical location of the target. For example, idiotypic regions of monoclonal antibodies that bind to cell surface antigens are particularly immunogenic (Benjamin et al. 1986). The downstream effects of binding to the target might also influence probability, e.g. cytokine release could enhance immunogenicity via an adjuvant effect (Routledge et al. 1995).

The impact of an anti-product antibody response that is able to cross-react with/neutralise an endogenous factor (e.g. erythropoietin, thrombopoetin) that has a unique function could be life-threatening and, clearly, represents the highest risk category. The consequences of a host anti-product antibody response to recombinant Type I interferons (IFN-α and IFN-β) appears to be limited by the existence of endogenous variants that perform a similar function. This is not the case for a Type II interferon such as IFN-γ (Rosenberg 2003). Accordingly, the consequences of a host immune response to IFN-γ that cross-reacts with the endogenous cytokine could be associated with a rather higher risk.

Question 3: What is the abundance of endogenous counterparts of the drug product?

Immune tolerance to cytokines present at relatively low levels appears to be partial (van der Meide and Schellekens 1997, Soos et al. 2003, Kyewski and Derbinski 2004), such that the levels of protein that are administered therapeutically could break tolerance. The existence of naturally occurring antibodies to endogenous cytokines might represent another level of immune regulation that is important to homeostatic control of the prevailing activity of the endogenous cytokine. So, administration of relatively high levels of the cytokine, particularly in the presence of factors (aggregates, adjuvants or neo-epitopes) that augment the immune response, might result in perturbation of the balance of this control.

On the other hand, if the endogenous counterpart is highly abundant, an immune response is (1) less likely to occur and (2) may be of lower consequence since the antibodies formed would have capacity to neutralise only a relatively small proportion of the endogenous protein. Moreover, high abundance of the endogenous protein may preclude detection of antibodies due to assay interference.

In the case of a deficiency syndrome, patients may recognise a human protein as 'non-self' due to lack of established tolerance. This may result in a high incidence of immunogenicity. Thus, the sponsor should discuss how the proposed drug exposure levels, and potential or measured levels of host anti-product antibodies, relate to the abundance of the endogenous counterpart.

Question 4: How is the product manufactured and characterised?

Immunogenic potential can be dependent on a variety of structural attributes of a recombinant human protein, as well as the way in which the product is formulated, presented or stored (Hermeling et al. 2004). In addition to rigorous control of the manufacturing process, this necessitates the application of suitably qualified analytical methods to detect presence of:

- aggregates that could cross-link/stimulate B-cell receptors via presentation of repeating motifs
- degradation products, e.g. truncated variants, or other structural modifications that present neo-epitopes
- incorrectly folded protein that contains modified conformational epitopes
- process-related contaminants that might act as adjuvants
- changes in the extent of post-translational modification that alter intrinsic immunogenicity or tendency for protein aggregation.

The sponsor should present a critical analysis of the potential impact of the manufacturing process, including the choice of cell substrate, on the immunogenicity of the protein. This should discuss the structural heterogeneity of the drug product relative to that of any endogenous counterparts. Use of transgenic production systems, e.g. for plant-derived monoclonal antibodies, will provoke regulatory questions about the risk of immunogenicity (and allergenicity) associated with atypical post-translational modifications (FDA 2002). This aspect must be addressed by a suitable risk management strategy (Gomord et al. 2005). Transgenic mouse models (Hermeling et al. 2005) might enable comparison of the probability of different product forms inducing a breaking of tolerance to a self-protein, although species differences in the antigen processing/presentation machinery limit absolute predictive power for the clinical scenario.

Major emphasis should be given to justification of the suitability of the formulation used for the drug product, as well as of the container/closure system. Moreover, alternate effects of structural modification/chemical derivatisation should be considered. For example, in the case of protein PEGylation, the presence of a PEG moiety with relatively large hydrodynamic volume might substantially reduce the recognition of immunodominant B/T-cell epitopes on the protein by lymphocyte receptors, thereby abrogating the intrinsic immunogenicity of the protein. On the other hand, reports of host immune responses directed to the PEG moiety of PEGylated proteins (Ganson et al. 2006) have alerted regulatory agencies to the need to monitor PEG-specific antibodies. This may necessitate development, prior to initiation of the clinical programme, of bioanalytical assay formats of different specificity.

Question 5: How is the product to be used?

A number of extrinsic factors associated with clinical application have been identified that may influence the probability of induction of a host anti-product antibody response (EMEA 2007, Strand, Kimberly, and Isaacs 2007). Accordingly, the sponsor will need to provide a critical discussion of the potential influence of these factors on the level of immunogenicity risk:

- route of administration
- concomitant medication/immune competence
- dose level and frequency
- patient factors, e.g.

  - HLA type
  - nature of underlying disease
  - Fc_yR polymorphism.

It is important to remember that these risk factors are not independent variables. Thus, exposure adjusted incidence of neutralising antibodies to epoetin decreased by 83% following the adoption of procedures to ensure appropriate storage, handling and administration of Eprex® to patients with chronic kidney disease (Bennett et al. 2004). As the authors pointed out, a confluence of factors, including a change to a formulation that could have been slightly less effective to protect the product against mishandling than an earlier formulation, appear to have contributed to an increased incidence of a very rare clinical syndrome (Pure Red Cell Aplasia) associated with breaking of immune tolerance to a self-protein (Chapter 6).

It is often this category of the risk assessment that is most important for the effective presentation of the *relative* risk of immunogenicity of a specific biopharmaceutical product. Use of a combination of factors, such as acute intravenous administration in patients who are immuno-compromised and whose disease is poorly controlled, may enable use of a product that has a significant probability of inducing an undesirable immune response. A good example might be a stent (device) product for angioplasty that is coated with a murine monoclonal antibody that can act locally to reduce the risk of re-stenosis of the vessel. If the murine monoclonal antibody-coated stent were to be applied on one or two occasions only, with the antibody covalently linked at very low levels on the stent surface, the risk associated with the immune response could be considered as negligible. Nevertheless, the sponsor will need to substantiate the immunogenicity-associated risk by appropriate monitoring for a host anti-murine IgG response during clinical studies.

Question 6: What is the extent of prior exposure to the product or to related products?

The persistence of immunological memory could impact both the probability and consequences of an immune response to a particular product. Delayed hypersensitivity reactions to infliximab were observed following re-infusion after a 2–4-year treatment-free period, and re-administration of abciximab was associated with an increased incidence of anti-product antibodies and reduced efficacy (Wagner et al. 2003).

Prior treatment with a monoclonal antibody that contains a common Fc region has the potential to enhance anti-isotypic/allelic responses against other monoclonal antibody products. For example, a serum sickness syndrome (Type III hypersensitivity) was observed in patients who had received a monoclonal antibody of different specificity but with a common IgG_1 Fc region (Strand, Kimberly, and Isaacs 2007).

Biosimilar medicinal products present a special case: for 'high risk' products, regulatory agencies may require a sponsor to evaluate the relative risk of induction of an immune response to the biosimilar product compared with the reference product (EMEA 2006b). Thus, for a biosimilar rhEPO, it will be necessary to present 12-month-exposure comparative immunogenicity data for subjects who had been previously stabilised on the Reference product, in addition to post-marketing surveillance within the context of an ongoing Risk Management Programme.

Question 7: What methods have been applied to measure anti-product immune responses?

The major focus of the regulatory assessment of immunogenicity risk to date has been on the methodology to detect a host anti-product antibody response. Standards for these methods rely substantially on an AAPS-sponsored initiative to publish a self-standing set of technical recommendations that represent the current 'state of the art' for both ligand binding and cell-based assay formats (Mire-Sluis et al. 2004, Gupta et al. 2007). Accordingly, sponsors do have clear guidance on bioanalytical assay expectations that are applicable during non-clinical and clinical development. Nevertheless, there are a number of assay design challenges that are discussed separately in this volume (Chapter 3). Also, from a data analysis perspective, sponsors will need to justify the selection of critical parameters, e.g. assay cut-point, based on study-specific assay performance.

The immunogenicity risk assessment should clearly describe how the bioanalytical methods are able to fulfil the fundamental criteria:

- To identify the 'at-risk' population; and
- To enable a thorough evaluation of the capacity of anti-product antibodies to bind both the product and endogenous counterparts.

The sponsor will need to describe anti-product antibody responses in terms of:

- incidence
- magnitude of binding response
- neutralisation capacity for product and endogenous counterparts
- timing of onset and duration
- identity of immunoglobulin class/sub-class.

A combination of methods (primary screen, confirmatory assay, cell-based assay for neutralisation, isotyping assay, etc.) will be required to generate the requisite data. The suitability of these bioanalytical methods must be justified by presentation of data that demonstrate the following:

- Specificity for the authentic drug product, related proteins and endogenous counterparts;
- Benchmarking of limit of quantitation relative to an appropriate positive control antibody;
- Optimisation of sample dilution factor relative to sensitivity, matrix effects and interference by residual drug product;
- Validity of assay cut-point to exclude false negatives whilst minimising false positives.

To date, regulatory agencies have not required bioanalytical methods to be fully validated for application to measurement of anti-product antibody response in non-clinical samples. However, FDA does require validation of bioanalytical methods for immunogenicity detection prior to proceeding into clinical studies. Bioanalytical methodology is the most common deficiency in the discussion of immunogenicity risk as presented in regulatory dossiers (IMPD, IND, MAA or BLA); the major deficiencies are discussed in a subsequent section of this chapter.

The priority is to be able to optimise sensitivity of the primary screening assay to enable earliest possible detection of binding antibodies that might represent a risk for long-term administration of the drug product. This implies 'real-time' monitoring of immunogenicity during early clinical studies, as far as this may be feasible. The focus of monitoring has been almost exclusively on the humoral response, since this is the easiest component of the immune response to measure, as well as reflecting the net outcome of antigen processing, presentation, co-stimulation of B- and T-lymphocytes and immune regulatory mechanisms. Although some guidance documents (e.g. EMEA 2007) refer to measurement of cell-mediated immune responses, as would be performed for many vaccine products, the sensitivity of such methodology to provide early detection of clinically relevant, *undesired*, immune responses to biopharmaceutical products remains to be established at this time.

Question 8: Are there any observations from non-clinical studies that indicate an impact of immunogenicity on pharmacodynamic markers?

Sponsors will need to apply suitably qualified bioanalytical methods to assay the time-course and magnitude of host anti-product antibody responses, in order to interpret the toxicokinetics associated with the repeat administration of a biopharmaceutical product (ICH 1995). The predictive value for human immunogenicity is highly dependent on the sequence homology between species – in many cases, the frequency of immunogenicity in animal models is rather high, reflecting the 'foreigness' of the human protein, and will be not be indicative of the response in humans. Nevertheless, observations concerning the impact of a host anti-product antibody response on pharmacodynamic parameters can be very useful in understanding the potential impact of immunogenicity. For example, the reversibility of an effect on biomarkers of function might reduce concerns about long-lasting neutralisation of an endogenous counterpart of the drug product (EMEA 2007).

Demonstration of a temporal relationship between appearance of host anti-product antibodies, reduction in AUC for the pharmacokinetic profile, reduction in pharmacodynamic markers, as well as reversibility of these effects following cessation of dosing (and, possibly, re-bound of the antibody response on re-administration) might indicate the scale of risk arising from an immune response. Specificity of binding for an endogenous counterpart of the product could confirm a need for caution in progressing into clinical studies, particularly if there were a high degree of inter-species sequence homology. An association with histological changes in a relevant target tissue might further contribute to an increased risk categorisation. Interestingly, non-human species do develop severe clinical symptoms that are reminiscent of those associated with autoimmune responses in humans (Randolph et al. 1999, Gao et al. 2004); therefore, such non-clinical data should be thoroughly assessed as part of the immunogenicity risk assessment.

Although transgenic mice have been useful for detecting the breaking of tolerance by structural variants of biopharmaceutical products (Ottesen et al. 1994, Hermeling et al. 2004), the complexity of these models precludes their routine application for evaluation of immunogenicity risk of novel biopharmaceutical products. This situation may change if stable germ-line transgenic mice that express functional components of the adaptive human immune repertoire become available.

Question 9: How is potential immunogenicity to be monitored/managed during clinical trials?

Because biopharmaceutical products may induce immune responses that have life-threatening consequences, albeit in rare circumstances, the sponsor must demonstrate that the design of a clinical trial gives due consideration to the following:

- Real-time monitoring of immune response, e.g. prior to/following each dose administration
- Treatment strategy for potential immune-mediated adverse events (infusion reactions and hypersensitivity response)

- Precautions against potential allergenic responses, e.g. skin testing prior to administration of plant-derived monoclonal antibodies
- Adequate duration of surveillance to detect antibodies formed after cessation of treatment, and for monitoring decline of detected antibodies
- Scheduling of blood sampling that minimises potential interference by residual drug product
- Correlation of host anti-product antibody response to clinical manifestations of hypersensitivity reactions
- Correlation between pharmacokinetic parameters, pharmacodynamic markers and antibody levels
- Validity of bioanalytical assay cut-point in patient population relative to that in healthy volunteers
- Application of additional bioanalytical assays, e.g. introduction of methods to detect IgM in addition to IgG.

Thus, the risk for human subjects could be substantially mitigated by exclusion of atopic individuals and by early detection of anti-product antibodies. Failure to develop bioanalytical methods of adequate sensitivity and/or specificity could result in a delay to initiate clinical studies for higher risk products. Conversely, a clear presentation of the analytical power of the assay methods, within the context of an immunogenicity risk assessment, could enable progression of investigational studies of products that are associated with a recognised risk of inducing a clinically significant anti-product immune response.

The timing of clinical sampling is not addressed with clarity in regulatory guidance. It is advisable to collect one or more pre-treatment samples to interpret the post-treatment measurements in relation to individual variations in background signal; in repeat-dose protocols, samples could be taken immediately prior to each administration; and a terminal sample should be collected at a time corresponding to 5 multiples or more of the estimated clearance half-life of the drug product, or at a time corresponding to a level of residual drug that is below the demonstrated threshold for interference in the assay; generally, if a humoral response is induced, it should be detected within 14–28 days of the last administration of the drug product, subject to potential interference by residual circulating drug.

Although anti-product IgM *could* be clinically significant, assays for IgM tend to have lower analytical sensitivity than assays for anti-product IgG, rendering the IgM measurement of questionable diagnostic value. Therefore, sponsors should not be obligated to develop assays to detect anti-product IgM, unless there is a substantiated clinical benefit. Equally, product-specific IgE is likely to be present at much lower levels than IgG, such that measurement of IgE may require depletion of the IgG fraction to avoid competition for the antigen.

Question 10: What is the estimated probability of a clinical immune response to the product?

Experience has demonstrated that most biopharmaceutical products are immunogenic in at least a proportion of treated subjects (Koren et al. 2002, Patten and Schellekens 2003). Therefore, it would be highly unlikely that a novel biological entity could be considered to have a zero probability of inducing a host immune response in humans. Consequently, this section of the risk assessment must rigorously review the empirical database relative to the levels of exposure to the drug product and, in particular, critique the limitations of the experience gained to date for extrapolation to a wider population.

The sponsor should indicate the incidence of human anti-product antibodies detected in earlier clinical studies, accompanied by a detailed description of the relevant extrinsic factors that might contribute to the level of immunogenicity. If such responses have been detected, the timing of their appearance and decline should be discussed relative to the dose level and frequency of administration of the drug product. The nature of the antibody response, including the capacity to neutralise the drug product and endogenous counterparts, should be critically discussed. The influence of concomitant medication on the incidence of immunogenicity should also be considered. Most importantly, the temporal relationship of the appearance of anti-product antibodies to (or lack of) (1) changes in pharmacokinetics of the drug product, and/or (2) changes in pharmacodynamic markers and/or (3) the appearance of clinical signs of an immune-mediated response should be assessed.

If no immunogenicity was detected in earlier clinical studies, the relevance of the patient population and the dosing regimen to the intended use should be discussed. The probability of an anti-product antibody response may then be estimated in terms of % incidence of binding/neutralising antibodies for a defined patient population, and assessed for a temporal association to immune response-mediated clinical sequelae (e.g. hypersensitivity reactions). Depending on the status of manufacturing process/formulation development, the potential impact of product changes on the probability of an immune response could also be presented.

Question 11: What are the possible/likely consequences of a clinical immune response to the product?

The clinical consequences of immune-mediated responses to biopharmaceutical products have been discussed elsewhere in this volume (Chapter 2) and summarised in some excellent review articles (Koren et al. 2002, Schellekens 2002b, Pendley et al. 2003). It has been recognised that these consequences can be categorised into a 'hierarchy of concerns' (Rosenberg 2003) that can enable a stratification of risk. In many cases, there is no apparent impact of anti-product antibodies on clinical safety or efficacy. Nevertheless, important effects may become evident following long-term administration to larger numbers of subjects. Therefore, the 'consequences' assessed must be carefully qualified by the extent of exposure of different patient subpopulations to the drug product.

The FDA has indicated that sponsors should anticipate adverse effects, and implement appropriate precautions, whenever a host antibody response to diagnostic or therapeutic monoclonal antibody products is detected (FDA 1997). Accordingly, the sponsor should discuss whether the induction of host antibodies to the drug product could lead to:

• modification of pharmacokinetic parameters
• changes in pharmacodynamic markers
• loss (or, possibly, enhancement) of efficacy
• appearance of a 'serum sickness' syndrome (Type III hypersensitivity, or 'immune complex' disease, mediated by IgG or IgM)

- anaphylaxis (Type I hypersensitivity; acute, systemic, severe allergic reaction, associated with de-granulation of mast cells or basophils that is mediated by IgE)
- infusion reactions (non-allergic type acute responses)
- autoimmune syndromes.

A combination of effects is quite possible. For example, in the case of infliximab, there appeared to be an association of anti-product antibodies with the incidence of infusion reactions, reduced plasma levels of infliximab and reduced efficacy (Baert et al. 2003). The impact of immune-mediated adverse reactions might be mitigated by palliative treatment/prophylaxis. Thus, although infliximab infusion was associated with acute reactions in approximately 5% of rheumatoid patients, these reactions were substantially prevented by adoption of suitable treatment parameters (Cheifetz et al. 2003).

Where possible, the sponsor should consider whether there could be a correlation between the levels of anti-product antibodies, the distribution between different immunoglobulin types (subject to analytical sensitivity to detect different isotypes) and potential adverse reactions.

Question 12: What is the overall risk for the target population, in balancing probability versus consequences of an immune response to the product?

In most cases, there will be considerable scope to balance overall risk by appropriate adjustment of the 'probability' and 'consequences' vectors. Although the limited number of subjects exposed in the pre-authorisation setting may not be adequate to provide a reliable probability estimate, a consideration of the nature of the product as well as the mode of use can enable a stratification of the risk. This risk level may then be refined during wider exposure to the drug product in the post-marketing setting.

Even if a product were associated with a relatively high (>30%) incidence of immunogenicity, and the product were intended for chronic use, the risk could be mitigated by a multitude of factors, such as:

- low risk of breaking tolerance to a self-protein based on structural considerations
- absence of endogenous counterpart having a unique function
- administration via intravenous rather than subcutaneous route
- low incidence of hypersensitivity reactions observed in clinical studies
- availability of suitability qualified bioanalytical techniques for biomarkers that could provide early detection of reduced efficacy
- other treatment options, including co-medication with immunosuppressive agents, which could be used in 'high-risk' subjects
- demonstration of effective control of product attributes that could influence potential immunogenicity, e.g. aggregation
- optimisation of product stability through comprehensive formulation development and appropriate choice of excipients.

It then remains further to minimise risk via presentation of an ongoing risk management programme in the final stage of the exercise.

Question 13: How will this risk be managed?

As stated at the beginning of this chapter, the estimated risk must be managed by one or more strategies: avoidance, reduction, retention and/or transfer. Such strategies can be very effective in managing adverse events arising from host antibody responses to chronic administration of biopharmaceutical products (Cheifetz and Mayer 2005) in non-life-threatening indications. This implies that there may be considerable scope for managing the clinical risk associated with the undesirable immunogenicity of biopharmaceutical products.

Various options could be adopted, for example:

- Avoidance of administration to healthy volunteers
- Exclusion of subjects due to HLA type
- Reduced rate of infusion (or stop completely)
- Shortened interval between infusions
- Use of pre-medication (e.g. steroid or non-sedating anti-histamine)
- Concurrent immunomodulation (e.g. azathioprine or methotrexate)
- Infusion of a combination of IV fluids, antihistamines and steroids in response to adverse reactions
- Switching to another agent (e.g. an alternate anti-TNF monoclonal antibody)
- Monitoring of vital signs during administration to provide early detection of infusion reactions
- Use of a dose regimen with maintenance infusions scheduled to induce tolerance.

Regulatory agencies will require, as part of a marketing authorisation application, the presentation of an effective risk management plan that provides appropriate surveillance of the probability and consequences of the immunogenicity of biopharmaceutical products. Most commonly, this would involve the establishment of a patient registry to identify 'at risk' patients/populations. In a number of cases, regulatory agencies have imposed a post-authorisation commitment to undertake an interventional study to generate additional data on the incidence of antibody responses and adverse events in a suitably sized cohort (which may depend on the incidence detected in pre-authorisation studies) for an adequate duration (e.g. 12–18 months). As associations with patient genotype become more evident, it may be logical to consider HLA typing as part of such post-authorisation studies.

13.5. Common Deficiencies

The majority of immunogenicity-related regulatory questions arising during the review of Marketing Authorisation Applications concern two aspects of the validation of the applied bioanalytical methods (primary screen, confirmatory assay and neutralising antibody assay), namely specificity and sensitivity.

13.5.1. Specificity

13.5.1.1. Use of Protein A/G as Immunoprecipitant

A radio-immunoprecipitation (RIP) assay often provides the most sensitive method to apply as a primary screening assay for anti-product antibodies. In most cases, Protein A/G has been used as the immunoprecipitant, and this raises the objection that IgM, IgA and IgG_3 isotype antibodies will not be detected. This objection could be countered by demonstrating adequate sensitivity of the RIP method to detect the most clinically significant IgG isotypes, coupled to a sample retention policy for 'look-back' analysis using an alternative method (e.g. BIAcore) if justified by clinical circumstances.

Sponsors should be aware that a regulatory agency might insist on the development of an assay format of broader immunoglobulin class/sub-class specificity but should remember that the attainment of broader specificity may lead to loss of sensitivity for IgG_1, IgG_2 & IgG_4. The use of Protein L may help to broaden the range of immunoglobulins that are detected in an RIP assay. If the clinical treatment regimen is relatively short, e.g. 28 days, there may be stronger justification for examining early responses using an assay format that is capable of detecting IgM.

13.5.1.2. Binding to Target Antigen, Related Proteins and Unrelated Proteins

Many assay validation exercises do not adequately address specificity. Most importantly, the relative reactivity against the endogenous counterpart of the drug product must be determined, e.g. using an immunocompetition format. In the case of a biosimilar medicinal product, it will be essential to demonstrate that an assay can detect antibodies to the test and reference products with comparable sensitivity. Immunocompetition experiments should include full titration curves with both the authentic product, proteins that are structurally related to the product, and the unrelated proteins, in order to validate an appropriate concentration for use as the competing antigen in the confirmatory screening assay.

13.5.1.3. Positive Control Antibody Versus Authentic Drug Product

Another aspect of specificity is the selection of a relevant positive control antibody. Sponsors will need to develop a positive control antibody preparation against the authentic product, rather than a related product. Thus, relying on a commercially available antiserum that has been generated against a related product is usually not adequate. Equally, use of a monoclonal antibody positive control should be avoided because this may bias the capacity of the assay to detect antibodies that might be poorly representative of the response to the different epitopes in the product.

13.5.1.4. Impact of Chemical Modification

In the case of a PEGylated protein, the presence of the PEG moiety might well reduce the immunogenicity of the protein. On the other hand, the modification could introduce immunogenic linker moieties, and the PEG itself may not be immunologically inert. Thus, there are several reasons why it is essential to generate a positive control antibody against the authentic product and to define the cross-reactivity of this antibody with the protein, linker and PEG moieties respectively.

13.5.1.5. Importance of Distinguishing Antigenicity from Immunogenicity

Appropriate reagents for immunocompetition might not always be available. One case in point is the difficulty of isolating plant glycans to test the immunogenicity of plant-derived biopharmaceutical products that contain non-human glycosidic linkages. Care has to be taken to avoid interpreting antigenicity, as represented by the binding of preformed antibodies to glycoprotein structures, as immunogenicity that is due to the plant glycan.

13.5.2. Sensitivity

Regulatory agencies will require an estimation of the binding/neutralising capacity of the anti-product antibody response, detected in the primary and secondary immunogenicity screening assays, as part of the validation of bioanalytical methods. This should enable an estimation of the mass/molar quantity of product bound/neutralised at a signal level that corresponds with the assay cut-point. While such a value has questionable meaning in absolute terms – since it may depend on the nature of the antibody response in an unrelated species/population receiving a different immunisation regimen, as well as the methods used to isolate and characterise the antibody preparation – it does provide a benchmark to calibrate the different assays that are applied during the course of a product development programme.

In routine practice, assay results will be reported as the titre corresponding to the assay cut-point. As the product progresses through clinical development, it may be possible to establish a human positive control antibody pool collected from responders in earlier clinical studies. It may not be necessary to affinity-purify the antigen-specific IgG to enable application of this positive control as the calibrant for the assay (Tacey et al. 2003), particularly if the assay titres can be related to appearance/severity of clinical adverse events or an impact on pharmacodynamic markers. Nevertheless, a regulatory agency will expect a definition of the capacity of a specific dilution of the positive control antiserum to neutralise a specified amount of the biological activity of the drug product/endogenous counterpart. This is because neutralisation of the activity of an endogenous cytokine can occur in the presence of a relatively low level of anti-product antibody (Thorpe and Swanson 2005).

Sponsors should expect to have to re-establish the assay cut-point as clinical studies are performed in different patient populations. The validity of the assay cut-point should then be confirmed by spiking the positive control antibody at the Lower Limit of Quantitation (LLOQ) into at least 20 individual untreated patient sera; as these samples represent true positives, these should register as an actual positive if the assay cut-point has been set correctly, enabling an acceptance criterion of 0% false negatives to be tested; the corresponding unspiked samples should generate a low ($\leq 5\%$) proportion of false positives.

13.6. Presentation

An immunogenicity risk assessment should be included within the overall clinical summary (Section 2.7.2.4 of Module 2 of the CTD format) of a marketing authorisation application. In addition, an analysis of the probability and consequences of immunogenicity could be included in the clinical pharmacology overview (Section 2.5.3). During clinical development, a summary of the immunogenicity risk assessment should be presented in the integrated summary of toxicological findings (non-clinical) and in the clinical benefit-risk analysis as relevant.

The sponsor could submit a descriptive analysis as an appendix to an IND, IMPD, BLA or MAA, cross-referenced from the main part of the dossier. An independent expert might author such a report. Sponsors should also consider developing a written immunogenicity risk assessment early in the development process. This will provide a structured framework for consideration of the pertinent risk factors and enable refinement of the development plan to address effectively the overall immunogenicity risk assessment. This document may then serve as a source reference for extracting the information required for the registration dossier, or for developing responses to regulatory agency questions.

13.7. Summary

An assessment of the risk associated with the potential for undesirable immunogenicity of therapeutic protein products can be structured by developing responses to a sequence of questions:

- What is the structural relationship of the therapeutic protein to endogenous counterparts?
- What is the target of the drug product and how unique is its function?
- What is the abundance of endogenous counterparts of the drug product?
- How is the product manufactured and characterised?
- How is the product to be used?
- What is the extent of prior exposure to the product or to related products?
- What methods have been applied to measure anti-product immune responses?
- Are there any observations from non-clinical studies that indicate an impact of immunogenicity on pharmacodynamic markers?
- How is potential immunogenicity to be monitored/managed during clinical trials?
- What is the estimated probability of a clinical immune response to the product?
- What are the possible/likely consequences of a clinical immune response to the product?
- What is the overall risk for the target population, in balancing probability versus consequences of an immune response to the product?
- How will this risk be managed?

The data to support this risk assessment will be accumulated throughout the life cycle of a biopharmaceutical product (Table 13.1) to enable an iterative refinement of the risk management plan via discussion with concerned regulatory agencies.

Acknowledgements: I would like to recognise the leading contributions of Amy Rosenberg, Tony Mire-Sluis, Gene Koren, Huub Schellekens, Robin Thorpe and Steve Swanson to the establishment of a solid foundation for the regulatory science of 'immunogenicity risk assessment' for biopharmaceutical products.

Table 13.1 Immunogenicity risk assessment during product development.

Development stage	Activity
Lead selection	• Evaluate intrinsic immunogenicity of lead candidates, including potential neo-epitopes 　○ In silico identification of promiscuous immunodominant B-/T-cell epitopes 　○ Ex vivo T-cell stimulation assays 　○ Relative immunogenicity/impact on biomarkers in pilot in vivo pharmaco-toxicology studies • Develop bioanalytical methods to measure anti-product antibody response • Prepare preliminary positive control antibody versus product candidate selected for development
IND enabling	• Qualify primary screening, confirmatory and neutralising antibody detection assays for application to non-clinical samples; validate for clinical applications • Evaluate impact of host anti-product antibody on toxicokinetic profile in relevant animal species • Define potential cross-reactivity versus endogenous protein/conserved sequences
Confirmatory efficacy/Phase III	• Validate additional bioanalytical methods as required • Implement human positive control antibody if available • Schedule blood sampling for antibody measurement to encompass potential early (IgM) and mature (IgG) responses, with appropriate duration of follow-up monitoring • Examine correlation between appearance of anti-product antibody responses, primary pharmacodynamics and adverse events • Develop strategy for managing potential immune-mediated clinical responses to product
Product registration	• Comprehensively describe the development and validation of bioanalytical assays, with particular emphasis on the specificity and sensitivity of methods to detect immune response to product • Critically evaluate immunogenicity signals with respect to all relevant intrinsic and extrinsic factors within the overall clinical benefit-to-risk risk assessment • Present plan for ongoing surveillance and management of immunogenicity risk
Post-marketing/ Risk Management Programme	• Accumulate data via a patient registry to refine the immunogenicity risk assessment in the wider clinical population(s) • If necessary, perform post-approval interventional cohort study to confirm association between the appearance of a humoral immune response to the product and clinical sequelae

References

Baert, F., Noman, M., Vermeire, S., Van Assche, G., D'Haens, G., Carbonez, A., and Rutgeerts, P. 2003. Influence of immunogenicity on the long-term efficacy of infliximab in Crohn's disease. N. Engl. J. Med. 348:601–608.

Benjamin, R., Cobbold, S., Clark, M. and Waldmann, H. 1986. Tolerance to rat monoclonal antibodies: implications for serotherapy. J. Exp. Med. 163:1539–1552.

Bennett, C.L., Luminari, S., Nissenson, A.R., Tallman, M.S., Klinge, S.A., McWilliams, N., McKoy, J.M., Kim, B., Lyons, E.A., Trifilio, S.M., Raisch, D.W., Evens, A.M., Kuzel, T.M., Schumock, G.T., Belknap, S.M., Locatelli, F., Rossert, J., and Casadevall, N. 2004. Pure Red-cell Aplasia and epoetin therapy. N. Engl. J. Med. 351:1403–1408.

Cheifetz, A., Smedle,y M., Martin, S., Reiter, M., Leone, G., Mayer, L., and Plevy, S. 2003. The incidence and management of infusion reactions to infliximab: a large center experience. Am. J. Gastroenterol. 98:1315–1324.

Cheifetz, A. and Mayer, L. 2005. Monoclonal antibodies, immunogenicity, and associated infusion reactions. Mnt. Sinai J. Med. 72:250–256.

Chirino, A.J., Ary, M.L., and Marshall, S.A. 2004. Minimizing the immunogenicity of protein therapeutics. Drug Discov. Today 9:82–90.

EMEA. 2006a. The European Agency for the Evaluation of Medicinal Products (EMEA). Guideline on Similar Biological Medicinal Products containing biotechnology-derived proteins as active substance: non-clinical and clinical issues, EMEA/CHMP/BMWP/42832/2005 (http://www.emea.europa.eu/pdfs/human/biosimilar/4283205en.pdf)

EMEA. 2006b. The European Agency for the Evaluation of Medicinal Products (EMEA). Guideline on Similar Medicinal Products containing recombinant erythropoietins, EMEA/CHMP/BMWP/94526/2005 (http://www.emea.eu.int/pdfs/human/biosimilar/9452605en.pdf).

EMEA. 2007. The European Agency for the Evaluation of Medicinal Products (EMEA). Draft Guideline on immunogenicity assessment of biotechnology-derived therapeutic proteins, EMEA/CHMP/BMWP/14327/2006 (http://www.emea.europa.eu/pdfs/human/biosimilar/1432706en.pdf).

FDA. 1997. US Department of Health and Human Services Food and Drug administration. Points to consider in the manufacture and testing of monoclonal antibody products for human use (http://www.fda.gov/Cber/gdlns/ptc_mab.pdf).

FDA. 2002. US Department of Health and Human Services Food and Drug administration. Draft Guidance for Industry on Drugs, biologics, and medical devices derived from bioengineered plants for use in human and animals (http://www.fda.gov/cber/gdlns/bioplant.pdf).

Ganson, N.J., Kelly, S.J., Scarlett, E., Sundy, J.S., and Hershfield, M.S. 2006. Control of hyperuricemia in subjects with refractory gout, and induction of antibody against poly(ethylene glycol) (PEG), in a phase i trial of subcutaneous PEGylated urate oxidase. Arthr. Res. & Ther. 8:R12 (http://www.arthritis-research.com/content/8/1/R12)

Gao, G., Lebherz, C., Weiner, D.J., Grant, R., Calcedo, R., McCullough, B., Bagg, A., Zheng, Y., and Wilson, J.M. 2004. Erythropoietin gene therapy leads to autoimmune anemia in macaques. Blood 103:3300–3302.

Gomord, V., Chamberlain, P., Jefferis, R., and Faye, L. 2005. Biopharmaceutical production in plants: problems, solutions and opportunities. Trends Biotechnol. 23:559–565.

Gupta, S., Indelicato, S.R., Jethwa, V., Kawabata, T., Kelley, M., Mire-Sluis, A.R., Richards, S.M., Rup, B., Shores, E., Swanson, S.J., and Wakshull, E. 2007. Recommendations for the design, optimization, and qualification of cell-based assays used for detection of neutralizing antibody responses elicited to biological therapeutics. J. Immunol. Method. 321:1–18

Hermeling, S., Crommelin, D.J., Schellekens, H., and Jiskoot, W. 2004. Structure-immunogenicity relationships of therapeutic proteins. Pharm. Res. 21:897–903.

Hermeling, S., Jiskoot, W., Crommelin, D., Bornaes, C., and Schellekens, H. 2005. Development of a transgenic mouse model immune tolerant for human interferon beta. Pharm. Res. 22:847–851.

ICH. 1995. International conference on harmonisation (ICH) of technical requirements for registration of pharmaceuticals for human use. ICH harmonised tripartite guideline S6 on Preclinical safety evaluation of biotechnology-derived pharmaceuticals, CPMP/ICH/302/95 (http://www.emea.europa.eu/pdfs/human/ich/030295en.pdf).

ICH. 2005. International conference on harmonisation (ICH) of technical requirements for registration of pharmaceuticals for human use. ICH harmonised tripartite guideline Q5E on Comparability of Biotechnological/Biological products subject to changes in their manufacturing process, CPMP/ICH/5721/03 (http://www.emea.europa.eu/pdfs/human/ich/572103en.pdf).

Jaber, A. and Baker, M. 2007. Assessment of the immunogenicity of different interferon beta-1a formulations using ex vivo T-cell assays. J. Pharm. Biomed. Anal. 43: 1256–1261.

Koren, E., Zuckerman, L.A., and Mire-Sluis, A.R. 2002. Immune responses to therapeutic proteins in humans – clinical significance, assessment and prediction. Curr. Pharm. Biotechnol. 3:349–360.

Kyewski, B. and Derbinski, J. 2004. Self-representation in the thymus: an extended view. Nat. Rev. Immunol. 4:688–698.

Mire-Sluis, A.R., Barrett, Y.C., Devanarayan, V., Koren, E., Liu, H., Maia, M., Parish, T., Scott, G., Shankar, G., Shores, E., Swanson, S.J., Taniguchi, G., Wierda, D., and Zuckerman, L.A. 2004. Recommendations for the design and optimization of immunoassays used in the detection of host antibodies against biotechnology products. J. Immunol. Method. 289:1–16.

Ottesen, J.L., Nilsson, P., Jami, J., Weilguny, D., Dühkkop, M., Bucchini, D., Havelund, S., and Fogh, J.M. 1994. The potential immunogenicity of human insulin and insulin analogues evaluated in a transgenic mouse model. Diabetologia 37: 1178–1185.

Patten, P.A. and Schellekens, H. 2003. The immunogenicity of biopharmaceuticals. In 'Immunogenicity of Therapeutic Biological Products', ed. Brown, F. and Mire-Sluis, A.R., pp. 81–97. Dev. Biol. Basel, Karger, 112.

Pendley, C., Schantz, A., and Wagner, C. 2003. Immunogenicity of therapeutic monoclonal antibodies. Curr. Opin. Mol. Ther. 5:172–179.

Randolph, J.F., Stokol, T., Scarlett, J.M., and MacLeod, J.N. 1999. Comparison of biological activity and safety of recombinant canine erythropoietin with that of recombinant human erythropoietin in clinically normal dogs. Am. J. Vet. Res. 60:636–642.

Roggen, E.L. 2006. Recent developments with B-cell epitope identification for predictive studies. J. Immunot. 3:137–149.

Rosenberg, A.S. 2003. Immunogenicity of Biological Therapeutics: a hierarchy of concerns. In 'Immunogenicity of Therapeutic Biological Products', ed. Brown, F. and Mire-Sluis, A.R., pp. 15–21. Dev. Biol. Basel, Karger, 112.

Rosenberg, A.S. and Worobec, A. 2004a. A risk-based approach to immunogenicity of therapeutic protein products, Part 1: considering consequences of the immune response to a protein. BioPharm International, November 2004, 22–26 (www.biopharminternational.com/biopharm/article/articleDetail.jsp?id=134110).

Rosenberg, A.S. and Worobec, A. 2004b. A risk-based approach to immunogenicity of therapeutic protein products, Part 2: considering host-specific and product-specific factors impacting immunogenicity, BioPharm International, December 2004, 34–42 (www.biopharminternational.com/biopharm/article/articleDetail.jsp?id=140695).

Rosenberg, A.S. and Worobec, A. 2005. A risk-based approach to immunogenicity of therapeutic protein products, Part 3: effects of manufacturing changes in immunogenicity and the utility of animal immunogenicity studies. BioPharm International, January 2005, 32–36 (www.biopharminternational.com/biopharm/article/articleDetail.jsp?id=146216).

Rosenberg, A.S. 2006. Effects of protein aggregates: an immunologic perspective. AAPS J. 8:Article 59, E501–E507 (http://www.aapsj.org/articles/aapsj080359/aapsj080359.pdf)

Routledge, E., Falconer, M., Pope, H., Lloyd, I. and Waldmann, H. 1995. The effect of aglycosylation on the immunogenicity of a humanized therapeutic CD3 monoclonal antibody. Transplantation 60:847–853.

Schellekens, H. 2002a. Bioequivalence and the immunogenicity of biopharmaceuticals. Nat. Rev. Drug Discov. 1:457–462.

Schellekens, H. 2002b. Immunogenicity of therapeutic proteins: clinical implications and future prospects. Clin. Ther. 24:1720–1740.

Shankar, G., Shores, E., Wagner, C. and Mire-Sluis, A. 2006. Scientific and regulatory considerations on the immunogenicity of biologics. Trends Biotechnol. 24:274–280.

Soos, J.M., Polsky, R.M., Keegan, S.P., Bugelski, P., and Herzyk D.J. 2003. Identification of natural antibodies to interleukin-18 in the sera of normal humans and three nonhuman primate species. Clin. Immunol. 109:188–196.

Strand, V., Kimberly, R., and Isaacs, J.D. 2007. Biologic therapies in rheumatology: lessons learned, future directions. Nat. Rev. Drug Discov. 6:75–92.

Tacey, R., Greway, A., Smiell, J., Power, D., Kromminga, A., Daha, M., Casadevall, N., and Kelley, M. 2003. The detection of anti-erythropoietin antibodies in human serum and plasma, Part I: validation of the protocol for a radioimmunoprecipitation assay. J. Immunol. Method. 283:317–329.

Tangri, S., Mothé, B.R., Eisenbraun, J., Sidney, J., Southwood, S., Briggs, K., Zinckgraf, J., Bilsel, P., Newman, M., Chesnut, R., Licalsi, C., and Sette, A. 2005. Rationally engineered therapeutic proteins with reduced immunogenicity. J. Immunol. 174:3187–3196.

Thorpe, R. and Swanson, S.J. 2005. Current methods for detecting antibodies against erythropoietin and other recombinant proteins. Clin. Diag. Lab. Immunol. 12:28–39

Van der Meide, P.H. and Schellekens, H. 1997. Anti-cytokine autoantibodies: epiphenomenon or critical modulators of cytokine action. Biotherapy 10:39–48.

Van Walle, I., Gansemans, Y, Parren, P., Stas, P., and Lasters, I. 2007. Immunogenicity screening in protein drug development. Expert Opin. Biol. Ther. 7:405–418.

Wagner, C.L., Schantz, A., Barnathan, E., Olson, A., Mascelli, M.A., Ford, J., Damaraju, L., Scaible, T., Maini, R.N., and Tcheng, J.E. 2003. Consequences of immunogenicity to the therapeutic monoclonal antibodies ReoPro® and Remicade®. In 'Immunogenicity of Therapeutic Biological Products', ed. Brown, F. and Mire-Sluis, A.R., pp. 37–53. Dev. Biol. Basel, Karger, 112.

Subject Index